Communicating Health

Communicating Health

MOHAN J. DUTTA

polity

First published in 2008 by Polity Press

Polity Press
65 Bridge Street
Cambridge CB2 1UR, UK

Polity Press
350 Main Street
Malden, MA 02148, USA

ISBN-13: 978-07456-3491-3
ISBN-13: 978-07456-3492-0 (pb)

A catalogue record for this book is available from the British Library.

Typeset in 10 on 12 pt Stone Serif
by Servis Filmsetting Ltd, Manchester
Printed and bound in Great Britain by
MPG Books Ltd, Bodmin, Cornwall

For further information on Polity, visit our website: www.polity.co.uk

To Ma and Baba

Table of Contents

List of Figures

List of Boxes

Glossary

Biomedical The most widely accepted model of healthcare that underlies the theories and practices of modern medicine.

Dominant The dominant approach in this book refers to the widely circulated health communication research and application that is based on mainstream ideas of what it means to be healthy and what are the best ways to address health problems informed by the biomedical model.

Dyad Two-person communication setting for interpersonal exchanges.

Epidemiology The study of distribution of disease patterns and the underlying reasons that govern these patterns.

Epistemology Part of philosophy which deals with knowledge and knowing.

Eurocentric Ways of thinking which are rooted in European value systems and European ways of knowing the world. Eurocentrism is connected to the Enlightenment project, which used the universal rationality of science to dominate over other ways of knowing.

Globalization Globalization refers to the global movement of economic commodities and communication across nation-states.

Heteroglossia The multiplicity of different worldviews and knowledge systems that co-exist.

Identity The sense of self of an individual; the way he/she sees himself/herself.

Ideology The stories and ideas through which dominant social actors maintain their control over the marginalized sectors of the world.

Marginalization The condition of being situated at the peripheries of mainstream society, without access to basic resources.

Medicalizing The medicalizing ideology looks at a disease as a problem that can be solved only through medicines and surgical treatments. In other words, the biomedical model is seen as the only viable solution to disease and illness.

Macro The occurrence of phenomena at social level and the explanations that account for these large-scale patterns.

Micro The occurrence of phenomena at individual, dyadic and small group levels.

Mobilization Collective communicative processes which bring the community together in its resistance to dominant structures.

Narrative The process of making a story and the story itself which is generated in the process.

Patriarchy Hierarchical organization of the social structures which privileges masculine norms and ideals and rewards masculine values.

Polymorphism The idea that multiple approaches and ways of knowing are complementary.

Redistributive justice Form of justice which addresses resource inequalities by seeking to redistribute economic resources within the social system.

Resistance Those processes that challenge the dominant structures and the control exerted by them.

Social capital Concept which refers to cohesiveness within a community and taps into features of social organization such as community participation, and norms of reciprocity, and trust in others, which facilitate mutually beneficial cooperation.

Acknowledgments

We become who we are owing to the sacrifices which continuous genera-tions of ancestors have made in order for us to be able to have a voice. This book is about rewriting a history of health communication from a viewpoint which is personal as well as political. I have learned early on, from my joint family who nurtured me to life, that what is personal is also political, and that politics is integral to the academic journey. I have learned from my family to speak from my heart, and to stand up in resist-ance to narratives of convenience. It is due to my family that I had suffi-cient faith in my voice as to want to speak, and sufficient commitment as to keep listening to what my own voice said. Hence this book is an homage to the voices of my family, community and culture that speak through me.

A big thank you goes to my teachers, who taught me the language through which I can now speak. Without you, I wouldn't know where to begin, where to end, or where to hang my thoughts in-between.

I thank my colleague Patrice Buzzanell, who has mentored me gener-ously during my formative years and has taught me the value of grace even as one engages in criticism. I also thank my colleagues Howard and Beverly Sypher, and Steve Wilson, for their friendship and for making Purdue an exciting place to work in, both intellectually and profession-ally.

Heather Zoller and Kimberly Kline have been invaluable collaborators on this journey, as they continued to ask critical questions in their own work and to provide points of entry for dialogue. My colleague and mentor Barbara Sharf has been, for me, an amazing role model as well as an immense source of support: she has read an earlier version of this man-uscript and provided detailed feedback, in spite of her very busy schedule. I would also like to thank my friend Teri Thompson for the faith she placed in me even before I had acquired my credentials, for her contin-ued support in the rigorous pursuit of health communication scholarship, and, not least, for her kindness and contaminating sense of optimism.

Without the visions of Collins Airhihenbuwa this book would not have been possible. Collins, thank you for igniting the spark in a young grad-uate student, almost a decade ago, to interrogate Eurocentric hegemony in health communication discourse. In those early days of graduate school – when I felt so unsettled by what seemed like the inherent racism of health communication programs that talked about development – your work gave me a language through which I could understand my feelings and emotions and give them a voice. Through your example, you have taught me the importance of continuing this work, which challenges our understandings of culture and the values that drive us to do what we do as health communicators.

Ambar, Iccha, Induk, Mahuya, and Rebecca – each one of you has contributed to this journey of discovery in ways that are profound. You have challenged me to think and rethink my work in new ways, and you have created new possibilities for the culture-centered approach. You have never shied away from engaging reflexively in work, although sometimes that task was painful. You have asked the difficult questions and walked along with me as we have grown together in our conversations, seeking to find the answers. The stuff of this book is very much a product of those late night talks and chats over coffee. I have full confidence that, as the next generation of culture-centered scholars, you will take this body of work to places that I haven't yet dreamt of, that you will continue to challenge this line of work with your critical eye and always keep open the possibilities of reflexivity. A special note of thanks goes to Ambar, for reading preliminary drafts of this manuscript and for sharing your insights. A big thank you goes also to my students who have enrolled in the "Culture and health" and "Culture and resistance" graduate seminars, where we debated many of these ideas.

I would like to thank my editor at Polity, Andrea Drugan, for showing faith in the value of this project and for providing invaluable feedback and detailed copyedits.

My grandmother, Nana, taught me to value life and to be committed to whatever I think is important in life. It is through you, Nan, that I came to appreciate the value of learning and to understand that learning is a journey that never ends – so that the best kind of scholarship is the one which never ceases to ask questions.

Finally, I dedicate this book to Baba and Ma. Baba, your dreams have taught me to dream. Your belief in me has given me the courage to put together this work, and to pursue those stories that speak to me from my heart. You taught me to value a good debate, to be politically engaged, and to make that politics a part of my academic commitment. Ma, your patience, love, and endless faith in my work made me believe that I could someday write a book. Both of you continue to be the pillars on which I stand.

Introduction

In recent years, the concept of culture has received increasing attention in health communication (Airhihenbuwa 1995; Brislin 1993; Dutta-Bergman 2004a, 2004b, 2005a, 2005b; Resnicow, Braithwaite, Dilorio, and Glanz 2002). The call to respond to the varied needs of multicultural societies is evident in the large amounts of funds available for multicultural interventions, and the growth in the number of multicultural health communication programs that seek to serve the needs of multicultural communities. These programs are being designed with the goals of being culturally sensitive, of responding to the diverse cultures in the global context, and of meeting a felt cultural need (Resnicow, Braithwaite, Dilorio and Glanz 2002). Furthermore, globalization processes have foregrounded the relevance of articulating the concept of culture in the context of health communication programs by questioning the universal narratives of healthcare embedded within the biomedical model (Airhihenbuwa 1995; Dutta-Bergman 2004a, 2004b, 2005a, 2005b; Dutta 2007; Dutta and Basu 2007; Dutta and Basnyat, in press). The locally situated nature of health communication processes has become particularly relevant in the context of a growing awareness of the diverse ways in which meanings of health and illness are constituted in diverse societies and cultures. As the grand narratives of health have been ruptured in the backdrop of an increasing realization that the *biomedical* model provides a limited viewpoint for engaging in issues of global health, there is also an increasing awareness of the need to open up the spaces of health communication to the voices of cultural communities.

Surveying the scope of the field, a new scholar might observe that health communication has become increasingly sensitized to the need to address these cultural shifts in the world. It might seem that the ways in which we traditionally conceptualize health and practice health communication have paved the way for a more humanizing approach by creating spaces for the discussion of cultures and for culture-specific health solutions. This book examines the response of health communication work to culture and suggests criteria for historically situating the study of culture in health communication. Its goal is to provide a historical overview of the ways in which culture has been used in health communication scholarship and to offer the culture-centered approach as an entry point for engaging with the culturally situated nature of health communication processes and meanings (Dutta-Bergman 2004a,

2004b). The historical overview of health communication scholarship using the concept of culture offers a trajectory for locating health communication scholarship and for comparing the various approaches to culture-based health communication (Dutta-Bergman 2005a; Dutta 2007). The culture-centered approach is juxtaposed in the backdrop of other approaches to culturally based health communication, demonstrating points of similarity and points of departure among these approaches. This comparison will ultimately equip the reader with both theoretical and methodological tools to examine the multicultural nature of the different approaches to health communication and to apply these tools in healthcare settings.

In discussing the culture-centered approach, the book suggests that the nature of how and what we communicate about health is embedded in our taken-for-granted assumptions about what it means to be healthy, what it means to be ill, and how we approach disease and illness. In suggesting this, the culture-centered approach is set up in opposition to the dominant approach of health communication, which represents the status quo and uses psychological cognitive theories to predict health attitudes and behaviors. The dominant approach is located within the biomedical model, with its focus on constructs and variables lent by this model, and with an emphasis on promoting and studying beliefs, attitudes, and behaviors within its framework. In the widely circulated biomedical model of health communication, health is treated as a universal concept based on *Eurocentric* understandings of health, disease and its treatment. Within this model, the way we come to see health is intrinsically built upon a Eurocentric *ideology* that privileges certain assumptions about health and downplays other approaches. The culture-centered approach locates this Eurocentric ideology by underlying the major approaches to health communication, and offers a criticism of the universal appeal of the dominant approaches that are built upon the culturally-situated Eurocentric notions of health and illness. The criticism of the Eurocentric ideology in health communication is based upon (a) criticism of the biomedical model that offers the foundation to much of the existing health communication scholarship (we will see this in greater detail in chapter 5), and (b) criticism of the basic premises of the health communication theories and applications that are widely circulated in the literature on cognitive behavioral principles (we will engage with these criticisms in chapters 1, 2 and 3). This criticism, both of the biomedical ideology underlying health practices and of the cognitive behavioral basis of health communication theorizing, offers openings for engaging culture in health communication scholarship in ways which are meaningful to the experiences of cultural communities hitherto marginalized; it also creates openings for alternative ways of knowing.

Therefore, in this book, the culture-centered approach is introduced as an alternative lens for understanding health communication. This approach is value-centered and is built on the notion that the various ways of understanding and negotiating the meanings of health are embedded within cultural contexts and the values deeply connected with them. Thus knowledge is embedded within value systems. These systems often remain hidden from the language of universal rationality in health communication scholarship; the culture-centered approach draws our attention to them. This approach questions the very values which underlie the universal logic of the biomedical model and of the cognitive–behavioral model, bringing out the hidden agendas embedded in the top-down frameworks underlying health communication and providing a critical entry point for interrogating them. As it does this, its emphasis is on looking at the erasure of the voice of those communities which have traditionally been rendered silent through treatment as subjects of health communication interventions doled out by the experts. Alternatively, the culture-centered approach proposes to build health communication theories and practices from the vantage point of cultural members, foregrounding their voices in the articulation of problems, the prioritization of problems, and the development of health solutions. The emphasis therefore is on creating opportunities for dialogue that bring out meanings of health articulated through the voices of cultural communities otherwise marginalized and silenced.

Ultimately, the goal of this book is to lay out the foundations for discussing the culture-centered approach and to create openings for its discussion in health communication. Chapter 1 introduces the reader to the concept of culture in health communication and provides a historical overview of the ways in which culture has been incorporated in health communication theory, research, and application. It examines the history of culture in health communication, studies the different models of health communication in the context of culture, compares the different strands of culture-based health communication work, and explores the applications of culture in health communication. Chapter 2 builds on the Introduction to discuss further the culture-centered approach to health communication by locating it in the backdrop of the *dominant approach* to health communication scholarship. After laying out the foundations and characteristics of the dominant approach to health communication, it explains the basic tenets of the culture-centered approach, which is followed by a discussion of its various applications in health communication theory, research, and practice. Chapter 3 examines and compares the theoretical foundations of the different approaches to the study of culture.

Chapter 4 offers a culture-centered overview of the relationship between culture, identity, and health. It suggests that this relationship is a complex and dynamic, so that the identities of cultural members play important roles in constituting health experiences of cultural members. Chapter 5 locates health and illness experiences in the different realms of healing and curing, thus making the dominant biomedical framework of healthcare into a culturally situated model and comparing it with other approaches to health and healing.

In chapter 6 we will engage with the topic of cultural marginalization and study the ways in which cultures are marginalized in health communication discourse and practices. More specifically, we will focus on what it means to be marginalized and on the kind of material and discursive conditions which create positions at the margins. We will further build on the topic of marginalization in chapter 7, to look at the health experiences of specific marginalized sectors. We will conclude the chapter by discussing marginalization in postcolonial and subaltern contexts.

Chapter 8 connects the culture-centered approach in health communication to the realm of the community. The emphasis on *social capital* examines the community-building and community-sustaining aspects of health communication, and connects the practice of culture-centered health communication to the sphere of community-organizing. Building on the notion of community-organizing, chapter 9 studies the ways in which resistance is enacted in culturally situated communities, and chapter 10 examines health communication processes in the area of globalization. Finally, chapter 11 demonstrates the pragmatic applications that might develop from the culture-centered approach.

Throughout the book, the culture-centered approach is used as a sensitizing lens for looking at the concept of culture and at the ways health communication scholarship has responded to culture. This approach will offer the foundation and criteria for investigating the various conceptualizations of culture in health communication and the various applications of health communication which have emerged from these conceptualizations. The rest of the introduction will provide a brief overview of the culture-centered approach, walking you through its basic principles. The goal of doing it is to equip you with a basic understanding of the approach, which should be used in reading the subsequent chapters. We will return to the discussion of the culture-centered approach in greater depth in chapter 2.

Culture-Centered Approach to Health Communication

What is the culture-centered approach to health communication? What are the basic tenets of the culture-centered approach to health communication? What does it mean to engage in culture-centered health communication scholarship? What are the characteristics of culture-centered health communication applications? The culture-centered approach is an emerging approach to health communication which questions the constructions of culture in traditional health communication theories and applications, examines how the latter have systematically erased the cultural voices of *marginalized* communities in their constructions of health, and builds dialogical spaces for engaging with these voices (Dutta 2006, 2007; Dutta-Bergman 2004a, 2004b). With its emphasis on interrogating the erasures in health communication discourse and application, the culture-centered approach primarily focuses on understanding health meanings and experiences in marginalized settings.

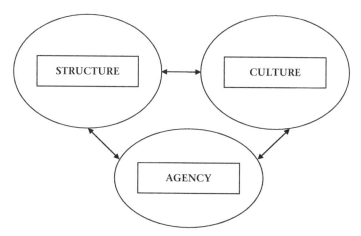

Fig. I.1 The culture-centered approach to health communication

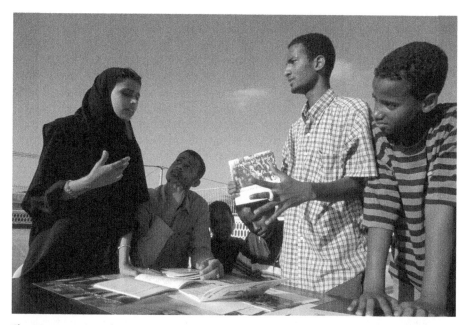

Fig. I.2 A meeting of peer educators in Africa. They educate young people about health issues, especially HIV and AIDS
© Giacomo Pirozzi @ Panos Pictures

As figure I.1 indicates, the culture-centered approach is built upon three key concepts and the interactions betweeen them: structure, culture, and agency). The intersection of structure, culture, and agency creates openings for listening to the voices of marginalized communities, constructing discursive spaces which interrogate the erasures in marginalized settings and offer opportunities for co-constructing the voices of those who have traditionally been silenced by engaging them in dialogue.

Structure

Structure, in this context, refers to those aspects of social organization that constrain and enable the capacity of cultural participants to seek out health choices and engage in health-related behaviors. Structures include elements such as medical services, transportation services, food, and shelter, which are essential to the healthcare of cultural members. Structure also refers to the ways the healthcare system is organized and its services are delivered, and to the organization of healthcare organizations. Structure is simultaneously constraining and enabling. On the one hand, it limits the opportunity for securing healthcare in marginalized contexts by determining the range of healthcare choices that are available or unavailable to cultural members; on the other hand, it creates opportunities for change by challenging the frameworks within which health is constructed. Structures are deeply connected with the material resources available to individuals and to the communities within which they live, and play out in the realm of the day-to-day healthcare choices in marginalized communities. Marginalized communities are those communities that have limited access to healthcare resources and to the various communication platforms which discuss healthcare policies and disseminate information on health. The emphasis on structure favors the orientation of the culture-centered approach toward the development of health communication theories and applications which are directed at marginalized healthcare settings (more on this in a later section). The role of structure in the realm of health communication is typically played out in the form of culturally situated health practices.

Box I.1   The story of Dr Maria Rodriguez

Dr Maria Rodriguez struggled with poverty as she grew up; her family barely had the money to make ends meet. Although Dr Rodriguez remembers a great deal of those days of struggle, she also has very fond memories of her trips to the church and of growing up in a closely knit family. As a second generation immigrant from Colombia, she also has vivid memories of her childhood and of the values that her grandmother taught her. She learned to respect her family and to recognize how important family is in one's life. As a medical student and, later, as a family medicine practitioner, Dr Rodriguez had a difficult time in understanding all the rules in the hospital system that limited the access family members had to patients, to interactions with physicians and to information about patients. She struggled with this sense of deep-rooted individualism in the medical system, as it clashed with her sense of family and of its role in the medical experience.

How would you interpret Dr Rodriguez's story from a culture-centered approach? What are the key elements of the culture-centered approach that play out in the narrative presented here? How do you suggest that culture, structure, and agency play out in Dr Rodriguez's experience?

Culture

The concept of culture, as embodied in the culture-centered approach, refers to the local contexts within which health meanings are constituted and negotiated (more on the various meanings and interpretations of culture in chapter 3). The emphasis here is on looking at the constitutive and dynamic nature of culture. In other words, culture provides the communicative framework for health meanings such that the ways in which community members come to understand health and illness are embedded within cultural beliefs, values, and practices. These beliefs, values, and practices are also contextual, and health meanings become localized within these contexts. It is this contextual nature of health meanings that contributes to the dynamic nature of culture, suggesting that cultural meanings continually shift. Culture is constituted by the day-to-day practices of its members as they come to develop their interpretations of health and illness and to engage in these day-to-day practices. Furthermore, cultural meanings provide the locally situated scripts through which structures influence the health choices of cultural participants.

Agency

Agency refers to the capacity of cultural members to enact their choices and to participate actively in negotiating the structures within which they find themselves. In other words, the concept of agency reflects the active processes through which individuals, groups, and communities participate in a variety of actions which directly challenge the structures that constrain their lives, and, simultaneously, work with the structures in finding healthful options. From a health communication standpoint, agency taps into the ability of individuals and of their communities to be active participants in determining health agendas and in formulating solutions to a variety of health problems, as these are perceived by the community. The emphasis, therefore, shifts to the community as an entry point for the articulation of knowledge. Participatory spaces are created and sustained that allow health communicators the opportunity to engage with the agency of cultural participants.

Interactions between structure, culture, and agency

The three concepts of structure, culture, and agency are intertwined. Structures within social systems are played out through the culturally situated contexts in communities. In other words, structural features gain meaning through the contexts of the local culture, thus creating a site for the articulation and sharing of meanings. Structural constraints become meaningful through the lived experiences of cultural members and through the sharing of these lived experiences. For instance, the structures that limit healthcare access in inner city United States are made meaningful through the culturally situated stories of residents in the inner cities as they discuss their daily lives and the struggles embodied in them (Abraham 1993). Simultaneously, culture offers the substratum for structure, such that structures are both reified and challenged through the cultural meaning systems that are in circulation within the culture. It is through the articulation of new meanings that cultures create points of social change. For instance, it is when cultural members in a marginalized context start sharing their stories of deprivation that greater awareness is created and opportunities are introduced for changes in the healthcare infrastructures (Wang and Burris 1994).

Agency is enacted in the lives of individuals and communities as they struggle with the structural constraints they face. Given the emphasis of the culture-centered approach on marginalized settings, much of the discussion of the approach relates to the lack of basic resources and economic capacities in these contexts. Agency offers an opportunity to situate the lives of marginalized individuals, groups and communities in the realm of their active engagement in living with, and challenging, the structures that constrain their lives. In other words, agency becomes meaningful in its relationship with the structures within which healthcare experiences are embedded. Members of marginalized communities continually interact with the structures within which they live, simultaneously working within these structures and participating in avenues that seek to change them. Ultimately, agency offers the opportunity for social change by challenging the structures that limit the healthcare capacities in marginalized communities.

It is in the realm of culturally situated meanings and actions that individuals enact their agency. In other words, culture provides the conduit through which agency is realized. The language for engaging in the discourses of health and the meanings of health that become possible are constituted in the domain of culture. It is through the culturally situated symbols that individuals communicate with each other, interact with the social structures, and come to organize collectively to address the structures. The interactions that individuals have with social structures are made meaningful through the lens of culture; therefore it is through the symbols that circulate in the culture that individuals enact their agency. Similarly, the ways in which individuals go about their daily practices of health are rendered meaningful through the symbols that circulate in the culture. Agency also offers an opportunity for changing culturally situated meanings as it is through their uses of discourse that individuals, groups and communities challenge the dominant cultural meanings and create new openings. Now that we have discussed the culture-centered approach and its basic configuration, the next section will discuss its roots, together with some of the concepts which are central to the ways we discuss and use it in health communication.

Roots of Culture-Centered Health Communication

The culture-centered approach draws much of its theoretical, methodological and application-based focus from critical theory, cultural studies, postcolonial theory and subaltern studies (see Dutta-Bergman 2004a, 2004b; Dutta 2007; Lupton 1994). Therefore the questions asked by the culture-centered approach, and the key concepts that inform it, draw from these disciplinary roots of the approach, which are represented by the four areas of study.

Critical theory

The culture-centered approach to health communication draws much of its impetus from critical theory. With its emphasis on questioning the ways in which knowledge gets articulated and talked about, the culture-centered approach locates knowledge in the realm of the concepts of power and control. It argues that the content of knowledge claims are embedded within the practices of powerful actors in social systems that have access to the spaces of knowledge. In this sense, knowledge is situated in the realm of the interests of powerful social actors, and the focus of critical theory is on examining how knowledge is used so as to ensure the control held by these dominant social actors.

Furthermore, drawing upon Marxist theory, critical theorists study the role of social structures in constraining the life experiences of the under-privileged classes. The critical lens focuses on studying the relationship between fundamental economic resources and the distribution of power within social systems. From this standpoint, knowledge is seen as a tool which is used for the purposes of controlling and managing the under-privileged social classes so that they may continue to supply the labor for capitalist economies, which in turn, serves as the basis for the profit secured by the owners of the capital.

The contents of knowledge claims are tied to the ways in which knowledge claims are made and to the positions of power from which they are made. Therefore the culture-centered approach locates knowledge as the subject of inquiry. As a first point of entry into talking about health communication, it looks at the ways in which knowledge claims are intrinsically tied to the positions from which they are made. To this extent, the culture-centered approach investigates the claims made in dominant health communication approaches and the ways in which these claims serve those in positions of power, thus primarily starting as a deconstructive exercise.

In addition to engaging with the concept of power, the culture-centered approach also draws upon the two concepts of *ideology* and *hegemony* in critical theory. Ideology reflects the taken-for-granted assumptions that help maintain the power structures; and hegemony refers to the ways in which the dominant actors retain their status of dominance without having to use coercive measures. In health communication, ideology and hegemony are intrinsic to the control exerted by the dominant social actors on the positions at the margins. The ideology of individual lifestyles, for instance, locates individual behaviors at the root of health problems without attending to the surrounding social and structural features of the environment that constrain the possibilities of health (Lupton 1994). Health campaigns are funded and implemented to curb the smoking habits of individuals, but they do not touch on the problem of regulating the tobacco industry and the marketing strategies used by it. Furthermore, transnational capital maintains its dominant status through hegemonic processes that ensure that global policies supporting the free market economy are supported, simultaneously sustaining conditions of poverty and inaccess to resources, which are often fostered by these unhealthy global policies (Kim, Millen, Irwin and Gershman 2000).

Drawing from critical theory, culture-centered health communication scholarship is engaged with questions of power, ideology, hegemony and control in the discourses and practices of healthcare (Dutta-Bergman 2004a, 2004b). It examines such discourses in terms of their maintaining the control of powerful social actors. From a critical standpoint, the goal of the culture-centered approach is to look at the dominant values in healthcare systems – values which underlie the ways in which these systems maintain the control of the powerful actors. Through the exploration of ideology and hegemony, attention is drawn to the health communication processes that maintain the privileges of the powerful social actors in healthcare systems and simultaneously exploit the poor, the working classes, women, racial minorities, and communities from the global South. The emphasis of the culture-centered approach on the concepts of ideology and hegemony are further complemented by the emphasis of cultural studies on the social constructions of knowledge and practices.

Cultural studies

Building on the questions of ideology and hegemony presented in critical theory, the domain of cultural studies is interested in how knowledge is socially constructed by powerful social actors. Aligned with the goals of critical theory, it keeps the focus still on power structures and the modes of their being maintained through the social constructions of discourse. A cultural studies approach to communicative practices locates these practices within the realm of power and studies how meanings are created and circulated in order to serve the interests of powerful social actors. That meanings are situated in the realm of cultural contexts drives much of the scholarship in cultural studies.

The culture-centered approach draws from cultural studies scholarship, with its emphasis on the social constructions of discourse and on the culturally situated nature of health narratives. On the one hand, this type of approach studies the social construction of meanings played out through the ideological devices employed by the dominant actors within social systems; on the other hand, it studies culturally situated health meanings and discursively explores the way these meanings are socially constructed by the local actors. For instance, a cultural-studies examination of the stigma of living with HIV/AIDS builds on the social construction of stigma and the ways in which meanings of stigma get attached to HIV/AIDS (Farmer 1999). The emphasis therefore is on agency and on the constitution of agency through the participants of the culture.

Postcolonial theory

Drawing from Said's influential work on Orientalism, postcolonial scholars are interested in interrogating the colonial agendas of knowledge structures. In other words, postcolonial scholarship explores how the dominant knowledge configurations serve colonial interests. From a health communication standpoint, a postcolonial approach interrogates the dominant health discourses that circulate globally. The interest here is to explore the dichotomies of the First and Third World, the North and the South, the West and the rest; and to see how these dichotomies play out in selecting who gets to decide the health agendas, who participates in the communicative processes leading up to it, and who gets to configure the communicative strategies for healthcare interventions. Simultaneously, based on a postcolonial lens, the culture-centered approach explores the communicative strategies through which points of dominance are created through the dichotomous categories of "primitive" and "modern" within the healthcare system. Questioning the values underlying this dichotomy exposes the political economy of health communication interventions that seek to maintain the dominant status of the North through the presentation of discourse which privileges it and locates the South in terms of absences tied to its so-called primitiveness, thus necessitating interventions carried out by the North. The categorization of the South/Third/Underdeveloped as "primitive" helps to maintain the privilege of the North/First/Developed world by creating and fostering conditions of dependence and need (Dutta-Bergman 2004a, 2004b; Dutta and Basnyat, in press; Escobar 1995).

Subaltern studies

As a discipline of inquiry, subaltern studies is interested in interrogating the erasures in the dominant configurations of knowledge (Beverly 2004; Guha 1988). Originally emerging from the ranks of historians, subaltern scholars were interested in what is absent from the mainstream articulations of history. With an emphasis on writing history from below, they asked how the writing of history and its products served the interests of the colonial powers and national elites. In doing so, they turned the lens on the dominant *epistemic* structures and questioned the underlying privileges of the elite that are maintained by these structures.

Questioning the absences in mainstream discourse offers opportunities for understanding how discourses are created, re-created, and circulated within social systems. The examination of the privileges and values of the dominant social actors, which are reflected in the ways knowledge is constituted, plays a critical role in defining the terrain for subaltern scholarship. The erasures also provide entry points for rewriting the narratives of knowledge through engagement with the voices of subaltern communities. Dialogues with subaltern communities offer opportunities for further co-constructing the discourses of knowledge through the voices of subaltern communities presented in the co-constructive process. It is worth noting that subaltern scholars seek neither to represent the subaltern nor to become absent from the discursive spaces. Rather, they present themselves as co-participants, reflexively aware of the privilege they embody in the discursive process. It is through the ownership of the privilege that subaltern scholarship enters into a relationship of solidarity with subaltern participants.

With its roots in subaltern scholarship, the culture-centered approach continually asks how dominant discourses of health communication erase the voices of certain groups and communities and create the conditions of subalternity (Dutta 2007; Dutta-Bergman, 2004a, 2004b). It focuses on examining the taken-for-granted assumptions in the dominant theories of health communication and their persistence in undermining the agency of cultural participants. The culture-centered approach claims that the undermining of the agency of subaltern groups is quintessential to the erasures of these groups from the dominant epistemic structures. Knowledge here is intrinsically connected to praxis, as the applications of health communication that are developed in mainstream social systems continue to erase the voices of subaltern communities by consistently categorizing them as the subjects of healthcare interventions. In this sense, the marginalized community or culture is located in a fixed category, imbued with "undesirable" characteristics, and interventions are developed to change the "undesirable" characteristics of the subaltern groups. By interrogating the absences of subaltern voices in healthcare policies, programs and evaluation strategies, the culture-centered approach creates discursive openings for co-constructing narratives of health through dialogue with subaltern communities. It proposes to bring about changes in healthcare policies and the way these policies are presented and represented through the voices of the subaltern participants engaged in dialogue with the culture-centered scholar. In the next section we will study the basic characteristics of the culture-centered approach.

Characteristics of the Culture-Centered Approach

Some of the key concepts that run through the culture-centered approach are the concepts of: (a) "power," "ideology," "hegemony," and "control," which demonstrate how health communication theories and research projects and applications serve the interests of the dominant social actors; (b) "marginalization," which reflects upon how conditions of subjugation are created and supported by the dominant practices of health communication; (c) "contexts" within which health experiences are realized and enacted; (d) the "stories" shared by cultural members about their health experiences, as being constituted in the realm of the structures as well as being about the possibilities of challenging these structures, within which health is constituted; and (e) "resistance," which reflects the ability of individuals, groups, and communities to challenge the dominant structures within which health is constituted, and offers opportunities for creating new discursive and material possibilities.

Power

As discussed earlier, power consists in the social, cultural and communicative practices through which the dominant social actors maintain their control over the social system. Power is deeply connected with the economic necessities of the dominant social actors. Furthermore, access to power is determined by economic access, such that owners of capital have greater power over those who provide the labor to the capitalist system. In order to maintain their power, dominant social actors employ ideological devices which create discursive spaces supportive of the control they hold. As discussed earlier in this chapter, the ability to maintain control over a social system without the use of coercive strategies is referred to as hegemony. The culture-centered approach is concerned with the way the ideology of healthcare serves the positions of power within social systems. It is also in the realm of power that conditions of marginalization are created and sustained.

Marginalization

Marginalization reflects an array of practices through which the social structures limit the resources and opportunities for participation in certain communities and cultures. Therefore, marginalized communities have minimal access to basic healthcare resources and to the mainstream communication platforms on which they could articulate their questions and concerns. Culture-centered theorists point out that mainstream health communication programs create conditions of marginalization by supporting the agendas of the powerful social actors and by simultaneously ignoring the health needs of subaltern communities (Dutta-Bergman 2004a, 2004b, 2005a, 2005b; Dutta and Basu 2007; Dutta and Basnyat, in press). Much of the emphasis of the culture-centered, approach is on studying the intersections between structure, culture, and agency in the realm of the experiences of these marginalized communities.

Context

Context refers to the locally situated nature of healthcare experiences, and is articulated through "thick" descriptions of the lived experiences of cultural members. Context taps into the dynamics and continuously contested nature of health communication such that health experiences become meaningful only when located in the perimeters of local context. Healthcare discourses and practices are continuously rendered meaningful through their engagement of the local contexts within which they become possible. The culture-centered approach engages with the local context through dialogues with the community members, thus bringing out opportunities for listening to the voices of marginalized communities (Dutta-Bergman 2004a, 2004b; Dutta and Basu 2007).

Stories

It is though stories that healthcare scripts are circulated. Stories are built upon shared cultural meanings and offer insights into the ways in which the culture constitutes its meanings of health, approaches health and illness, and engages in healthcare practices. Cultures pass on certain health meanings through a community of participants, and the culturally situated stories provide points of meaning-making to cultural participants (Airhihenbuwa 1995). It is within these communities that stories offer lessons about health, what it means to be healthy, what it means to be ill, and what actions to take in response to illness. It is also through stories that new meanings of health are articulated and change is brought about through the introduction of new possibilities into the discursive space. The culture-centered approach permanently draws our attention to the stories through which culture continues and yet transforms.

Resistance

Resistance reflects an array of communicative practices through which the dominant structures are challenged. In the area of healthcare, marginalized communities resist dominant structures in various ways, which range from the micro-practices of resistance to the macro-practices of resistance. Micro-practices of resistance include practices such as refusal to take medications prescribed by doctors, refusal to get a child immunized, or refusal to take certain preventive measures as prescribed by the dominant paradigm. Macro-practices of resistance include transformative acts which seek to change the social system. Examples include hunger strikes designed to oppose unhealthy global policies, participation in protest marches to discuss the lack of doctors with policy-makers, *gheraous* at the local hospital etc. (Dutta-Bergman 2004b; Dutta and Basu 2007; Dutta and Pal, in press).

Conclusion

In conclusion, the culture-centered approach offers an avenue for opening up the dominant framework of health communication to communities and contexts that have so far been ignored, rendered silent and been treated simply as subjects of health communication interventions. By examining how we communicate in our traditional health interventions and the linkages between these interventions and the dominant value systems, the approach offers us opportunities to question the inherent biases in our modes of thinking about health and of going about promot-ing it in communities. In the realm of the media, the culture-centered approach specifically examines the distribution of media structures in sub-altern contexts and how the mainstream media marginalize the voices of certain cultures and communities. Furthermore, by engaging in questions of agency, the culture-centered approach creates openings for the voices of those communities that have traditionally been silenced by mainstream media platforms. These points of engagement with subaltern contexts create opportunities for social change in the healthcare system. The culture-centered approach, therefore, is mainly concerned with the possi-bilities of social change through communication.

In the realm of interpersonal relationships in healthcare, the culture-centered approach offers us opportunities for examining physician–patient relationships and for conceptualizing ways in which such relationships might be informed by notions of culture. It also expands the nature of rela-tionships in healthcare settings by looking at alternative ways of healing and curing. In the area of healthcare organizations, the culture-centered approach creates avenues for looking at how mainstream health organ-izations marginalize the health experiences of subaltern communities. Furthermore, healthcare organizing challenges the status quo through its emphasis on processes of organizing subaltern communities. It does this with the goal of changing unhealthy social and economic structures which constrain the healthcare experiences of subaltern communities. In mass media contexts, the culture-centered approach deconstructs the dominant mass mediated campaigns targeted at changing target behaviors. It also interrogates the role of global mass media in promoting the ideology of biomedicine.

Throughout the book, we will explore the various ways in which culture informs our manners of talking about health, the health messages we develop, and the healthcare applications we engage in on a daily basis. We will explore the issue of how healthcare identities and relationships are culturally situated; the different cultural approaches to health, illness, and healing; the various ways in which local communities are marginalized in their healthcare experiences; and the possibilities, brought about by the culture-centered approach, for challenging the unhealthy structures sur-rounding the health of marginalized communities. Ultimately, the goal of the culture-centered approach is to suggest points for a structural transfor-mation which should open up new possibilities for equitable and accessi-ble healthcare. To this end, the book concludes with suggestions for a praxis in health communication based on the culture-centered approach.

Points for reflection

- What are the goals of the culture-centered approach? How do these goals inform the ways in which we practice health communication?
- Consider the health experiences of Sarah, a 41-year-old single woman with three children living in rural Ohio. Sarah was recently fired from her

part-time job, and currently does not have health insurance cover for her medical expenses. Which aspects of the culture-centered approach help you to understand Sarah's health experiences? How?

- You have recently been hired as an outreach worker for a health services clinic promoting condom usage among Hispanic migrant farm workers in Kinnesaw, Kansas. In one of your assigned readings for a class in college on culture and health, you came across the concept of the culture-centered approach. Discuss the ways in which you would incorporate the approach in your work.
- What is marginalization? In the context of healthcare, what factors in social systems contribute to marginalization? How? Please discuss in detail the ways in which dominant health communication approaches create conditions at the margins.
- What are the ways in which marginalized communities enact their agency? Please discuss.

1 Culture in Health Communication

Chapter objectives

In this chapter, we will:

- examine the history of culture in health communication
- study the different models of health communication
- compare the different strands of culture-based health communication work

How did culture emerge as a concept in health communication, and how does culture get used in health communication theories and applications? In our discussions in this chapter, after reviewing the major health communication theories, we will connect our discussion of these theories to the dominant and culture-centered approaches to health communication. As articulated in the introduction, closely aligned with the biomedical model, the dominant approach focuses on utilizing cultural variables to develop more effective health communication solutions (more on this in chapter 2); and the culture-centered approach is a critique of the dominant approach that focuses on the erasure of cultural voices in dominant discourses and seeks to engage with these voices as entry points for dialogue. Locating the current scholarship on culture-based health communication in the realm of its historical roots will offer the foundation for discussing the culture-centered approach to health communication in chapters 2 and 3. Throughout the present chapter, the discussion of the different approaches to health communication will draw upon the critical and cultural underpinnings of the culture-centered approach outlined in the Introduction.

Box 1.1   The story of Suzanne

Suzanne has recently graduated with a PhD in Health Communication from a prestigious US university, and has received a tenure-track position as an assistant professor at a research university. Although she has never really traveled much to other parts of the world, she is very interested in issues of global health. The topic of global health has a great deal of funding potential and Suzanne thinks this would be a great opportunity for her to set up a program of research. She expresses this interest to her Department head and is assigned to teach a course on "Gender, Development, and

Health." She has quite a few women who she thinks come from somewhere in the Middle East (she does not know where from exactly . . . both of these students are actually from Pakistan) and feels uncomfortable having them in class because they wear *burquas*. Being a feminist, she feels that women should not have to cover their heads, and especially not in the US. She is further aggravated by the Middle Eastern women after her Head of Department calls her to his office letting her know that there has been a complaint lodged against her for being culturally insensitive in her classroom by talking about the "primitive cultures" of the Muslim world when she addressed the topic of honor killings in her lecture day on "Gender and Health." She is quite confident that those women are the ones who probably complained. This infuriates her as she feels that the climate of political correctness in the academy has gone too far – one can't even address "primitive cultures" and call them for what they are. She further feels that one can't even discuss the real health problems in the Third World. After all, she only wants to help these women and others like them, who are oppressed by their men. Based on your reading of culture in health communication, how would you interpret Suzanne's attitude toward her Pakistani students? What do we learn about Suzanne from this encounter? What do we learn about the values of Suzanne and what are the similarities and differences between these values and the values of dominant health communication projects that use the concept of culture?

Historical Overview

The role of culture in health communication started to receive increasing attention in the 1980s, with the acknowledgement of the shifting demographic patterns within the US, and with the emerging understanding that health communication efforts needed to respond systematically to the shifting cultural landscape in order to be effective; this created the climate for multicultural health communication efforts (Brislin and Yoshida 1994; Resnicow et al. 2002). The emphasis on multicultural populations within the US was set in the backdrop of the criticism of health promotion efforts in the global South that questioned the universalist assumptions of the health communication programs targeted at the global South and emphasized the necessity to incorporate an understanding of culture in international health communication efforts (Airhihenbuwa 1994, 1995; Airhihenbuwa and Obregon 2000). This criticism was keenly aware of the negative ramifications of the top-down approaches which did not take local cultures into account. Advocating an urgency to situate culture and context at the core of public health communication practices, Airhihenbuwa noted (1995: x):

> It has become common practice in the field of public health and in the social and behavioral sciences to pay lip service to the importance of culture in the study and understanding of health behaviors, but culture has yet to be inscribed at the root of health promotion and disease prevention programs, at least in the manner that legitimates its centrality in public health praxis.

In the decade following this observation, health communication theorizing and practice has taken a turn towards incorporating culture in health communication (see Dutta-Bergman 2004a, 2004b, 2005a, 2005b; Dutta 2007; Dutta and Basu 2007; Ford and Yep 2003; Harris et al. 2001). Scholars have increasingly vouched for a need to develop communication frameworks grounded in the culture and context of those who are at the heart of health promotion efforts (Airhihenbuwa and Obregon 2000; Airhihenbuwa, Makinwa and Obregon 2000; Dutta-Bergman 2004a; Dutta and Basu 2007). Airhihenbuwa (1995) writes that health is a cultural construct and health theory and practice must be rooted in cultural codes and meanings, inherently tied to values. These values make up the transient framework of a person's everyday living. Embedded in and influenced by these values are notions of community rules, traditions, health beliefs, socio-economic ability, societal power structures, education, religion, spirituality, gender roles and exposure. Helman (1986: 71) adds that in every human society beliefs and practices related to health are a central feature of culture: "both the presentation of illness, and others' response to it, are largely determined by socio-cultural factors."

This growing awareness of the cultural differences globally is based on the understanding that there are many different ways of perceiving and interpreting health across different cultural groups, and, in order to become effective, health communicators needed to become aware of these cultural differences (Hammerschlag 1988). Cultural differences were conceptualized as barriers to effective health communication efforts, and the goal of the health communicator was to develop communication programs that would address these barriers and overcome them. Health communicators now faced the challenge of identifying the barriers to effective communication and of incorporating them into successful messages that would target these barriers.

In responding to the concept of culture, the literature in health communication suggests some important constructs that have been developed for the purposes of assisting the health communicator (Huff and Kline 1999a; Resnicow et al. 2002). These constructs include *acculturation* and *assimilation*; *ethnocentrism*; and *cultural competence*. Each of these concepts was brought into health communication for the purposes of guiding the health communication scholar and his/her work, and suggested methods for modifying the existing concepts of health communication so as to take culture into account. Furthermore, responding to the call issues by Airhihenbuwa (1995), the PEN-3 model and the culture-centered approach emerged as two key approaches that attempt to place culture at the center of theorizing and application development rather than as an afterthought.

Acculturation and assimilation

The literature on acculturation explores the ways in which multicultural populations adjust to the cultural values and mores of a dominant culture (Resnicow et al. 2002). Acculturation reflects the degree to which an individual migrating into another culture gives up the traits of the home culture and adopts the traits of the dominant culture (Locke 1992). According to Locke, immigrants typically may be categorized into one out of four groups, on the basis of their levels of acculturation into the dominant culture. The "bicultural" individual functions equally well both in his/her home culture and in the dominant culture; the "traditional" individual is defined as someone who holds on to most of the traits of his culture of origin; the "marginal" individual seems to have lost contact with traits from either culture; and the "acculturated" individual seems to have given up most of the traits of his culture of origin and has adopted the traits of the dominant culture. Locke points out the importance of addressing the level of acculturation of the target audience in order to develop meaningful health promotion messages.

Like acculturation, assimilation relates to the degree to which the members of a multicultural population merge and mingle with the dominant culture. The idea of assimilation taps into the notion that cultural assimilation is critical to important health outcomes. The dominant culture is taken for granted as the normative ideal, and immigrant communities are evaluated on the basis of their adherence to the broader cultural standards; the more assimilated the community is, the better equipped it is to succeed in the dominant culture. Much of the health-promotion work that emerges out of this line of thought seeks to teach skills to multicultural communities with the goal of assimilating them into the broader community.

Ethnocentrism

Ethnocentrism reflects the social, cultural and individual trait of remaining closed to other cultures, which are considered outside cultures (Ferguson 1991). In other words, ethnocentrism refers to cultural insularity. In this sense, the goal of health communication programs is to counter the ethnocentrism of healthcare professionals, so that they can provide better and more effective healthcare services to their multicultural clients and stakeholders.

Cultural competence

The idea of cultural competence captures the degree of adeptness displayed by healthcare professionals in handling the cultural mores and rituals of other cultures they interact with daily (Campinha-Bacote 1994). A highly culturally competent healthcare professional is well equipped to pick up the nuances of other cultures and to respond to them. The goal of health communication efforts dealing with the notion of cultural competence is to train healthcare professionals and to evaluate them in terms of their competence.

What we see in the emerging efforts toward incorporating culture into health communication scholarship is an increasing awareness of the

Box 1.2   The story of Ibasa

Ibasa migrated with his mother Jameela in 1998 to Minneapolis, after his family was left homeless during the civil war in Somalia. Since moving to the US, Ibasa and his mother have enrolled in vocational training classes and joined a local church directed at acculturating Somalis. Ibasa has also received invitations to multiple health trainings and health workshops at the local community health center. However, Ibasa has been skeptical about joining these training programs, because he has heard from his Somali friends how these workshops talk about the importance of family planning and keep pushing the idea of contraceptive choice.

He feels uncomfortable with this, as contraception does not fit well with his values and beliefs. One of his friends at work, Sam, told him the other day that he should forget about his old values; "the quicker he is able to forget them, the better he will be." Sam had said, "Ibasa, become an American. Forget the old dreams. . .they are standing in your way. This is a new land of opportunities." However, Ibasa still struggles.

What does Ibasa's story teach us about the experiences of acculturation? What are the possible advantages of acculturation? What are the possible drawbacks of acculturation?

cultural differences that constitute health experiences. An awareness of these cultural differences improves the existing approaches to health communication by incorporating the concept of culture; the goal is to adjust the health messages to the cultural beliefs, mores, and rituals. Knowledge of the cultural differences allows the health communicator to develop further messages and communication strategies that are sensitized to these differences. Furthermore, notions such as acculturation, assimilation, and cultural competence conceptualize culture as a static entity, which may be extracted to articulate differences. By contrast, the concept of culture driving the PEN-3 and culture-centered approaches is dynamic and context-based (to be discussed later).

Discussion point 1.1

- What is health communication to you?
- How would you define culture?
- Now examine your own values and beliefs about culture. Where did you learn your concept of culture? What does your concept of culture tell you about yourself and the world you live in?

Models of Health Communication

The models discussed in this section have been instrumental in guiding health communication interventions. Whereas some of these models have explicitly debated, and engaged with, the concept of culture, other models have implicitly assumed the role of culture in health communication.

Theory of reasoned action (TRA)

Having been applied in the realm of multiple health campaigns, TRA explains volitional human behavior, proposing that one's intention to perform or not to perform a behavior is a result of that person's attitude toward the specific behavior and of her perception of the evaluation of the behavior by important others (Ajzen and Fishbein 1980; Fishbein and Ajzen 1975). The attitude of the individual results, in turn, from her salient beliefs about the outcomes of the behavior in question. Two critical components define the participant's state of belief toward the behavior: her belief strengths and her belief evaluations. Similarly, the individual's motivation to comply with salient others in her social network, accompanied by the normative beliefs regarding the target behavior ascribed to these salient others, produce her subjective norms. Central to the conceptualization of the theory of reasoned action is the role of beliefs in the formation of attitudes and subjective norms.

The theory suggests that individuals systematically identify and weigh outcomes in order to form attitudes. In other words, beliefs lie at the core of the persuasion process, and health campaigns which target behavior change need to address the beliefs of the audience in the first place. Campaign planners have attempted to induce change in the target population by adding a new belief, by increasing or decreasing the favorability or unfavorability of an existing belief, and by increasing or decreasing the belief strength, depending upon the nature of the behavior.

The persuasive process documented in the theory of reasoned action is primarily based on information. The rationally acting receiver of the message is able to evaluate all possible outcomes, weigh them and make a decision based on a cost–benefit analysis. This model of rational choice becomes particularly problematic in the case of certain choices: choices made on the spur of the moment, or choices which don't involve deliberate cognitive evaluation. The centrality accorded to cognition and belief-based evaluation is founded on an individualistic epistemology where the locus of choice is the individual. The enactment or non-enactment of the behavior is a result of individual-level processes that precede the behavior.

Consider, in this light, a collectivistic culture where the emphasis is on collective identity. The behavior then gets located in the characteristics of the collective and becomes a part of the collective being. Although proponents of the theory of reasoned action might argue that subjective norms explain the role of the collective in individual decision-making, it may be counter-argued that subjective norms are driven by an individual-motive orientation and therefore are fundamentally unable to capture the locus of decision in the collectivity. The rational actor model espoused in the theory of reasoned action also does not capture the socio-cultural context of a behavior. Structural resources and access to them might be critical to the development of an understanding of health communication in marginalized contexts.

The health belief model (HBM)

Widely used in predicting the adoption of preventive health behaviors (Bond, Aiken and Somerville 1992; French et al. 1992; Gillam 1991; Witte et al. 1993), the health belief model is yet another model located in the individual and in his rational choices of preventive behaviors. Six components are central to the development of the health belief model: severity, susceptibility, benefits, barriers, cues to action and self-efficacy (Janz and Becker 1984; Mattson 1999; Rosenstock 1974). These six components situate the preventive behavior in the realm of a certain health outcome such as HIV infection, cancer, heart disease etc. The model positions the individual's likelihood of engaging in the health behavior within the realm of perception. Perceptual processes filter the way an individual evaluates the proposed preventive behavior and the outcomes associated with it.

Whereas perceived severity refers to the individual's assessment of the outcome associated with the preventive behavior, perceived susceptibility focuses on the individual's assessment of the extent to which he/she is likely to succumb to the negative outcome. Benefits include the individual's beliefs regarding the effectiveness of the proposed preventive behavior in reducing the vulnerability to the negative outcomes (Mattson 1999; Rosenstock 1966). Barriers decrease the individual's ability to engage in the preventive behavior; they are described as the evaluation of potential negative consequences that might result from the enactment of the espoused health behavior (Mattson 1999; Rosenstock 1966). Self-efficacy taps into the amount of confidence individuals have in their ability to perform the health behavior; it positively predicts the adoption of the preventive behavior (Mattson 1999). Cues to action are the specific stimuli that are needed to trigger the appropriate health behavior (Janz and Becker 1984; Mattson 1999). When exposed to a health threat and both the perceived threat and the efficacy are high, the individual attempts to control the danger by adhering to the recommendations of the message; when the perceived threat is high but efficacy is low, individuals are motivated to control the fear through defensive avoidance or denial.

Critical to note here is the emphasis on cognitive evaluations as precursors to the adoption of the healthy behavior. The model does not accommodate the communicative practices in alternative discursive spaces where a systematic evaluation of the target behavior does not precede health practices. It also does not accommodate those cultural situations where the behavior is located within the broader culture and its practices. As articulated earlier, a key antecedent of behavioral intention in the health belief model is perception. What gets left out from the model is the reality of the contextual scenario that surrounds the individual and the risks that encompass her life. On the other hand, the perceptions generated in the audience might not actually tap into the real risks faced by the individual members, but reflect and propagate instead the biases of the sender of the message.

In addition to propagating Western hegemony through the creation of risks that are alien to the lived experiences of the members of the culture, the health belief model fails to look for the origins of a behavior in those places beyond the individual that might actually hold the key to the enactment of the behavior – for instance lack of money, which prevents individuals from lower socio-economic areas from eating regularly, let alone buying fruits and vegetables. In addition to addressing the perceived severity or susceptibility associated with a particular behavior, campaign planners often choose to address directly the benefits or barriers associated with a behavior through communication materials such as leaflets, brochures, advertisements, letters, and the like.

A communication-based approach which addresses the question of benefits or barriers by providing information does not fundamentally question the key structural elements of barriers, those which fundamentally impede the enactment of behavior in particularly deprived parts of the world, where individuals don't have the basic capabilities of life such as food, clothing, and shelter. What I am arguing here is that a communication campaign informed by the health belief model which attempts to provide solutions for severity, susceptibility, benefits and barriers through leaflets, television shows, or radio programs is a trifling exercise in futility. Such communicative ventures don't even come close to capturing the real barriers, which severely constrain people's abilities and define their lived experiences centrally. It is only after equipping individuals and communities with the basic capabilities of life that we could start talking about higher-order health behaviors such as getting mammograms, not smoking cigarettes, having safe sex, and so on.

For instance, individuals in rural Pakistan might drink unsafe water, not because they choose to do so, but because they don't have access to any other form of water. Even if access to clean water is created in the community, individual community members might not be willing to drink it because of the long lines they have to stand in to get it (and hence lose valuable time that could have been spent earning money). Instead of taking a Eurocentric and parochial approach to communicating in the context of international health, communication scholars need to address the role of communication as a conduit for capability building. How can communication be harnessed for addressing those structural barriers which severely limit the lives of individuals? How can communication be used as a conduit in the realm of capability building?

Yet another important element to note is the defining role of culture in creating a lens through which health practices are envisioned and practiced. Although the individual might operate as the vehicle through which a certain behavior is enacted, cultural practices much stronger than his/her personal evaluations of that behavior might hold the key to understanding it. These cultural practices might be located in the social cement as opposed to being located within the individual. The important role of culture might be particularly evident in the realm of habitual behaviors, where the enactment of the behavior is based upon an existing script, without a thoughtful and systematic assessment each time.

The extended parallel process model (EPPM)

The extended parallel process model posits that the evaluation of perceived threat and perceived efficacy related to a specific intervention determine the pathway taken by the target audience after exposure to a message (Witte 1992, 1995). The extended parallel process model primarily focuses on fear appeals and suggests specific guidelines for their construction. Two primary pathways are available to the audience member upon exposure to a threatening message: the pathway taken will depend upon the level of perceived threat and perceived efficacy. As mentioned above, when exposed to a health threat, and when both the perceived threat and the efficacy are high, the individual attempts to control the danger by adhering to the recommendations of the message, that is, engaging in the preventive behavior that minimizes the danger; when the perceived threat is high but the efficacy is low, individuals are motivated to control the fear through defensive avoidance or denial, not adopting the recommended action.

Witte (1992) outlines a mechanism for the operation of fear appeals. She points out that audience members first evaluate the perceived threat of the hazard. If the perceived threat elicited by the message is low, the individual is not motivated to process the message further; however, if and when the perceived threat is moderate to high, the individual moves on to the second appraisal: that of the efficacy of the recommended action (ibid.). In situations when both the perceived threat and the perceived efficacy of the recommended action are high, the message recipient is prompted to follow the recommended action; "individuals respond to the danger, not to their fear" (p. 338). However, on processing a message triggered by perceived high threat and not being convinced about their ability to deter the threat, individuals use a defensive mechanism to cope with their fear; they "respond to the fear, not to the danger" (ibid.). Since its introduction in the 1990s, the extended parallel process model has enjoyed a great deal of attention. Prevention campaigns using fear appeals have focused on combining threat producing messages with messages that seek to increase the response efficacy and the self-efficacy of the target audience along with the creation of perceived threat (severity and susceptibility).

However, much like the theory of reasoned action and the health belief model, the extended parallel process focuses on the individual. The emphasis is on the trajectory taken after exposure to the message. Ignored in the conceptualization of individual response is the surrounding context within which the individual might be embedded while viewing, reading or hearing the message. The recipient is highlighted; the media environment within which the message is received is ignored. A college student watching a fear-based message all by himself/herself in his/her dorm room will perhaps respond very differently to the message from when he/she is exposed to it amidst a group of friends at the student union. Or take, for instance, the case of audience exposure to a fear-inducing advertisement right after they have watched a television program inducing some positive emotion (a situation comedy). The viewer might be likely simply to avoid the message in order to maintain his/her positive emotional state (Kamins, Marks and Skinner 1991; Shapiro, MacInnis and Park 2002). Similarly, Mitchell (2001) demonstrates that sad moods generate greater perceptions of susceptibility and severity. What I am trying to articulate here is that the experience of fear is highly subjective and situation-driven; how a recipient responds to a fear appeal is perhaps greatly related to the context within which he/she is exposed to the message. By simply highlighting the basic elements of a message, the extended parallel process model fails to take into account the role of the context in driving the reception of the message. It is important to point out that the EPPM is likely to find support when studied in a laboratory setting; the student is exposed to the single message and a response with high internal validity is elicited. However, the artificiality of the very laboratory setting fundamentally removes the contextual factors that surround the reception of a message and, therefore, suffers from problems of external validity. These issues of external validity are important, since fear appeals are almost always embedded within the context; the loss of the surrounding context is not something that could be written off in the limitations section of a study on message effects. The highly contextualized nature of media consumption is particularly critical in collectivistic cultures, where individuals consume media in family and community settings, necessitating the development of measurement tools that capture the media consumption context (Davenport Sypher et al. 2002). For instance, research documenting the listenership of *Tinkha Tinkha Sukh* documented that community members formed informal groups which later became formalized into radio clubs that listened to the program as a group and subsequently discussed its content; these radio clubs actively participated in their local and surrounding communities, spreading the message of the social change project (Papa et al. 2000). The example of *Tinkha Tinkha Sukh* documents the interpenetration of the intrapersonal, interpersonal, mediated, group and community levels of communication.

The emphasis on the individual also locates the behavior in individual choice. As argued earlier in this chapter, theorizing the roots of health behaviors in individual choice reflects the individualistic orientation of the theorists who have worked on, and developed, these health communication theories. This emphasis on the individual ignores the role of the collective, which many a times shapes and directs a behavior. The meanings associated with the behavior and the behavioral outcome might very well be located in the social cement, the collective fabric of the community. In such instances, the individualistic messages of behavior change might fundamentally run counter to the values of the collective. The proposed behavior might not be able to co-exist in harmony with the values and goals of the collective.

In other instances, although a message might be created to assure the individual of the efficacy of a particular behavior and of his/her ability to engage in the behavior, such assurances created through the message might simply be false. In other words, the perceptual changes in efficacy introduced through a message might not reflect the real efficacy of the individual about to engage in the behavior. The message-based intervention might not really tap into the "real" structural and socio-cultural barriers faced by individuals in the community. These barriers might actually need to be addressed through policy changes and through the implementation of programs which seek to remove the barriers instead of communicating to people through messages. Worth pointing out here is the fact that many of the structural barriers experienced in marginalized populations, which are typical targets of health interventions, might not be overtly related to the specific behavior being proposed, or might not present themselves directly to the scrutiny of the external observer (Mony et al. 1999; Sarkar et al. 1997). For instance, the *Sonagachi* project in Calcutta recognized that an HIV/AIDS campaign in a severely resource-undernourished high-risk sex worker community would fail if it simply focused on distributing condoms and generating behavioral change through message design (Jana et al. 1998; UNAIDS 2000). Instead, the project emphasized the imminent contextual risks such as lack of access to money, arguing that the women in the community might need so much to sell their bodies to earn just enough money that they may agree not to use condoms if threatened or forced into this position by a paying client (The Synergy Project 2002; UNAIDS 2000). The sex workers of Sonagachi formed a consumer's cooperative called the Usha Multipurpose Cooperative Society, which would "help the sex workers save money and avoid the exorbitant interest charged on small loans by money lenders in the area" (Jana et al. 1998; UNAIDS 2000: 70). Recognizing the strong interlinkage between economics and safe sex practices among sex workers, the *Shakti* project in Bangladesh offered skills training in alternative modes of supplementing income, such as embroidery and sewing (UNAIDS 2000). On a similar note, the *SWEAT* project in South Africa fostered the development of exit programs, support programs, job creation schemes, and skills training programs for sex workers, while the *Prerana* project in India provided education, shelter, health and vocational training to the children of sex workers (The Synergy Project 2002).

Furthermore, although Witte (1998a, b) argues that the extended parallel process model is an improvement over earlier models and theories of health communication because it takes into account the role of emotions in information processing, it is worth pointing out that much of the experience of emotions is dependent upon cognitive appraisal. In the EPPM, the recipient's experience of a particular emotion (fear) is contingent upon his/her appraisal of the threat and subsequent evaluation of the efficacy. In other words, the experience of emotion is contingent upon cognitive appraisal.

Also, mostly ignored in the EPPM is the role that a highly negative emotion might play in deterring cognition (Shapiro, MacInnis and Park 2002). Witte (1992, 1998a, b) suggests that the individual recipient of the message will move from stage one, appraisal of the threat, to stage two, appraisal of the efficacy. In other words, a sufficient level of perceived threat will push the individual to move to the second step of figuring out the alternative ways of minimizing the threat. Once again, in this very sequencing of cognitive appraisals, Witte (1992) fails to note the response of an audience member to a highly threatening message where any form of cognitive appraisal is beyond the reach of the individual because too much fear has been built up (Shapiro, MacInnis and Park 2002). Although the recipe for controlling fear through efficacy evaluation and subsequent threat control might indeed be present in the message, the fear elicited might be substantive enough to prevent the individual from cognitively considering the efficacy component proposed in the message.

Finally, the fear appeal-based research has traditionally ignored the ethical issues related to the arousal of fear in target populations, especially among resource-deprived and marginalized individuals that are already voiceless. How ethical is the application of fear appeals in an attempt to induce behavior change in a population which already lives amidst fear and hopelessness? How ethical is it to use a fear appeal to target homeless shelters with individual-based messages of avoiding drugs? Instead of providing hope and bettering the lives of these deprived individuals, one might argue that fear appeals contribute further to their hopelessness, despair and negativity. The use of fear appeals to promote a particular behavior, which is laden with the cultural values of the message designer, almost verges on the use of coercive force to attain behavioral change. While on the one hand fear appeals might fundamentally violate the values of a people, on the other hand they might create a false appraisal of risks – one based on the value system of the message designer. These risks might not really reflect the real risks faced by a community.

Now that I have discussed three important campaign theories and problematized them, in the next section I will interrogate alternative articulations of social change projects.

Health as locus of control

Rotter (1966) has defined locus of control in the context of the explanations which various individuals give of their behaviors, positing that an internal locus of control is associated with the belief that individual behavior is causally related to outcomes, while an external locus of control is associated with the belief that outcomes are determined by external factors such as luck, powerful others, and fate. While the internal locus of control, this body of research suggests, is linked with information seeking (Lefcourt and Wine 1969), with autonomous decision-making, and with having a sense of well-being (ibid.), the external locus of control is linked with depression (Naditch, Gargan and Michael 1975), anxiety (Feather 1967), and being less able to cope with life stressors (Sandler and Lakey 1982). A plethora of studies in health psychology attest to this difference, positing that internals are better able to perform healthful life choices than externals (Bearinger and Blum 1997; Nir and Neumann 1991; Stewart and Streiner 1995). While Third World countries of Asia, Africa and Latin America are consistently classified as externals, many European nations and the northern United States are categorized as internals (Wrightson and Wardle 1997).

Critical to note here is the Eurocentric value judgment imposed on the comparative framework: while an internal locus of control is healthy and normal, an external locus of control is unhealthy, abnormal, deviant, something that should be changed through institutional enterprise. While cultures with an internal locus of control are happier, those with an external locus of control are depressed and unable to cope with life stressors. Also important to note is the idea that the Western nations of the world consistently emerge as cultures with an internal locus of control, by comparison to the external locus of control in the Third World. It looks as though the construct gives us an insight into the poverty, the filth, the dirt and the underdevelopment in the Third World, helping us understand such depravity in the context of the lack of agency and enterprise on the part of the people from that culture. By doing so, the research agenda of the "locus of control" justifies the colonizing Western intervention to uplift the poor and downtrodden, to take up agency on their behalf, and to enlighten them to practices of the modern world. Perhaps, locus of control also serves as an excuse for the failure of the multi-million international campaigns: after all, the agency-less externals are difficult to uplift and enlighten.

A similar construct widely in circulation in the cross-cultural health communication literature is fatalism. Fatalism is defined as "the perceived lack of control over one's environment, health, and day-to-day activities" (Casey 1994, as quoted in Witte 1995: 239). African, Asian, and Hispanic cultures are typically clustered together as highly fatalistic cultures and it is articulated that such cultures don't value prevention and planning ahead because they are propelled by the belief that health is a part of God's plan (Klessig 1992; Witte 1995). Witte (1995) posits that disempowerment lies at the heart of a fatalistic worldview. She writes: "people who believe that they have no control over their health will have no motivation to engage in health promotion or disease prevention activities," and recommends that program planners consider methods of addressing the fatalistic attitudes of target populations in developing their health communication campaigns. Fatalism is located in the cultural beliefs of a population and is treated as a barrier that needs to be overcome by the health communication campaign. In her discussion of fatalism, Witte points to the powerlessness and silencing of Third World women. Particularly critical are her descriptions of agency-less, disempowered women of the Third World; women that are victims of a strong patriarchical social system of a savage world. Important to note here are the similarities in the articulations of Witte and those of modernists, presented in the introduction to this paper. The scripting of the Third World inhabitant as a sterile subject stripped of agency is further narrated in social cognitive theory.

Social cognitive theory

Informed by Bandura's social cognitive theory (1986), international and cross-cultural health communication applications have articulated the role of self-efficacy in interventions. Self-efficacy refers to the extent to which people believe in their abilities to achieve a certain outcome. Bandura (1986) suggested that self-efficacy taps into people's assessments of their capabilities to organize and execute a specific course of action in order to attain a specific goal. Bandura argued that self-efficacy influences the "choices individuals make, their aspirations, how much effort they mobilize in a given endeavor, how long they persevere in the face of difficulties and setbacks, whether their thought patterns are self-hindering or self-aiding, the amount of stress they experience in coping with taxing environmental demands, and the vulnerability of depression" (ibid., p. 257). The concept of self-efficacy has been applied to a wide range of health issues, suggesting that individuals are better able to attain healthful goals when they have a high level of self-efficacy. These individuals believe in their ability to change their behaviors and attain a healthy life. On the other hand, it is stated that individuals with a perception of low self-efficacy are less able to attain healthy goals because of their lower likelihood of believing in themselves and their abilities.

Once again, critical to note is the conceptualization of self-efficacy in a value-laden framework. The health behavior is located in the individual and in the choices he/she makes. The emphasis on the individual's sense of his/her assessments does not take into account the real barriers to his/her action and his/her real capabilities, which might be embedded in the resources available in her/his environment. Self-efficacy locates capability in the perceptions of individuals, transforming capability into a psychological construct, a thing of the mind. I counter-argue against this position and propose that efficacy is not simply located in the individual but also in the presence of fundamental resources in his/her environment. Self-efficacy is an integral element of the structure that surrounds the individual. By treating self-efficacy as an audience-orientation variable (read psychological variable, a thing of the mind) without taking into account the actual resources of the environment, the proponents of self-efficacy run the risk of losing the pivotal structural context in developing an appropriate understanding of the culture.

Much of the decision-making in the realm of health in Third-World countries happens way beyond the reach of individual actors. In addition, in certain collectivist cultures, the healthy activity is located in the broader culture, and not in the individual. While cultures with limited resources might report on the lower end of the self-efficacy scale, members of such cultures might indeed demonstrate a high level of ability to comprehend their life situation and develop a sophisticated sense of the world. In this context, an application of the idea of self-efficacy on the host population becomes an exercise in Western epistemology, by way of judging the world through the lens of the West. Self-efficacy becomes yet another construct in categorizing the world into normal and deviant groups, without understanding the socio-structural contexts that often underlie health behaviors, without developing an understanding of the basic resources that define and constrain the capabilities of the individual, and without fundamentally questioning the value-laden nature of the categorical schemes we develop in health communication theorizing, research, and practice.

Diffusion of innovation

Diffusion refers to the process through which an innovation is communicated to the members of a social system through the use of certain channels (Muhiuddin and Kreps 2004; Rogers and Kincaid 1981; Rogers 1995). An innovation is defined as an idea, practice or object that is perceived to be new among individuals and other units of adoption. In the context of health promotion and prevention messages, the health attitude, belief or behavior is considered to be the innovation (Muhiuddin and Kreps 2004). Diffusion of health-related ideas has been widely studied (ibid.). The diffusion model has been widely and successfully used to study the spread of population control programs and for the purposes of developing interventions (Rogers 1995). Intervention-based diffusion studies have been conducted that measure the success of contraceptive-related education programs and the nature of the adoption of these programs. Intervention-based health promotion efforts using the diffusion framework seek to maximize the exposure and reach of innovations, strategies, or programs (Oldenburg, Hardcastle and Kok 1997).

   In the diffusion framework, an innovation is perceptual; in other words, an attitude, belief or behavior is considered to be an innovation to the extent that it is perceived to be new among the members of a social system. The extent to which an innovation is diffused within a population depends upon its relative advantage and its compatibility. Relative advantage refers to the degree to which an innovation is perceived to deliver advantages to the members of the social group. Furthermore, compatibility taps into the extent to which the proposed innovation fits with the existing norms of the system. In the domain of health behaviors, it is important to consider the ways in which the normative ideals of a community fit with the proposed innovation (Rogers 1995).

   Rogers outlines five main steps in the diffusion of innovations: (a) knowledge; (b) persuasion; (c) decision; (d) implementation; and (e) confirmation. Knowledge reflects the state when the individual becomes aware of the innovation, gains information about it and understands its functions. Persuasion refers to the stage where the individual or the group develops a favorable or unfavorable attitude toward the innovation. Decision reflects the state in which the individual or the group engages in activities that lead to a choice of either adopting or rejecting the innovation. Implementation refers to the stage when the innovation is put to use; and confirmation occurs when the individual or group that has already adopted the innovation seeks reinforcement about their choice of adoption. The diffusion process typically occurs in a time-ordered sequence, such that knowledge leads to persuasion, which in turn leads to decision, followed by implementation and then confirmation. There are however, instances when exceptions to this sequence might occur.

Communication is critical to the diffusion of innovation, and is primarily conceptualized in the realm of the channels that may be used in order to disseminate the message (Rogers 1995). Channels are the means through which messages get communicated to the members of the audience, and are typically classified into mass media channels and interpersonal communication channels. Diffusion is a social process and interpersonal channels play a critical role in the dissemination of the innovation (Rogers 1995). Most people depend upon other individuals in their social networks, who have adopted the innovation and can convey subjective information about its benefits. These important others in the social network, who determine the nature of diffusion of the innovation, are referred to as opinion leaders. Opinion leaders are those individuals who provide information and advice about innovations to others in the system. In other words, opinion leaders are key players in shaping the attitudes and beliefs of others in the social system.

Taken for granted in the diffusion of innovation literature are questions about the fundamentally value-laden nature of innovations. Who gets to decide what is an innovation? Who gets to be positioned as the innovator? Who is positioned as the receiver or the target audience of the innovation? Inherent in the diffusion of innovation framework are power differentials that dictate the flow of innovations. Eurocentric innovations are almost always imposed upon Third-World spaces with the goal of uplifting them. The terrain of power distribution is so largely uneven that it is almost impossible for us to imagine health innovations from elsewhere being diffused into dominant spaces. For instance, whereas USAID-sponsored diffusion programs in Bangladesh might seem legitimate and commonplace to the health communication student and scholar, to envision a health innovation planned by a Bangladeshi aid organization and implemented in the US would seem almost illegitimate. It is critical to interrogate the basic nature of innovations and look beyond the altruistic health claims for them, as the diffusion of innovations is inherently intertwined with exercises of power that often silence and erase alternative possibilities of health, just as they impose a dominant set of practices (often Eurocentric) that come to be accepted as the desirable parameters of health under the modernist paradigm.

Entertainment–education

Building on the early diffusion of innovation work, entertainment–education models have been widely circulated in the recent years to address a wide range of social issues in different parts of the world (Singhal and Rogers 1999 and 2002; Vaughan et al. 2000). Primarily based on the strategic placement of educational content in entertainment messages, the entertainment–education approach has been used to promote gender equity, family planning (Storey et al. 1999; Vaughan, Regis and St. Catherine 2000), and HIV/AIDS prevention (Piotrow et al. 1997; Singhal and Rogers 1999; Yoder, Hornik and Chirwa 1996) in a wide variety of countries including Nepal, India, Gambia, Philippines, Tanzania, Mexico and Peru (Singhal and Rogers 1999; Davenport Sypher et al. 2002). Entertainment–education strategies capitalize on the popular appeal of entertainment media to introduce socially relevant themes to the target population, seeking to achieve changes in audience knowledge, audience attitudes, and audience behavior (Singhal and Brown 1996; Singhal and Rogers 1999). Fundamentally, the purpose of the entertainment–education approach is to "contribute to directed social change" (Singhal and Rogers 1999: 9) and supporters of the approach believe in the ability of popular media to change cultural mores and to motivate prosocial behaviors (Singhal, Rogers and Brown 1993; Storey et al. 1999).

Almost all entertainment–education models embody the one-way flow process. Population Communications International (PCI) was one of the early initiators of the entertainment–education model, transferring the entertainment–education soap opera strategy to Third World countries such as India, Kenya, and Tanzania (Singhal and Rogers 1999). Subsequently the Johns Hopkins University Center for Communication Programs (JHU/CCP) utilized the entertainment–education model to reach more than thirty countries through over sixty projects (ibid.). Both Population Communications International and Johns Hopkins University's Center for Communication Programs, the two pivotal senders of messages in the entertainment–education context, were Western organizations with values that deeply reflected those of the Western world. Although local elites and national governments were involved in the process of developing the entertainment–education programs, the agenda was already decided by the Western interventionist (ibid.). The initiative and the thrust for the campaign were generated in the West.

Patrick L. Coleman and his colleagues at the Johns Hopkins University orchestrated health campaigns with the theme of sexual responsibility in Mexico and other Latin American countries, the Philippines, and Nigeria; David O. Poindexter, then president of the Population Control Institute, played an instrumental role in the development of *Hum Log* in India, *Twende na Wakati* in Tanzania, and *Tinkha Tinkha Sukh* in India. The entertainment–education programs launched in distant parts of the world became tools of Western hegemony that partook in the process of universalizing Western values and Western ways of looking at the world. In other cases, these programs became tools for propagating the combined product of national governments and Western ideologies. Let's take for instance the case of *Hum Log* in India. Initial support for *Hum Log* from Prime Minister Indira Gandhi was generated in the 1980s; in her tenure as prime minister, Gandhi and her son Sanjay gained notoriety for the forced sterilization policy. During Gandhi's regime, poor and lower middle-class men were coerced into sterilization, which paved the way for a reign of terror.

Addressing the critical question of values inherent in entertainment–education programming, Singhal and Rogers (1999: 219) argue that "the educational issues promoted by past entertainment–education are of unquestionable value, such as HIV/AIDS prevention. Who would want individuals to contract HIV/AIDS?" Notice the idea, implicit in the above quotation, that the very questioning of entertainment–education programs is problematic. Who, in their right minds, would question the values of a preventive effort? In rhetorically phrasing the question of HIV/AIDS, the authors oversimplify alternative interrogations of an ideologically-laden enterprise and systematically preempt alternative possibilities. Although perhaps the prevention of HIV/AIDS is an important priority, other imminent risk factors that threaten a culture might need greater attention. HIV/AIDS prevention may well be important, but it is perhaps even more important to make sure that the citizens of a nation-state have access to the fundamental resources of life such as food, clothing, and shelter. In cultures and countries plagued by famines and floods, it is critical to question any preventive effort in the context of the risks faced by members and fundamentally to trace the values that determine the prioritization of such efforts.

The argument that one-way flow models of entertainment–education also serve as conduits for imposing Western values and worldviews on Third World countries is further supported by the commercialization of Third World spaces, achieved through the use of entertainment–education. Entertainment–education programs serve as the conduits for introducing commercialized and globalized values into the Third World space. Celebrating the commercialization of *Doordarshan*, the state-sponsored television in India, Singhal and Rogers (1999: 101) write:

> Hum Log launched the era of commercially sponsored programs on Doordarshan. A sponsored television program is one for which an advertiser pays the production costs of a program, in return for several minutes of spot advertisements, before, during, or immediately following the broadcast . . . Commercial interests can be served without sacrificing social interests . . . The product advertised was Maggi 2-minute noodles, a radical consumer innovation in India . . . Hum Log represented a turning point in the commercialization of Doordarshan.

According to the authors, the introduction of Maggi in India demonstrated the combined power of strategic marketing, program planning and television diffusion in launching a new product on the Indian market. Alien to the Indian way of life (since noodles were perceived to be a Chinese product), Maggi became a part of the Indian household through its clever marketing strategy and advertising on Humlog. With the slogan "Fast to cook, and good to eat", Maggi opened up the Indian discursive space to a new mantra: convenience. Interestingly enough, unquestioned in Singhal and Rogers' celebration of the commercialized Indian television space are the fundamentally Westernized values and economic interests that inherently underlie commercialized television (supported by advertising), or the values that drive a life of convenience and fast foods. The case study of Humlog and Maggi brings to surface the basic problem of entertainment–education: its programs serve as the tools of globalization, of capitalism and of Western imperialism. They impose a monolithic set of Western values on other parts of the world, which open up the doors of countries suffering from starvation and poverty to commercial products of the free market economy. Meant to create pro-social change, entertainment–education becomes the machinery for the oppression of the poor and downtrodden in the Third World, colluding with other machineries of Western oppression such as the World Bank and the International Monetary Fund.

Western values are imposed on the Third World not only through the message content in the entertainment–education programs, but also through the choice of channels to carry their messages. Most entertainment–education programs since the early 1970s have relied on traditionally Western media types such as television, radio, and recorded music. These channels of entertainment are Western in their very nature, having been invented in the West. Missing from the discussion of entertainment channels for carrying educational information is the discussion of local or folk forms of entertainment that are quintessential to the many third-world cultures discussed and addressed in the entertainment–education campaigns. For instance, missing from the much-covered discussion of entertainment–education in India are discussion of the street plays (*patha nataks*), theaters (*jatras*), street demonstrations (*michil*), street stories (*patha kotha*), folk songs, folk dances and fairs that define some of the many cultural outlets of the culturally rich Indian landscape. Surely plentiful in the Indian landscape and yet missing from the discursive space of the modernization projects of entertainment–education are the indigenous forms of communicating art and entertainment that are unique to India, that are embedded in the socio-cultural space, and directed toward transformative politics that seeks to change the unhealthy structures. While television and Maggi noodles communicate to the upper class and middle class of the Indian population, they surely remain a distant cry from those in the far-away villages of Kalahandi and Kashipur, where villagers die of starvation.

Also fundamentally problematic in the conceptualization of entertainment–education is the naïve idea that entertainment holds the panacea to the basic problems that underlie health inequities in the world. The determination of the solution within an entertainment context trivializes the problems faced by the deprived populations in Third World nations

and abdicates the national government's responsibility in solving the critical resource needs faced by the people of the nation. The locus of the
problem is the individual, his beliefs, attitudes, cognitions and behavioral
intentions. Missing from the theoretical conceptualization of entertainment–education programming are the contextual and environmental
factors which encompass the individual and which seriously impede or
promote certain behaviors. Also, similar to other approaches in health
communication, the entertainment–education model is based on the conceptualization of the receiver as a rational actor.

Yet another criticism of the entertainment–education approach lies in
the episodic nature of the approach. The solutions proposed are, typically,
short-term and are measured over a short-term period. As a consequence,
the results of such efforts are typically either marginal or short-lived,
without really offering sustainable changes in the community. Hornik
and McAnany (2001) pointed out that, while in many cases population
changes could not be directly attributed to media campaigns, in other
instances the change in the population due to the media program
returned to a baseline level after the media program ended. In other
words, program effects seemed to last "only as long as the programs were
operating at a high level" (p. 464). The review conducted by Hornik and
McAnany suggests the need to conduct long-term campaigns with long-
term goals that seek to make fundamental changes in the population on
the basis of population needs. Instead of the myopic approach of funding
agencies on immediate outcomes, what is necessary is a commitment to
building the fundamental resources and capabilities of a community over
a long period of time. Sustainability of health programming needs continuous attention as we consider ways of improving health in the marginalized sectors of the globe.

Finally, the entertainment–education approach is linear. It assumes that
communication flows in a linear manner and that communicative
processes are linear. The linear model of communication effects espoused
in the entertainment–education model ignores "the complexity of social
change processes that require interaction, deliberation, and action by
members of the social system" (Papa et al. 2000: 33). This linearity reflects
the Western bias of health communication scholarship, which has systematically focused on media-centered health communication efforts
without really understanding the relevance of developing social structures, community contexts, and local narratives within which health
meanings can be continuously contested and negotiated.

For entertainment–education to respond to the real needs of the people
of at-need groups, the one-way flow model has to be replaced by a two-
way flow, where both interactants can learn something new from each
other in the relationship. The emphasis should be on developing a meaningful and profound relationship without the thrust of achieving campaign objectives within short-term periods. Perhaps the emphasis should
be on capability-building and harnessing communication to equip community members with the ability to articulate their voices, determine

their choices as a collective and secure those basic resources that are critical to their livelihood. Perhaps, rather than emphasizing the diffusion of certain health practices, the focus should be on developing meaningful communicative spaces where health issues might be articulated and contested. Only when the gates of communication have been opened and both parties have made attempts at developing an honest communication process could we talk about health communication campaigns in international settings that are meaningful to the local communities.

Social marketing models

Social marketing is based on the use of marketing principles for the development of health communication programs. In other words, the goal of social marketing is to use the basic concepts of marketing in the realm of socially relevant ideas and issues (Lefebvre and Flora 1988; MacStravic 2000; Kotler, Roberto and Lee 2002). Social marketing, based on the idea of consumer orientation, uses audience analysis, formative research, channel analysis, and process evaluation in order to market a health behavior (product) at a given price (what has to be given up, or lost, so as to practice the proposed health behavior), by using the right communication channels to market the product (place) and by using the right strategies/materials to market it (promotion). Social marketing programs respond to the call for culturally appropriate health messages by taking into account the inputs from the target audience in developing health campaign messages. Formative research provides inputs for effective messaging strategies in diverse cultures. In other words, the process of engaging in formative research, i.e. of gathering data as inputs for the development of communication strategies for the campaign, is considered to make a social marketing program culturally responsive by taking into account the cultural inputs of the target audience. The social marketing model moves toward acknowledging the role of culture by highlighting its inputs into the communication strategy. In some instances, representatives from the target culture are included in focus groups and in feedback teams, in order to guide the campaign and ensure that the campaign messages are culturally appropriate for the community.

The PEN-3 model

The PEN-3 model builds on the cultural criticism of the existing models of health communication, to suggest that health promotion efforts need to be responsive to the concept of culture. The PEN-3 model offers "a space within which cultural codes and meanings can be centralized in the development, implementation, and evaluation of health promotion programs" (Airhihenbuwa 1995: 28). This framework locates health behavior in the domain of the social and the cultural, addressing questions on health that extend beyond the biological. Context is situated at the core of analyzing health behaviors and cultural texts are accommodated in the construction of health meanings, such that culture becomes an enabler in the process of empowerment that is driven from within the spaces which are the foci of health campaign efforts. Structured on the PEN-3 model, Airhihenbuwa, Makinwa and Obregon (2000) lay out a culturally meaningful framework of HIV/AIDS campaigns. It centralizes culture, structural capabilities, gender roles and spiritual values of a community – as these concepts are articulated by community members – and combines these contextual factors in a collaborative exercise with policy-makers in an effort to promote health and HIV prevention.

The culture-centered approach

The culture-centered approach builds on the criticism offered by Airhihenbuwa (1995) and Dutta-Bergman (2004a, 2004b) to the dominant models of health communication (Dutta-Bergman 2004b, 2005a, 2005b; Dutta and Basu 2007). Privileging the narratives that emerge through conversations with members of marginalized communities, this approach highlights the interaction between culture, structure and agency in the way health communication is theorized at the margins. Structures constrain and limit the possibilities of health among underserved populations. Examples of structures include micro-level resources such as community medical services, community modes of transportation, channels of communication, and health-enhancing resources such as food, clean spaces, and spaces for exercising; meso-level resources such as points of policy implementation, avenues of civil society organizations, and media platforms; and macro-level resources such as national and international political actors and points of policy formulation, and national and global health organizations.

Agency is enacted in its interaction with the structures and embodies communicative actions and processes that challenge, navigate, and attempt to change these structures. This line of thinking foregrounds the importance of understanding articulations of health by engaging participant voices (Airhihenbuwa 1995; Dutta-Bergman 2004a; Ford and Yep 2003). These new articulations present opportunities for social change by suggesting new interpretations for, and thus challenging, the dominant articulations of social reality and cultural and behavioral norms. The culture-centered approach underscores the importance of the participation of community members in the articulation of health problems as a step toward achieving meaningful change (Guha 1988; Guha and Spivak 1988). In doing so, it emphasizes dialogue and mutual understanding, locating the agency for examining health practices in the culture being studied, not in the researcher/interventionist and in the institutional practices that inform his or her research practice.

Cultural context is located at the core of the culture-centered approach, emphasizing the meanings that are co-constructed by the researcher and by the cultural participants. Narratives of health become meaningful when understood in terms of culture. The interplay between

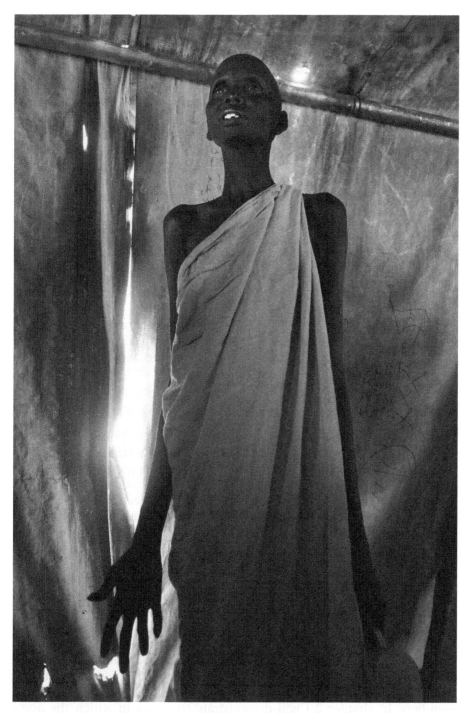

Fig. 1.1 A tuberculosis (TB) patient in a clinic run by Médecins Sans Frontières in Sudan
© Sven Torfinn @ Panos Pictures

structure and agency is realized and contested in this realm. On the one hand, cultural contexts embody the role of structure in constraining and defining the possibilities of health; on the other hand, transformation of meanings in these cultural contexts offers openings for changing the structures that constrain the possibilities of health in marginalized communities. Note that the focus of the culture-centered approach is not on "empowering" from the outside the marginalized subjects of a health campaign, as this very stance once again assumes the implied expertise of the researcher and exhumes the community member who participates in the campaign of his/her agency. The emphasis is on understanding existing forms of participation in communities, so that the latter become agents of social change in any health promotion effort that is directed at them.

Discussion point 1.2

- What do you understand by structures? Think about a specific health issue which is important to you. How do you think structure influences this particular health issue?
- With respect to the specific health issue and the structures you identified, comment upon the role of communication in reinforcing the structures. How do you think communication can be deployed in order to challenge the structures?

Culture in Health Communication

Worth noting so far is the increasing relevance of the concept of culture in health communication programs. With the increase in multicultural populations within the US and with the increasing global flows, health communicators have called for more work which should engage with the concept of culture (Airhihenbuwa 1995). In this section I will suggest that there are two distinct strands in health communication scholarship and health communication applications that include the concept of culture: the dominant approach, also referred to as the culturally sensitive approach, and the culture-centered approach (Dutta-Bergman 2004a, 2004b, 2004c, 2005a, 2005b; Dutta 2007). Although these two approaches have been widely circulated in the recent literature on cultural applications of health communication, they are certainly not exhaustive in tapping into the range of possibilities for health communication efforts that are responsive to culture (more on this in chapter 2).

In the dominant approach, culture is treated as a static set of values, beliefs, and practices; the culture-centered approach refers to culture as dynamic and transformative, constituted through the voices of cultural members. In chapter 2 I will demonstrate the ways in which the dominant approach and the culture-centered approach drive health communication theorizing and the development of health communication applications. I will then compare these two different strands in health communication scholarship, which have recently received attention, with regard to their applications of the concept of culture in the development of health communication programs (Dutta 2007).

Our understanding of these different strands of scholarship will equip us with a categorizing scheme for understanding the different approaches to the use of culture (this will be developed in greater detail in the next section), and the ways in which these approaches may evolve into health communication theories. The dominant approach to culture (or the cultural sensitivity approach) uses the concept of culture as a static entity, and culture is incorporated into health communication programs with the goal of making them more effective. In this sense, the focus is on adapting pre-existing health communication concepts to the different cultures in which these concepts are tested. However, the culture-centered approach treats culture as a dynamic entity which is contextually constituted, continuously contested, and communicatively negotiated. Taken in this sense, culture consists in the meanings constructed by cultural members. Culture-centered theorizing in health communication emphasizes the voices of cultural communities, examines the ways in which these voices have been erased by the dominant discourses of health communication, and suggests alternatives to these dominant discourses by engaging with the voices of cultural communities.

Discussion point 1.3

- Please pick a particular health issue that is of interest to you. How would you go about developing an application based on the dominant approach to health communication? Please outline the steps that you would take.
- How would you respond to the same issue utilizing the culture-centered approach? How exactly would you proceed? How would you evaluate the application you develop?

Applying Culture in Health Communication

The nature of health communication applications utilizing the concept of culture depends upon the theoretical framework they draw upon (Dutta-Bergman 2004a, 2004b; Dutta 2007). In other words, the overarching theoretical positioning of culture-based health communication influences the ways in which health communicators go about developing health communication applications, and the ways in which they evaluate the success or failure of these applications. For the practitioners of the dominant approach to health communication, the goal of health communication applications is to identify cultural variables, to develop measures for these variables, and to utilize these variables for the purposes of predicting health beliefs, attitudes, and behaviors. In this sense, health communication interventions focus on utilizing the concept of culture in order to become more effective. For instance, the health belief model can

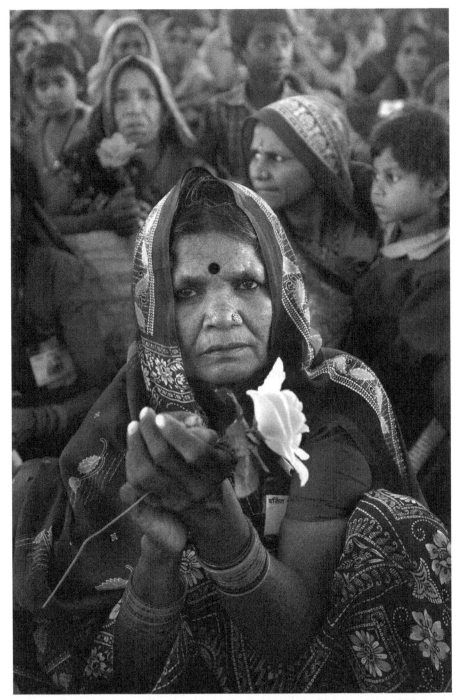

Fig. 1.2 A Dalit woman with a flower attends the 2006 Vanangana conference in Chitrakoot. Vanangana, a women's group dedicated to human rights issues, receives strong support from the Dalit community
© Ami Vitale @ Panos Pictures

measure the cultural barriers to a particular behavior (say, getting a mammogram) and then develop messages that address this barrier. Similarly, according to the extended parallel process model, appropriate cultural cues might be identified in order to develop more effective fear appeals that would work well with the target population.

In contrast to the dominant approach to health communication that studies culture as a variable and uses it to predict certain behaviors and outcomes, the culture-centered approach looks at culture as a dynamic and fluid entity, and, hence, emphasizes the meanings that are co-constructed by cultural members through dialogues with health communication scholars (Dutta-Bergman 2004a, 2004b, 2005a, 2005b; Dutta 2007; Dutta and Basu 2007; Dutta and Basnyat, in press). In order to imagine new possibilities of health through dialogue, the emphasis of the culture-centered approach is on creating communicative spaces, even as it draws attention to their continually shifting nature. The spaces, as sites of contestation of health meanings and agendas, are themselves contested and continuously negotiated.

Conclusion

The goal of this chapter was to (a) provide you with a historical overview of the concept of culture in health communication, (b) compare the ways in which different approaches to health communication utilize the concept of culture, (c) examine the different theoretical roots of the culture-based health communication approaches, and (d) compare the different health communication applications that emerge from these approaches. We have so far seen how the different models of health communication applied in the dominant framework treat culture primarily as a static set of values and beliefs, as compared to the culture-centered approach, which looks at culture as dynamic, transformative and continuously constituted through relationships and meaning-making from the cultural members. In this regard, it is also important to point out that, although I suggest the distinctions between the dominant and the culture-centered approaches for the sake of theoretical clarity, there are multiple instances where health communication theories and applications shift back and forth between these two approaches, or may simultaneously draw from the tenets of both. In other words, there is a large possibility for gray areas which defy the neatly packaged categorization scheme proposed in this chapter and throughout the book.

Now that we have set up the different models of health communication and examined the points of comparison among them, in the next chapter we will take a closer look at the culture-centered approach and locate it in the backdrop of other approaches to health communication.

2 The Culture-Centered Approach to Health Communication

Chapter objectives

In this chapter, we will:

- examine the dominant paradigm of health communication
- examine the theoretical roots of the culture-centered approach
- compare the dominant paradigm and the culture-centered approach

So far, we have looked at the various approaches to health communication and at the ways in which these approaches lay out the concept of culture, either explicitly or implicitly. This chapter builds on the discussion of the culture-centered approach to the study of health communication presented in the Introduction and in chapter 1. More specifically, it answers the questions: What is the culture-centered approach? Why do we need a culture-centered approach to the study of health communication? We will begin by reviewing the basic tenets of the traditional approach to health communication scholarship, which may also be described as the dominant paradigm of the field. The dominant paradigm refers to the status quo, the way things are typically done, the set of practices that constitute the discipline, the conventional standards that suggest what it means for it to be a discipline, and the gatekeeping practices that define what is acceptable as disciplinary scholarship and what is not.

In this chapter I will provide an overview of the field of health communication and place it in the backdrop of the culture-centered approach. In doing so, I will first examine the key strands in what has come to constitute health communication scholarship. I will then summarize the criticisms that have been offered with reference to the dominant paradigm of health communication. These criticisms will offer the framework for putting forth the culture-centered approach, suggesting why we need such an approach, what are the voids in our current theorizing it seeks to address, and how we might go about theorizing and practicing the culture-centered approach in health communication.

Interrogating the Dominant Paradigm

The dominant paradigm responds to the concept of culture by suggesting the ways in which cultural concepts may be incorporated into the bio-medical model and into health promotion interventions in order to make

Box 2.1   The story of Minoti

Minoti is a 46-year-old Bengali woman from the district of Bankura in West Bengal, India. She earns her living as a paddy grower, selling the paddies grown in the fields to middlemen who pay cash for the paddy purchased. As a farmer, Minoti depends upon the monsoon season to have a good produce. When discussing her access to healthcare, she recalls that one year when the scorching sunlight burnt the crops, the drought was heavy and there was hardly any water to irrigate the crops. That year the produce was bad and she did not have much of an earning. It was also that year that her son Shontu was bitten by a cobra when he was crossing a paddy field. Minoti and her husband Boloram took Shontu to the *ojha* (spiritual healer), who would suck the poison out of the 8-year-old boy.

them more effective. Why, then, do we need alternatives to the dominant paradigm? Minoti's story narrated here provides us with an entry point for engaging with the need to think about alternatives.

Why did Minoti and Boloram decide to take Shontu to the *ojha* instead of taking him to the state-sponsored local hospital that was located approximately 25 miles away from their home? What does the decision of the parents tell us about their values and views on health and healing? One way of answering these questions is to suggest that Minoti and Boloram are illiterate and superstitious, not having the knowledge to take their son to a doctor who practices modern medicine. However, another approach to the same situation would be to converse with Minoti and Boloram, to engage with them in dialogue with the goal of understanding what happened. As pointed out in chapter 1, this act of engaging in dialogue with cultural members lies at the heart of the culture-centered approach. The culture-centered approach suggests that, in order to gain a profound understanding of what really happened in the life of Minoti, we need to begin by creating spaces for those voices in our work that we have systematically silenced through our expertise and elitism.

Inherent in the dominant paradigm are certain taken-for-granted assumptions about what it means to study something, the tools that may be used to study it, and the criteria that may be applied to evaluate the manner of conducting the study. The dominant paradigm is built upon the dialectical relationship between inclusion and exclusion. Certain assumptions, conceptual frameworks, and methodological tools constitute the disciplinary body of knowledge. These markers filter what is included, the tools that are used and, more fundamentally, who gets to provide the explanations and make the predictions. Simultaneously, a variety of other interpretations, definitions, approaches, and tools are excluded, together with the absence of many voices that do not have access to these tools and to the accompanying conventional practices.

Every dominant paradigm is built upon a set of shared meanings about that paradigm: the questions that are typically asked, the methodological tools that are typically used to answer these questions, the ways in which studies are conducted and reports are written, and the criteria against which these studies are evaluated. These questions, tools and criteria are defined, developed, and refined by the scholars within the discipline, by the body of experts who serve as the producers and gatekeepers of disciplinary knowledge. In other words, a dominant paradigm is located within a meaning community – the community of scholars and practitioners who have come to define what it means to theorize and practice within the discipline. In the realm of health communication, then, the dominant paradigm supplies the set of questions, tools and criteria which are activated by the community of communication scholars engaged in understanding, describing and/or explaining health communication phenomena and practices. These questions, tools and criteria, however, are not devoid of values. The culture-centered approach to health communication foregrounds these very values, which are inherent in how health communication is traditionally studied and understood.

Culture here is defined as a complex web of meanings (Geertz 1973), intertwined with the shared values, beliefs and practices that run through the strands of a community (Helman 2001). The question of culture provides an alternative set of criteria for the evaluation of the taken-for-granted assumptions, conceptual frameworks and methodological tools that are systematically employed in the dominant paradigm of health communication scholarship. The goal of the culture-centered approach is two-fold. On one hand, it seeks to locate in the culture the dominant paradigm of health communication that pushes certain universal truths about health; in this way it demonstrates that taken-for-granted Eurocentric values related to health have systematically shaped the universal questions asked within the field of health communication, the tools which have been applied to solving the problems, and the universal criteria used to evaluate the success of health communication interventions. This, in turn, has influenced the types of universal policies and applications that have often been developed, implemented and talked about in the health communication literature. On the other hand, the culture-centered approach seeks to nurture a space where voices of cultural members may be brought to the forefront in order to articulate the questions that are meaningful to them. In doing so, the culture-centered approach privileges the dialogue between the researcher/practitioner and the community as a way of knowing (Dutta-Bergman 2004a, 2005a, 2005b). It is through this dialogue that problems are articulated and solutions are developed.

Discussion point 2.1

- What is, to you, the dominant paradigm of health communication?
- How has the dominant paradigm of health communication come to influence you and the work you do?
- What taken-for-granted assumptions do you bring to the table when thinking about your understanding of health communication processes?

Health Communication

Health communication refers to the study of communication pheno-mena in healthcare settings (Thompson 2003). The area of health communication may be divided into two streams of scholarship: (a) process-based and (b) message-based perspectives on communica-tion. The process-based perspective examines a variety of communica-tion processes that are enacted in healthcare settings, with an emphasis on the ways in which health meanings are constructed, negotiated, resisted and sustained. For instance, the process-based approach to the study of safe sex might focus on the question: how do college students negotiate the use of condoms in intimate relationships? Scholars applying the message-based perspective focus on the impact of health messages on healthcare delivery and individual health outcomes, with the goal of developing and evaluating messages that achieve desired outcomes. Therefore the message-based approach to the safe sex issue might ask the question: how can messages be designed to encourage college students to use condoms in intimate relationships? Both per-spectives have been applied to examine health communication pro-cesses and messages in the interpersonal, mass-mediated, organizational, and social and community realms, although much of the existing health communication research has emphasized the message-based per-spective, focusing on the production of effective messages to achieve desired outcomes.

Interpersonal communication scholarship examines provider–patient interactions, communication with friends and family members, and social support issues in the realm of health (Thompson 2003). These issues have been approached from both the process and the message-based perspectives, although a predominant proportion of the research in the area has focused on messages (Albrecht and Goldsmith 2003). For instance, in the area of HIV/AIDS, interpersonal scholars have studied the health effects of comforting messages; they have also studied the ways in which individuals seek and provide comfort in their relationships (Brashers 2001). Health communication scholars exploring communica-tion in the interpersonal context have also systematically examined the doctor–patient relationship, exploring the role of communication skills on the nature of the relationship (Cegala and Broz 2003; Street 2003). Outcomes measured in this literature include satisfaction, compliance, duration of the interaction and the like.

Mass communication scholars have been historically interested in studying the effects of mass-mediated messages on individual health (Murray-Johnson and Witte 2003; Salmon and Atkin 2003). Much of the mass communication scholarship has focused on communication cam-paigns and on the intended dissemination of communication activities targeting an audience segment within a specified period of time with the goal of generating desired outcomes in the target population (Rogers and Storey 1987). Providing an overview of the campaign literature, Salmon and Atkin (2003) state that the campaign design team needs to begin by identifying the focal segments of the population whose health-related practices need to be changed, and by defining a set of focal behaviors that the campaign seeks to change. In their review of campaign theories, Murray-Johnson and Witte (2003) point out that the health belief model, the theory of reasoned action, social cognitive theory, the theory of planned behavior and the extended parallel process model provide important guidelines for message design. In addition to theories of health communication campaigns, media theories have also explored the effects of mass media agendas on the audience's agenda of critical health issues; the framing of health issues on mass media; and the cultivation of health beliefs among heavy viewers of television programs (Kline 2003).

Scholars approaching health communication from organizational perspectives have interrogated health communication processes and effects in organizational settings (Lammers, Barbour and Duggan 2003). The message-based approach in organizational settings has focused on developing workplace interventions targeted toward changing beliefs, attitudes, and behaviors of individual workers within the organization (Chenoweth 1994; Geist-Martin, Horsley and Farrell 2003; Harris 1994). Employee assistance programs (EAP) are often offered by organizations with the goals of improving employee job performance, family life and health (Shain and Groenveld 1980). These programs identify troubled employees, motivate them to resolve their troubles and provide access to counseling and treatment services (Sonnenstuhl and Trice 1986). In addition to providing treatment options, EAPs also offer health promotion programs that address prevention-related issues (Chenoweth 1994; Geist-Martin, Horsley and Farrell 2003; Harris 1994). Other health communication scholarship has explored organizations that offer healthcare services such as private practices, hospitals, parish nursing, hospices and so on (Lammers, Barbour and Duggan 2003).

Box 2.2   The story of Sarah

Sarah was a Peace Corps volunteer before joining the Department of Public Health at Emerald University, one of the leading public health institutions in the US. Emerald University runs several projects in developing countries and Sarah is currently enrolled in a course on "Health in the Third World." She has learned about the epidemiological issues in the Third World and the ways in which these issues might be solved through public health interventions targeted at promoting contraceptive use. However, these simplified toolkits and linear models don't really appeal to Sarah because they don't really fit with her life experiences while working for the Peace Corps in Uganda. Theoretically, though, she doesn't know how to articulate her viewpoints, or even where to begin. She recently contacted you because you had told her that you are enrolled in a course on "Culture and Health." How would you guide Sarah? What theoretical points of entry would you suggest to her?

Critiques of the Dominant Paradigm

Biases of domination

The dominant paradigm of health communication scholarship is built upon the expert position of health communication scholars and the object positions of the participants they study (Foucault 1988). Inherent to this enterprise is an assumption of expertise on behalf of the scholar – an assumption that she/he has the tools and the knowledge to examine the beliefs, values, and practices of those who are researched and, subsequently, to offer interventions for altering these beliefs, values, and practices. The "expert" exists in a dialectical relationship with the "researched." In other words, it is the existence of the object position of the research participant that allows the enterprise of research, providing topics for scholarly investigation and sites for the development and empirical testing of applications. These positions of the expert and of the research subject are predicated on power; those with access to power get to construct conceptual maps, develop problem configurations, and implement solutions in the target community – a community which typically exists at the margins of the power configuration and hence must serve as the object under investigation.

It is important to question this expert–object relationship in the context of the geographic, socio-economic, racial, and gendered lines along which it plays out. For instance, most of the scholarship in international health communication demonstrates a demarcation in the geographic distribution of expertise; campaigns are typically conceptualized, designed and implemented by the centers in the First World and are directed toward the Third World. This First–Third distribution pattern might be substituted by a North–South divide, where the northern nations of the world have systematically been the manufacturers of health knowledge and health applications targeted at the southern nations of the world. Similarly, the area of physician–patient communication, where a large percentage of services directed toward women are offered by men, demonstrates gender inequities. Most of the interventions targeting African Americans and Hispanics within the United States are designed, conceptualized and implemented by Caucasian scholars trained in theoretical approaches that have typically been articulated by other Caucasian scholars. For instance, the three key theories of health communication campaigns, theory of reasoned action, health belief model and the extended parallel process model were developed by Caucasian scholars working in North American universities. Similarly, typically middle- and upper-middle-class academics at North American universities pursuing funded research serve as the gatekeepers and practitioners of health interventions targeting lower socio-economic communities.

These unequal distributions of expert–object positions across space, race, socio-economic status and gender create inherent biases associated with the positions of privilege of health communication researchers within academia and outside it. These are the dominant biases of the field; they constitute the conceptual maps used in the study of health communication phenomena. Health communication theories and applications generated and empirically tested by middle- or upper-middle-class Caucasian men in North American universities suffer from the biased values and beliefs associated with the positions of privilege of these researchers within and outside the academic world. Therefore such theories and application can be better understood when located in the context of the values and beliefs associated with these positions of expertise and privilege.

Individual-level focus

The conceptual frameworks used in health communication have most often suffered from a bias associated with the predominant value of individualism in Western cultures (Dutta-Bergman and Doyle 2001; Triandis 1995). Health communication has traditionally been studied at the individual level, being conceptualized and empirically tested there. In other words, the individual has served as the object of theory development, guiding the methodological and practical choices of both scholars and practitioners (Airhihenbuwa 1995; Dutta-Bergman 2004a, 2004b, 2005a, 2005b; Lupton 1994; Wallack 1989).

This individual-level focus is perhaps linked to the historical roots of the discipline of communication in psychological research, particularly in persuasion research such as conducted by Lazarsfeld, Hovland, and Laswell (Delia 1987). For these scholars, who have often been identified as the founding fathers of the discipline of communication, the study of communication involved the design and development of messages which could have the maximum effect on the target audience. The goal was to persuade; to get the target audience to shift its beliefs, attitudes, and behaviors so as to agree with the intended objectives of the persuader.

The persuasion-based approach continues to dominate much of the health communication scholarship in the area of campaigns (Dutta-Bergman 2005a, 2005b). Campaign theories such as the health belief model, the theory of reasoned action, and the extended parallel process model focus on crafting most effective messages in order to persuade the individual to engage in a behavior. The locus of the problem therefore is the individual and his/her behaviors. The individual-level focus excludes other key factors from the realm of health, for instance cultural context, structural context, community context, and so on. Take, for instance, the ways in which HIV/AIDS is conceptualized as a problem in the dominant paradigm. In the exponentially growing body of health communication literature on HIV/AIDS campaigns, campaign theorists and practitioners focus on the individual's sexual behaviors, seeking to persuade him/her to engage in safe sex practices such as abstinence, using condoms or disclosing HIV/AIDS identity. Absent from the articulation of this problem are factors such as socio-economic status, access to resources, shifting cultural norms, community-wide decision networks, issues of gender inequity and relationship negotiation, and so on, which are central to the negotiation of safe sex.

Similarly, the individual-level focus is also observed in studies on inter-personal communication in healthcare settings. For instance, the individual's communication skills are investigated in the literature on patient communication styles (Bain 1979; Beisecker and Beisecker 1990; Stewart 1984; Street 1991; Street et al. 1995). Communication skills explored in this literature have primarily focused on information exchange (Cegala 1997; Cegala, Coleman and Warisse 1998; Cegala et al. 1995). Information exchange has further been categorized into information seeking, information verification and information provision (Cegala, Coleman and Warisse 1998). The research on information seeking has pri-marily focused on the questions that patients ask their providers (Cegala et al. 2000; Cegala, Post and McClure 2001; Dow, Verdi and Sacco 1991; Rost et al. 1991; Roter 1977; Socha McGee and Cegala 1998). Similarly, scholars studying information provision have focused on the expression of concerns, on the clear and competent reporting of symptoms, and so on, all on the basis of the notion that the efficiency and effectiveness of information provision have significant impact on the length of medical interviews, on the cost of healthcare, and on healthcare quality (Cegala, McClure et al. 2000; Dugdale, Epstein and Pantilat 1999; Goold and Lipkin 1999). These scholars refer to the pragmatic relevance of such skills to the managed care system in the US, ensuring high quality and cutting costs simultaneously (Cegala and Broz 2003). Information verifying skills are used by individuals in order to check on information in daily conver-sations, and are particularly important in task-oriented communication, where accurate understanding and reception of information is essential to accomplishing a coordinated objective (ibid.).

A variety of interventions arising out of this literature has been devel-oped and implemented with the goal of training patients in communica-tion skills (ibid.). For instance, a meta-analysis conducted by Anderson and Sharpe (1991) suggested that the most effective training interven-tions include modeling and/or practice components. They suggested that most patients need to see someone asking questions, providing complete and clear information, and negotiating treatment options, and, subse-quently, to have an opportunity to practice these skills with a feedback, in order to learn them most effectively (Cegala, Marinelli and Post 2000; Cegala et al. 2000; Cegala, Post and McClure 2001; Dow Verdi and Sacco 1991; Kaplan et al. 1989). The outcomes measured in these interventions include individual-level behaviors such as asking more questions, provid-ing more information, and/or being more compliant. Other outcomes include time of interaction, cost effectiveness, and so on.

But the individual-level focus shifts attention away from the very rela-tionship between physicians and patients that this body of literature seeks to address. Although relationships are based upon two or more individu-als who enter into an exchange, it may be argued that a relationship is more than the sum of the individual characteristics and skill sets of the individuals entering into the exchange. In instances where communica-tion researchers code the characteristics of communication between the provider and the patient, they break up the communication into individual characteristics and link these characteristics to outcomes rather than attempting to understand the relationship holistically. Questions remaining unexplored in this area include: What are the structural constraints on physician–patient relationships? What are the ways in which managed care constrains the nature of these relationships? How do cultural values inform the character of physician patient relationships? How does power affect the physician–patient relationship? How does the relationship between providers and patients change over time, especially with respect to their contextual location in the cultural environment? Factors such as community, culture, and structure, which are simultaneously at play in the realm of health communication, remain unexplored.

Cognitive bias

The dominant approach conceptualizes health communication in the realm of rational action on the basis of the underlying beliefs of individuals (Airhihenbuwa 1995; Dutta-Bergman 2005a, 2005b; Lupton 1994). Therefore, it focuses primarily on changing the thoughts and beliefs of the target audience on the basis of the delivery of effective messages that seek to address these beliefs, thus creating a pathway for the enactment of the behavior (Witte 1995). This cognitive approach is founded on the notion that information influences action by changing the underlying beliefs and attitudes. The informed audience will know how to practice the recommended health behaviors, on the basis of changes in the belief structure induced through information-heavy messages.

In the area of health communication campaigns, cognitively-oriented theories such as the theory of reasoned action (TRA), the health belief model (HBM) and the extended parallel process model (EPPM) have dominated the development of both health communication theorizing and health communication applications. According to the theory of reasoned action, the individual's beliefs about the proposed behavior and his/her evaluations of the importance ascribed to the behavior by significant others influence his/her attitude toward the behavior in question and the likelihood of engagement in it. Note in this case that the beliefs and subjective norms are filtered through a cognitive frame. The formation of attitudes here is a product of the thoughtful evaluation of the advantages and disadvantages of the behavior and of what important others think about the behavior.

Similarly, the health belief model addresses the role of perceptions about the severity of the outcomes, about the individual's susceptibility to the condition, about benefits of the recommended behavior, about barriers to practicing it, about self efficacy, and about response efficacy – all seen as antecedents of behavior adoption. In instances where the perceived severity and susceptibility are high, the individual perceives herself to be at threat. The combination between a high level of perceived threat, a high level of perceived self-efficacy – that is, belief in one's ability to engage in the behavior – and the behavior's response efficacy – that is, ability to prevent the outcomes – leads to the adoption of the recommended behavior. Once again, note in this case that the individual goes through a large number of steps of rational analyses to arrive at the decision to adopt a behavior.

Decontextualized bias

Health as conceptualized in the dominant approach is typically removed from the context that surrounds it (Dutta-Bergman 2004a, 2005a, 2005b; Melkote, Muppidi and Goswami 1995). Health communication theories in the area of campaigns target an individual behavior that becomes the focus of the designed and implemented messages (Salmon and Atkin 2003). In such a scenario, the behavior is isolated from a variety of contextual factors within which it is typically enacted. For instance, to go back to the example of safe sex used earlier in this chapter, the singular emphasis on promoting condoms during sexual encounters typically misses out on elements of the context such as the bar or night club where sex may be initiated and negotiated, the dyadic nature of the negotiation of safe sex, or the perceptions associated with the desire to use condoms. In other words, the promotion of condoms is embedded within the setting, in the relationship expectations of the partners engaging in sex, in the messages available to them in the immediate context, etc. Similarly, a safe sex program targeting sex workers is decontextualized when condom use is singularly promoted without regard for elements of the structural context, for instance the lack of financial resources and the inability to negotiate condom use because of this dependence on money.

The single behavior emphasis also misses out on the measurement context within which behaviors are typically enacted, creating artificial conditions for the testing of theories. Take for instance a campaign design that seeks to study the effect of perceived susceptibility on behavioral intention. The participant is shown a public service announcement, followed by the self-reported measurement of his/her outcomes. The measurement of the public service announcement (PSA) as an individual stimulus removes the contextual environment within which PSAs are typically consumed. These PSAs are usually embedded within programming and therefore need to be studied in the context of other programs that accompany them. Similarly, research participants need to be engaged in their natural settings rather than being studied as individuals responding to different messages. Media consumption often happens collectively, when members of a community watch a program together. In such instances, the measurement of the response of an isolated individual is a far stretch from the day-to-day scenario of collective viewership of programming.

Status quo bias

Another criticism of the dominant approach to health communication focuses on its systematic omission of the structural contexts that encompass the health experiences of individuals, groups, and communities (Airhihenbuwa 1995; Dutta-Bergman 2004a, 2005a, 2005b; Lupton 1995b). The emphasis on the individual operates simultaneously with the absence of structural factors that encompass the health experiences of individuals (Dutta-Bergman 2005a, 2005b). For instance the theory of reasoned action, the health belief model, and the extended parallel process model all target the individual and his/her behavior. The objective is to shift the underlying beliefs and perceptions associated with that behavior, so that the behavior may be encouraged within the community. Similar tendencies are observed in the organizational study of health communication, where employee assistance programs (EAPs) emphasize the need to identify individuals with drawbacks, who are then subjected to workplace interventions aimed at making them more productive workers.

By focusing on the individual, the dominant approach serves the status quo, ignoring the roles of structural readjustment and redistributive justice in the realm of health experiences of individuals in the marginalized sectors of the world. Dutta-Bergman (2004a, 2004b, 2005a; Dutta, 2007) states that theories of health communication ought to put poverty and the lack of basic resources at the heart of theorizing; basic capabilities need to be taken into account in order to develop meaningful health interventions. In his work with Santalis, Dutta-Bergman (2004a, 2004b) engaged in dialogue with this marginalized sector of the Indian population, calling for the need to address corrupt medical practices and unequal resource distribution strategies – a need which emerged from the conversations with cultural members. The conversations with Santalis suggested the need for engaging in political processes in order to change the structures surrounding the health experiences of the members of communities.

Control bias

Intertwined with the status quo position of the dominant approach is its desire to control the health experiences of the target audience (Lupton 1995b). The strand of health communication scholarship described in the last few sections is built upon this notion of control (Dutta-Bergman 2004a, 2004b). Control refers to the development and implementation of communication strategies directed at a target audience such that the beliefs, attitudes, and behaviors of that audience might be changed. The goal here is persuasion on the basis of the problem and solution configurations as conceptualized by the senders of the message.

This bias toward control is also played out in the testing of health communication theories, which often reflects the cultural values of the Western scientific enterprise that privileges the experimental condition. A singular behavior is often picked as the object of healthcare interventions, and narrowly defined measures are used to examine whether that behavior has changed as a result of the campaign. Control is similarly evident in the realm of provider–patient relationships, where multiple studies build upon the creation of spurious settings, designed to test the effectiveness of communication training strategies directed at providers and/or patients. Strategies seeking to train providers serve as the *panopticon* under which provider communication in the workplace may be assessed. In addition, the very objective of teaching communication skills to patients is based on the desire to control, so that desired outcomes as conceptualized by the message developers may be achieved. Such form of control also becomes a way of streamlining patient behavior and of minimizing deviations from the norm.

The Culture-Centered Approach

Central to the culture-centered approach is the understanding that communicating about health involves the negotiation of shared meanings embedded in socially constructed identities, relationships, social norms, and structures. These identities, relationships, social norms, and structures are mutually interdependent. For instance, the experience of illness articulated by a breast cancer patient is intrinsically connected with her identity as a colleague, spouse, mother, and so on; her relationship with family members, colleagues, and healthcare providers; her membership in the demographic community (for instance a church group), the breast cancer support community, and other forms of community such as the workplace community; and her interactions with structures such as clinics, hospitals, health insurance systems, and so on (Sharf, Geist-Martin and Ray 2003). It is important to note that these different levels of communication experiences are interdependent. In other words, the manner of the breast cancer patient's communications with her family is intertwined with the way she constructs her identity as a breast cancer patient, which, in turn, is linked with her experiences as she navigates the healthcare system. Therefore healthcare interactions and experiences may be observed in a variety of intertwined settings which form a complex web of negotiated meanings.

The concept of culture that drives the culture-centered approach foregrounds the active participation of community members in the construction of shared meanings and experiences; culture is constituted through this act of participation and therefore is actively constructed by its members (Dutta-Bergman 2004a, 2004b, 2005a, 2005b). It is through this active participation that they create shared meanings, values, and practices; these meanings, values and practices, in turn, constitute the culture of the community. Culture is comprised of traditions that are passed on from one generation to the next, and also of changes that are introduced into it as members engage with structures that surround their daily lives. Hence culture is simultaneously stable and dynamic, drawing from the past, constituting the present, and changing through the interactions with various social structures. Essential to this conceptualization of culture is the association between structure and agency; structure provides the constraints for human action, and it is within these constraints that community members must enact their agency, thus constituting a culture built upon shared meanings, values, and practices (Giddens 1990).

The culture-centered approach provides an alternative entry point for theorizing about, and practicing, health communication by suggesting that communication about health is played out in the relationship between structure and the agency of the participant. On the one hand, structures define the realm of possibilities in the context of health; on the other hand, it is through the enactment of agency in relationship with structure that individuals, communities and societies come to experience health. This line of thinking and application development foregrounds the importance of understanding articulations of health by engaging participant voices, particularly in the context of the marginalized sectors of the world (Airhihenbuwa 1995; Dutta-Bergman 2004a, 2004b, 2005a, 2005b; Ford and Yep 2003). The culture-centered approach underscores the importance of the participation of community members in identifying health problems as a first step toward achieving a change which is meaningful to community members; therefore, communicative spaces need to be created and sustained that foster opportunities for dialogues (Guha 1988; Guha and Spivak 1988). Note the emphasis on meaningful change, with meanings being located in the realm of the community and not in the realm of health outcomes imposed by external experts, on the basis of their expert knowledge.

Sketching out the fundamental tenets of the culture-centered approach, Dutta-Bergman (2004a: 259) states:

> The culture-centered approach to health communication emphasizes dialogue and mutual understanding, locating the agency for examining health practices in the culture being studied, not in the researcher and the institutional practices that inform his/her research practice. Cultural context is located at the center of the culture-centered approach, emphasizing the meanings that are co-constructed by the researcher and the cultural participants.

The culture-centered approach stresses the need to develop programs in ways that are consistent with a people's and community's cultural framework (Airhihenbuwa 1995). The stance embodied in the culture-centered approach is respect for the capability of the members of marginalized communities to define their health needs and to seek out solutions which fulfil these needs. Voices of community members are presented through the dialogical engagement with the community. In this context, the researcher does not claim to be the expert on the so-called lay theories articulated by the participants, nor does he/she seek to remove himself/herself completely from the dialogue, knowing that this is neither possible nor desirable. The voices of marginalized communities are therefore played out through the dialogues between the researcher and the community members. This perspective takes us outside the realm of wanting to change people and to teach them how to better live their lives through one-way transmission-based models, to a framework that is built on the goal of developing an understanding of people and of their cultures (Beverley 1999; Dutta-Bergman 2004a, 2004b; Foss and Griffin 1995; Mokros and Deetz 1996).

The culture-centered approach suggests a shift in the role of the researcher – from an interventionist who plans and executes campaigns to a listener and a participant who engages in dialogue with the members of the community. For Freire (1970, 1973), engaging in dialogue involved a fusion of identities among the participants on the basis of the absence of subject–object distinctions, where the sense of self and world is developed through the interactions among the participants. The researcher moves from his/her objective position outside the field to that of a participant engaged in dialogue; reflexivity becomes a critical tool. The very process of engaging in dialogue introduces into the discursive space key ideas that have typically been omitted or taken for granted; the voices of cultural participants become a part of the discursive space through this process of dialogue. Noting the moral commitment required for the dialogical process to occur, Freire (1970: 46) articulated that "being dialogic is not invading, not manipulating, not imposing orders. Being dialogic is pledging oneself to constant transformation of reality." Fundamental to the articulation of the culture-centered approach is the notion that members of communities actively participate in interpreting the social structures that encompass them, in making sense of these social structures, and in interacting with them on a daily basis. The culture-centered approach seeks to narrate these stories and to achieve social change by the very introduction of the marginalized voices into the discursive space.

Culture can be conceptualized as a process which is in a continuous state of production and reconfiguration through communication, leading to "a complex social, economic and political structure characterized by a system of values that influences attitudes, perception and communication behaviors and practices in a given society" (Airhihenbuwa 1995, as cited in Ford and Yep 2003: 248). For Geertz (1973), culture is an "acted document" (p. 218), it is "public" (p. 218), it consists of "socially established structures of meaning" (p. 219) and webs of significance within which the human being is suspended. Culture can be construed as the living framework of individuals and of their collectives – a learned/learning experience, a process of evolving, living, learning, adapting, orienting, thinking, communicating, producing knowledge – within which "every individual and social group operates" (Ford and Yep 2003, p. 248).

It is this context of life that the culture-centered approach celebrates. The context is highlighted in the conversations between the researchers and the cultural participants; the voices of the participants guide the meanings that are constructed in the discursive space. Cultural participants engage actively in dialogue, to identify the issues that are critical to the community; these configurations of the critical problems drive praxis instead of the problem being defined by external entities. In this case, opportunities of learning are not only opened up for the participating members of the culture, but also for the researcher/scholar who engages in dialogue with the culture. The traditional construction of the receivers of the message is expanded, moving from the realm of the communities targeted for the diffusion of innovations to the inclusion of funding agencies, policy-makers, researchers/scholars, community members and other stakeholders involved in the project, who continuously switch between the roles of sender and receiver as they engage in dialogue, identify problems and propose solutions to these problems.

This approach to health communication is embedded in the logic that the very effort to empower, to build skills, to create participatory public spheres assumes the absence of agency on the part of the cultural participants. By drawing from the extensive body of scholarship on subaltern studies, it demonstrates that members of marginalized spaces have historically participated in socio-cultural and political processes in challenging, shaping and coping with the structures that have encompassed their existence (Guha and Spivak 1988). In the culture-centered approach, the emphasis is not on creating skills, so that community members can be empowered through the campaign after being taught communication skills (see for instance, Storey and Jacobson 2004). Rather, the emphasis is on understanding existing forms of participation in communities which have been traditionally treated as devoid of agency. The culture-centered approach begins with the understanding that participatory forms of communication have long existed in communities across the globe, even in those marginalized spaces which have typically been conceptualized in Western discourse as passive recipients of interventions.

The important role of participation in marginalized spaces can be seen in the works of subaltern studies scholars who have extensively documented participation in peasant societies (Guha and Spivak 1988). Ample evidence is found in this body of scholarship that testifies to the agency and active participation of the peasant class, a class that is often treated as the passive recipient of campaign messages of enlightenment. The culture-centered approach provides a starting point for including, in the discursive space of knowledge, those voices which have typically been treated as an object of campaigns in much of the international and development communication work, in spite of the growing emphasis on the participatory rhetoric aimed at distinguishing these campaigns from the traditional one-way flow models.

Theoretical origins

The culture-centered approach draws its theoretical roots from postcolonial and subaltern studies (Beverley 1999, 2004). Postcolonial scholarship theorizes about the historically contingent nature of knowledge in the realm of European imperialism. The location of the colonies at the margins of the European centers of knowledge which sought to control the practices of these colonies through the deployment and management of knowledge is the subject of postcolonialism. In postcolonial scholarship, knowledge is theorized in terms of its relationship to the colonial history within which its production is rooted, and it is located in a postcolonial world where boundaries are blurred, identities are continually shifting, and relationships are in flux. The object position of the post-colonial participants and the subject position of the expert are predicated on a colonial history that defines these positions; and the postcolonial approach interrogates this relationship.

Subalternity deals with the position of being erased, of being under, of not having been recognized (Spivak 1988). The field of subaltern studies articulates the need for alternative scholarship, which seeks to dislocate the socio-spatial relationship embedded in the traditional production of knowledge about the colonies and their peoples which emanates from the European centers. Responding to the Eurocentric renderings of history, subaltern studies scholars have focused on writing "history from below" (Spivak 1988). Their efforts have emphasized alternative explanations as offered by the subaltern classes.

The subaltern studies effort, in essence, problematizes the value-free writing of history and locates history in the backdrop of the political goals, agendas and values of those writing it. Therefore the alternative writings of history in subaltern studies emphasize the dialogue with sub-altern voices as a necessary step toward such writings. It is on the basis of this dialogue that the researcher and the community members come to engage in the co-construction of knowledge. In the context of health communication scholarship, subaltern writing attempts, by engaging in dialogue with subaltern voices, to foreground the existing biases in the dominant articulations of knowledge and to dislocate the dominant phrasing of what it means to communicate about health. The subaltern roots of the culture-centered approach suggest the importance of the sol-idarity between the researcher and the community in which he/she par-ticipates. It is this solidarity that forms the basis of a dialogical platform, where the researcher engages in conversations with members of the com-munity. These conversations bring forth conceptual maps for under-standing health communication processes and for the development of solutions that make sense to the community.

Discussion point 2.2

- What are the fundamental tenets of the culture-centered approach? Do you agree or disagree with these tenets? Why? Why not?
- What are the ways in which you might use the culture-centered approach in your work? Outline the specific steps you might take in order to incorporate the culture-centered approach in your research and applications of health communication.

Characteristics of the Culture-Centered Approach

With its emphasis on locating culture at the center of theorizing, the culture-centered approach may be identified by some key characteristics. Some of them include voice and dialogue, structure, context, space, values, and criticism; these characteristics provide the conceptual framework for understanding what the culture-centered approach is. In addition, they also provide a scheme for demarcating the dominant approach to health communication from the culture-centered approach. This demarcation is important in order to prevent the co-optation of the participatory principles of the culture-centered approach by the dominant paradigm (Gramsci 2003).

Voice and dialogue

One of the central commitments of the culture-centered approach is to the voice of the subaltern participant (Beverley 1999). The experiences of other cultures are articulated through dialogical engagement (Bauman 2000; Giddens 1986). The culture-centered approach seeks to introduce the voice of local communities into the ways in which issues of health are understood, interpreted and communicated. The very act of engaging subaltern voices is a way of writing health communication from an alternative perspective, demonstrating the gaps in current theory and practice, and showing alternative strategies that might be adopted in health communication. These alternative strategies emerge from the dialogic engagement with communities. An example of such an alternative theory-building is my work with Santalis in the areas of Bengal and Bihar in eastern India (Dutta-Bergman 2004a, 2004b). In this line of work, my conversations with Santalis articulate theories of health that are inherently different from the conceptual maps imposed by the dominant paradigm of health communication. For instance, Santalis talk about health being intrinsically intertwined with nature; they see the loss of health as coming together with the increasing deforestation and urbanization projects of modern India. The notion of health conceptualized in this realm offers a different vantage point from the biomedical, psychosocial and behavioral models that privilege modernity and fail to interrogate it.

Subalternity is marked by its absence from the dominant discourse. It is the state of being omitted, of being looked over. Airhihenbuwa (1995) discusses the subalternity of African cultures in the dominant health discourse when he points toward the minimization of the oral tradition in conceptualizing communication. Much of the published health communication literature in subaltern spaces is presented in the way of top-down health interventions targeting subaltern participants. In these interventions, messages are designed by actors at the center to convince the target audiences to adopt a proposed behavior. For instance, the Center for Communication Programs at Johns Hopkins University systematically works with the United States Agency for International Development (USAID) to plan, execute and evaluate population control programs in the Third World. The center–periphery location is defined by access to power; those geographical spaces with access to power conceive and implement the messages, whereas the positions at the peripheral locations of power serve as target audiences of messages.

The emphasis of the culture-centered approach is on creating a communicative space for dialogue with the subaltern participants. It is important to note that this emphasis is not on representing the subaltern position or on being a spokesperson for the subaltern. Rather, the culture-centered perspective is built upon dialogical engagement between the researcher and the community. Central to this dialogical engagement is the commitment to friendship with the subaltern communities. Instead of attempting to provide solutions through interventions, the culture-centered approach focuses on gaining a sense of understanding of subaltern perspectives based on these dialogues with the community. What is privileged here is the process of engaging in the dialogue. The researcher is as much a part of this dialogue as are the subaltern participants she/he engages in dialogue with. It is through this engagement that the culture-centered perspective brings about an understanding of how health meanings are constructed in communities. For instance, in his research with the Hmong residents in Chicago, Dwight Conquergood (1982a, 1982b, 1988, 1989) explored the ways in which these residents came to understand what it means to be healthy.

It is important to note that the communicative space fostered in the culture-centered approach is also a reflexive space for the researcher, who can locate his/her cultural values in the dialogue. By locating himself/herself within the dialogical space, the researcher demonstrates a commitment to the co-construction of meanings rather than taking the position of an objective observer from outside. This placement of the researcher within the discursive space is critically different from that of traditional health communication approaches, where the researcher takes the objective position of the omniscient observer, who can document the practices of a culture on the basis of his/her superior abilities (Bauman 2000; Giddens 1986). As opposed to a commitment to the method of absence of the author (Giddens 1986), he/she begins with the understanding that, in order to engage in dialogue, it is critical to be present in the discursive moment and that there is no way out of this presence. It is through his/her presence in the discursive space that the researcher comes to understand his/her own values, beliefs, and ideologies, which inform his/her understandings of the interaction.

This privileging the voice of the subaltern participant is rooted in the emphasis placed by the culture-centered approach on understanding human agency. Agency refers to the capacity of human beings to interact with structures in order to create meanings; such meanings provide scripts for interacting with the structures, for sustaining these structures, and for transforming them. Therefore agency is both stable and dynamic. On the one hand, it connects to the roots of the culture, providing continuity with the past, documenting the ways in which cultural members live their daily lives negotiating the structural contexts that surround them. On the other hand, it provides an avenue for resistance, for attempts at changing those structural processes that limit the health-related capabilities of individuals. Once again, we see instances of both types of agency in my work with the Santalis in Bengal and Bihar. Participants talk, simultaneously, about the ways in which they ration their use of medical services so as to make it possible for their children to have access to the best healthcare in a resource-deprived environment, and about their participation in political processes with the aim of changing the corruption of the medical system (Dutta-Bergman 2004a, 2004b).

Structure

Structure refers to those organizations, processes and systems in society which determine how that society is organized, how it functions, and how individual members within it behave with respect to each other, to social organizations, and so on. By centralizing the dialogue with subaltern participants, the culture-centered approach creates a space for conceptualizing the ways in which structure constrains human agency, and the ways in which it facilitates the enactment of human agency. As a central focus, agency provides the theoretical ground for articulating structure, and structure provides the setting for the enactment of agency. Agency exists in a dialectical relationship with structure, being made possible because of the existence of structure, and continually working, at a variety of micro- and macro-levels, to negotiate the constraints imposed by structure and to change the structural processes that limit its enactment. Structure defines the limits of human action, at the same time creating the scenario for the enactment of human agency.

In the realm of the culture-centered approach, the emphasis is on gaining a sense of understanding of those structural processes in healthcare settings which limit the possibilities of health for community participants. Structure is articulated through the discursive engagement with members of the subaltern sectors. For instance, discursive co-constructions with women living in poverty indicate that access to, and availability of, healthcare are critical problems facing these women (Marshall and McKeon 1996). In addition, existing healthcare services are underused because of limited financial resources; focus on more basic needs such as food, clothing, and shelter; transportation and child care problems (ibid.).

Communicationally, structures constrain human action by setting up communicative barriers: for instance the homeless report facing a series of communicative barriers such as being mistreated by the hospital staff, being asked to fill out forms or not receiving directions about the steps to follow, and such. In this instance, the marginalized state of having minimal access to healthcare as a homeless person is communicatively enacted and reinforced through the ways in which the healthcare system treats the homeless. In other instances, structures create conditions of stigmatization which continue to construct those at the margins as inferior, primitive, and passive recipients of interventions targeted at them.

As suggested earlier, structure exists in a dialectical relationship with agency. In my work with the Santalis, the participants have talked about ways of changing the system. In their conversations, they have outlined two different approaches to challenging the structure. In the first instance, they talked about learning the tools of the system in order to gain access. They discussed sending their children to school and making sure they were educated, so that family and community members could find better access to a variety of resources, including healthcare. In addition, they also talked about the ways in which the corrupt practices of those in power needed to be challenged. Toward this end, they discussed participating in political processes in an attempt to change the structure.

Context and space

Context refers to the local and immediate surroundings within which cultural members make choices. The structures and processes at the macro-level are played out through micro-level contexts within which health meanings are continuously created and recreated. These contexts are part of the day-to-day life experiences of community members, and are characteristics of the local community within which the participants live their lives. Localized contexts surround health meanings, health values, health beliefs, and health practices, and exist in a continuous flux with the broader structures surrounding them. These contexts connect individual members to the cultures within which they live, and simultaneously offer opportunities for enacting cultural change through the practices adopted by individuals in response to them.

Contexts are intertwined with the structures within which communities are embedded, providing a local interface through which the structure constrains the life experiences of the community member. For instance, the Hmong community in the United States is embedded within the broader structures of immigration and poverty. These structures, in turn, constitute the local contexts within which the life experiences of the members of the Hmong community are enacted. The local contexts include language issues, cultural practices, religious practices, minimal access to healthcare and so on – which are enacted through the interactions with structural markers such as immigration policies and authorities, community hospitals and hospital staff, the welfare system and social workers. In another example, Burke (1976) observed that Asian female immigrants in Birmingham had higher suicide rates than in their countries of origin, pointing out that language difficulties for women, the expectation to remain at home, and cultural conflicts between the values of home and those at school or workplace contribute to this. In this instance, the local context of language difficulties, expectations to stay at home and culture conflict exist within the broader structure of immigration.

The contextual experience of health, the negotiation of health meanings, and the interactions with structures also may be located spatially. The health experiences of marginalized communities are typically located at the geographic margins of the healthcare system. For instance, members of rural communities are often marginalized by the geographic location at the margins of urban and suburban healthcare systems. In

Dutta-Bergman's work with the Santalis in West Bengal (2004a, 2004b), the geographic location of the participants in distant villages which are not connected by roads is central to the experience of inaccess to health-care resources. In other instances, the location of participants in the Third World (a geographic position at the margins) makes them the target audience for interventions conceptualized, implemented and evaluated by members of the developed world.

The dominant and the marginalized communities typically exist in center–periphery relationships; those at the center have access to positions of power and get to have a say on issues of policy and implementation, whereas those without access serve as target audiences. The spatial location at the margins are typically accompanied by marginalizing practices such as attempts to reform, to control and to transform. Those at the spatial margins typically experience communicative marginalization through the enactment of a variety of strategies; their voices typically remain unheard, as experts at the center continue to plan and implement interventions targeted at them. Therefore one of the goals of the culture-centered approach is to foreground the spatial distribution of power in the way we communicate about health. The spatial exploration of power distributions focuses on questions such as: Who gets to speak? Who is silenced? What communicative strategies are used for the purposes of silencing? What communicative strategies may be put in place, to resist the acts of silencing? What is the relationship between power, space, and positions of authority in the healthcare system? These questions offer starting points for politicizing the study of health communication and for suggesting strategies for interrogating the dominant approach to health communication. One of these strategies is the centralization of values in health communication scholarship.

Values

The culture-centered approach suggests that values are central to the ways in which we conceptualize the problems we consider to be important and the corresponding solutions we develop to these problems (Dutta-Bergman 2004a, 2004b, 2005a, 2005b). The extent to which something is a problem depends upon the lens we bring to bear on the problem. The problem is never free of this cultural lens. Health communication typically involves the privileging of certain values and the omission of certain other values from the discursive space. Take for instance the problem of sanitary hygiene, as defined by the Western approach, and locate it with respect to the sanitary practices documented in many communities in South Asia, for instance in India, Pakistan, and Nepal. In these communities, individuals use public spaces to defecate and then cleanse themselves using public water. To the Western eye, this is a public health problem that ought to be remedied by building latrines and teaching hygienic cleaning practices (Storey and Jacobson 2004; Dutta and Basnyat, in press). However, the simplistic focus on building latrines does not take into account the structural constraints embedded in such communities. Furthermore, an alternative problem articulation from the cultural perspective looking at Western hygiene would emphasize the "poor" Western quality of cleaning habits, which do not include using water after defecation. In certain South Asian contexts, the practice of using paper towels is inherently unhygienic, because paper does not completely cleanse the body. In addition, the typically taken-for-granted Western practice of using toilet paper may be thought of as environmentally unfriendly, adding to deforestation and contributing to pollution. The problematization of this behavior might call for a health campaign which promotes the use of water instead of toilet paper as a means of cleaning. As this example demonstrates, problem definitions are inherently located in cultural values and in the criteria linked with these values.

Yet another example in the realm of value-based problem configurations is the definition of population growth as a global resource problem. In the realm of the dominant discourse, which takes as a desirable standard the nuclear family with two children, alternative articulations regarding large family sizes either seem implausible or are painted as deviant, primitive, or abnormal. However, if large families built on the values of sharing and caring are centralized as the norm, nuclear families with two children might be looked at as manifestations of the selfish tendency to save and to optimize material enjoyment. The typical message of population control programs, which discusses the joys of well-planned nuclear families, might be seen as epitomizing individual greed and materialism.

Cultural values are not only intertwined with the way we define health problems, but also with the types of solutions which are proposed to these problems. As a result, these solutions become sites of political contestation, engaging different stakeholder groups with different goals and interests. In the dominant paradigm, it is this very contestation that is challenged. The objectivity and universal standards of science are mobilized to support a particular solution being pushed. Take for instance the problem of population control, as defined by key agencies which carry out these health promotion programs. The distribution of condoms is often normalized as the standard solution in the dominant public health discourse, in spite of the availability of options such as abstinence or waiting to have sex until one is married.

Criticism

The culture-centered approach provides a critical framework for interrogating the dominant theories and practices in health communication by suggesting the need to articulate the values that have driven the dominant paradigm, and by locating these values in the realm of the dominant ideology (Dutta-Bergman 2004a, 2005a). The criticism of the dominant paradigm offered by the culture-centered approach is an effort to return the gaze that has typically been cast on the subject position of the subaltern participant. It is an attempt to subjectivize the producer of knowledge and to uncover the dominant interests active in constructing certain truths; essentially, it is an effort at locating the political interests in health communication. The subaltern groups that have typically been treated as objects of study provide a conceptual space for interrogating the scholarly practices of the European "knowers" who have historically been placed outside the realm of values open to discussion and revision. The uncontested position of the knower and the universal appeal of scientific rationality have been turned into a subject of study: what questions has the knower asked? What tools has he used? To what conclusions has she arrived on the basis of these tools, and what have been the political implications of these conclusions?

Therefore, by centralizing culture in health communication, Europe has become a subject of study, providing the focal point for investigating the origin of the scholarly values and practical impulses in health communication. When we locate European values in a cultural frame of reference, the otherwise privileged and taken-for-granted assumptions for categorizing the world start coming under scrutiny. These values no longer remain as desirable universals, but become contextually embedded in cultures and their practices. Airhihenbuwa (1995) provides an excellent example of the universal logic in value framing when he discusses the so-called "limitation" of the languages of African cultures, in that they treat as brothers and sisters relatives who are traditionally addressed as nephews, nieces and cousins in Western cultures. He points out that this is perhaps a deliberate construction in African cultures, which capture the intimacy of a sibling relationship – something that is typically absent in the individualistic Western cultures, which are built upon the notion of defining boundaries in interpersonal spaces. Similarly, he questions the notion of "extended" families in Western discourse, where the nuclear family is the norm; an alternative approach, which takes the extended family as the norm, would lead to the categorization of the typical Western family as the "constricted family."

By situating the study of health communication culturally, the culture-centered approach suggests that the very articulation of problems, development of solutions, and choices of theoretical and methodological tools are embedded in culture. As a result, who we are as scholars and practitioners deeply influences the questions we ask when given a certain problem configuration at the general level. Similarly, the politicians, funding agencies, and non-governmental organizations which actively shape our research agendas are embedded in a cultural system and serve certain goals that are politically determined. For instance, the objective of USAID to fund population control programs is tied to the logic of creating secure spaces for the transnational hegemony and of creating new markets for transnational corporations (Dutta 2006).

The cultural lens provides the script for indicating which aspects of the problem will be highlighted and which aspects will be backgrounded or omitted, and for suggesting the explanations that will be provided for a phenomenon. In other words, the study of health communication is embedded in culture, and one cannot step out of cultural values and norms just because one has decided to do so. The location of the scholar and the practitioner in a cultural landscape casts doubts on her capacity to suggest health solutions from an objective position of expertise. Take for instance the rise in unsafe sex as a problem defined by funding agencies. For someone who has been culturally trained to look for explanations of phenomena at an individual level, questions such as (a) why individuals are engaging in unsafe sex; (b) how we can develop messages to persuade them to engage in safer sex; and (c) what psychological processes underlie the decision to have unsafe sex might make sense. However, for someone who has been culturally trained to think about collective norms as guidelines for action, the following questions might make greater sense: (a) what are the cultural norms around safe sex? (b) how is safe sex culturally negotiated? – and (c) what are the cultural rituals surrounding sex? In yet other value orientations, which are more directed toward structural factors, questions such as (a) what are the socio-economic incentives for engaging in unsafe sex? (b) what are the organizational processes in schools that facilitate unsafe sex? (c) what are the structural incentives for spaces such as bars and night clubs, which facilitate unsafe sex? – and (d) how can we change unsafe structures through policy regulations? – might seem more plausible. In other words, the very same problem might be conceptualized in a plethora of ways, depending upon the lens we bring to bear on it. Accordingly, the solutions might look very different depending upon the value position of those who suggest these solutions. The objective position of the European knower/campaign planner/development agent/funding agency/policy-maker is problematized by, and is imbued with, the values which that person brings to the study of a health phenomenon.

Discussion point 2.3

- What are the characteristics of the culture-centered approach? How do these characteristics differentiate the culture-centered approach from the cultural sensitivity approach?
- The culture-centered approach discusses the possibilities of engaging the voices of marginalized communities. Discuss.

Conclusion

The culture-centered approach to theory and practice suggests that the field of health communication is intrinsically intertwined with the values we bring to the study of health processes and messages. Inherent in these values are the biases and ideological apparatuses of knowledge production embedded in the way health communication has been traditionally studied and practiced. Starting to interrogate these traditional ways of conceptualizing and practicing health communication not only provides us with an understanding of the questions which have been asked, but also directs us toward those questions which have not been asked in the dominant approach to health communication. The centralizing of values simultaneously offers a space for criticizing the dominant approach on the basis of the value positions it espouses, and for building alternative theories of health communication through dialogical engagement with members of cultural communities.

3 Theoretical Approaches to the Study of Culture

Chapter objectives

In this chapter, we will:

- examine the different theoretical approaches to the study of culture
- analyze the relationship between theory and application in culture-based work
- compare and contrast the different culture-based health communication approaches

In chapter 2 we looked at the culture-centered approach to health communication and delved into its characteristics. In the present chapter we will locate this approach in the backdrop of other approaches to culture in health communication. In order to do so, we will look at a categorization scheme which lays out the fundamental criteria for studying the different approaches to cultural health communication. The presentation and comparison of these approaches will provide a framework for understanding what we mean by culture when discussing it in the context of the culture-centered approach and how this conceptualization differs from the others that are applied in health communication scholarship. Ultimately, the purpose of this chapter is to provide an understanding of the theories of culture and of the applications of such theories as they relate to the culture-centered approach, and simultaneously to provide a sense of what, in the domain of the culture-centered approach, culture is not.

The chapter will begin with an overview of the communication scholarship which examines culture. An integrated categorization scheme will be offered to equip you with an understanding of the different approaches to culture in the study of communication, and, more specifically, health communication. Based on the presentation of these different approaches to the study of culture, commonalities and differences inherent in these approaches will follow. Drawing upon this overview, the culture-centered approach will be compared with the dominant approach in health communication.

Communication and Culture

Both communication theorists and practitioners have acknowledged the relevance of culture to health communication in the last two decades

Box 3.1   The story of Carmen

In discussing the death of her daughter Carmen, Mrs Renee Morton discussed poignantly the difficulties her daughter had faced in going to the hospital located in central Los Angeles. Carmen was incapacitated by stomach pains that had started around Christmas, and did not have the money to pay for the approximately $65 round trip it would take her to get to the hospital. So she decided to wait out her stomach pain and thought that it would gradually disappear. By the time Renee decided to take Carmen to the Mercy hospital in central Los Angeles, it was too late, Dr Hallowell announced. Carmen was now waiting for her death, waiting in silence, waiting in pain, and waiting for it all to be over.

Why did Carmen die within a healthcare system that is one of the most expensive healthcare systems in the world? Why would Carmen's inability to afford $65 for each trip to the hospital be critical to her inability to access healthcare? Carmen and Mrs Morton's story documents the health experiences of individuals living in marginalized communities.

(Airhihenbuwa 1995; Brislin 1993; Dutta-Bergman 2004a, 2004b, 2005a, 2005b; Lupton 1994, 2003; Resnicow et al. 2002). The concept of culture has gained particular importance in the context of the discussions of globalization, immigration, and changes in US demographic characteristics, with health communicators wanting to develop multicultural health programs which address the needs of diverse audiences. Scholars and practitioners alike have become interested in the concept of culture, so that health communication theories can be developed in multicultural settings and applications can be better developed by practitioners.

The experiences of Carmen and Mrs Morton demonstrate how health is construed at the intersection between culture, structure, and agency. It raises the following questions: How do health experiences emerge at the intersection between structural forces in social systems and the cultural meanings through which these structures are interpreted? How do individuals make sense of the structures they experience in their day-to-day lives? How do they engage with such structures? The way we approach such questions depends upon the fundamental framework guiding our theorizing, research, and application development. How culture, structure, and agency are interpreted depends upon the overall framework that guides these approaches.

The different approaches to culture presented in this chapter draw upon two classification schemes, which intersect orthogonally to generate an integrated categorical framework with four different approaches (see figure 3.1). The first classification scheme is based upon the distinction between the predictive models of culture and the models of cultural understanding. In the predictive approach, culture is a container of beliefs, values and practices, whereas the models of cultural understanding conceptualize culture as an active process of meaning-making embedded in the local context (Dutta 2007). Whereas the predictive model focuses on prediction and

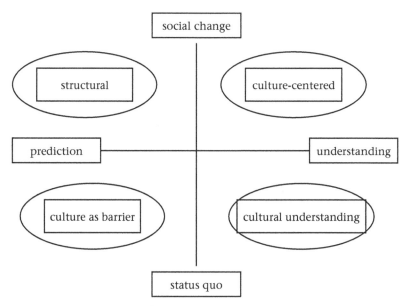

Fig. 3.1 Approaches to the study of culture

control, the understanding-based model focuses on meanings and the descriptions of these meanings. In other words, these two important yet vastly different threads of scholarship in the area of culture in health communication draw upon their respective goals – of explaining communicative phenomena by cultural variables and of understanding communicative phenomena in cultural contexts. The different goals of the two approaches set up very different theoretical assumptions, methodological tools, and conceptual bases for application development in health communication.

Yet another manner of categorizing the different approaches to the study of culture proceeds by examining the ways in which such approaches engage culture in order to achieve health applications that support the status quo or question the inherent power relations in cultures which create conditions of marginalization and poor health (Dutta-Bergman 2005a, 2005b; Lupton 1994). Under this classification scheme, health communication theory and research are examined with respect to the extent to which they support the dominant biomedical model of health communication and the status quo, emphasizing individual-level change in behaviors and de-emphasizing the social, cultural and economic factors that are pivotal to health or focus on the role of structural readjustments and of resource mobilization in improving health conditions. These two categorizing schemes, prediction versus understanding, and social change versus status quo, provide the axes for developing an integrated categorical framework for the classification of health communication research and application in the area of culture (see figure 3.1).

Predicting versus understanding

Studies of culture that focus on predicting communication practices in the realm of culture conceptualize culture as a variable, as a stable container of values, beliefs and practices that are enclosed within a determined boundary. In predictive approaches of this kind, culture is typically defined by a marked boundary (such as nationality) and by clearly demarcated indicators which are typically stable within one culture and vary systematically across several (such as ethnicity or immigrant status), and is characterized in terms of certain stable patterns (such as values and beliefs). The goal is to examine the relationship between culture and the communication variable at stake. The predictive power of culture is the topic of interest, typically based on the questions: How much variance in the communication phenomenon of interest is explained by culture? How much variance in a health outcome is explained by a certain cultural characteristic? A specific aspect of the culture is extracted for comparison. Such approaches, which emphasize explaining communication by culture, typically compare multiple cultures in order to develop a comparative framework.

Cultural characteristics that are typically used to categorize cultures include individualism–collectivism, power distance, uncertainty avoidance, and masculinity–femininity (Dutta-Bergman 2005a). These characteristics are applied universally, to create a categorization scheme for cultures such that they may be assigned a certain score on the basis of their level of individualism–collectivism, power distance, uncertainty avoidance, and masculinity–femininity. Individualism–collectivism refers to the extent to which cultures value independence, autonomy, and personal freedom, as opposed to valuing relational harmony, group cohesiveness and so on. Power distance refers to the extent to which cultures value hierarchical norms in relationships. Uncertainty avoidance reflects the degree of comfort which the cultural members feel in dealing with uncertainty. Finally, masculinity–femininity refers to the level of emphasis on masculine and feminine values in the culture. Health communication interventions based on the predictive model attempt to develop solutions related to these cultural characteristics, which have been predetermined by categorizing schemes. In studies of individualism–collectivism, for instance, communication researchers have used this feature to explain the amount of variance in the preference for certain messages in health settings.

In other instances, scholars have studied constructs such as health locus of control for the purpose of explaining the role of culture in communication and health outcomes (Pérez-Stable et al. 1992). Locus of control refers to the extent to which cultural members perceive themselves to be in control of their health behaviors and health outcomes. Cultures with internal locus of control consider health to be in the hands of individuals and resulting from their choices, whereas cultures with external locus of control typically place health among external factors beyond individual control. Cultures with external locus of control are also described as fatalistic because they invest external entities with the primary responsibility of health. Therefore health interventions typically attempt to alter the locus of control of externals in order to make them take charge of their lives and engage in the prescribed behaviors. Research on physician–patient relationships, for instance, seeks to convert patients into internal locus of control individuals, so that they may have better health results.

In contrast to the effort of studying the predictive power of culture on certain communication variables, health communication studies which emphasize cultural understanding foreground the meanings and interpretations of health constructed by cultural members through communication (Hahn 1999). Such an approach is typically located within the interpretive paradigm of health communication scholarship. Culture interpenetrates the meanings co-constructed by the researcher and the cultural participants. Therefore understanding is located in the communication between the researcher and the cultural participants. It is through the process of engaging in conversations with the cultural participants that the researcher or practitioner comes to have a sense of understanding of the culture and of its health meanings.

Such an approach, which seeks to develop an understanding of the culture, asks the question: How do cultural members communicate with each other? How do they understand the meanings of health? How do they negotiate these meanings? In the area of health communication, scholars who deal with the topic with the purpose of developing an understanding of the culture approach the culture with open-ended questions rather than with predetermined constructs that may be imposed on it from outside. Methods of understanding typically include qualitative ones, such as in-depth interviews or focus groups, with an emphasis on developing grounded theories of health from within the cultures. Such efforts at understanding emphasize the role of communication in developing cultural understandings; communication simultaneously informs culture and is informed by culture. With reference to the physician–patient relationship described earlier, scholars applying the interpretive approach seek to understand how members of a culture communicate with physicians, how they ask questions and provide reports, and how they come to understand the physician–patient relationship. In the realm of health interventions, an interpretive approach would begin by engaging in conversation with the cultural members, to gain an in-depth view on the cultural understanding of the behavior proposed to be promoted in the community. It would then engage with cultural members in creating meaningful messages, which resonate with the community.

Discussion point 3.1

• What are the advantages and drawbacks of predictive approaches to culture in health communication?

- What are the advantages and drawbacks of the understanding-based approaches to culture in health communication?
- Which of these two approaches seems more appealing to you? Why?

Status quo versus social change

Status quo refers to the existing patterns of beliefs, attitudes and behaviors that operate within a certain structural formation in society. It refers to a predetermined configuration of access and health experience, which is based on the unequal distributions of power in society (Lupton 1994, 2006). Approaches to culture that support the status quo focus on altering values, beliefs, attitudes and behaviors at the cultural level in order to generate conditions of greater health for the target culture on the basis of dominant values in biomedicine. Greater health is achieved via the widespread adoption, at the individual level, of the prescribed behavior drawn from the biomedical model. Therefore health communication practices that support the status quo seek to alter individual behavior as a means of improving the health condition of the individual, without addressing the structural contexts within which health is located (Dutta-Bergman 2005a).

Health communication research and application which demonstrate such an approach in the cultural context focus on using communication strategies in order to stimulate a process of acculturation, in order to create more culturally sensitive physician–patient interactions so that outcomes may be improved, or in order to create health campaigns that are culturally sensitive and hence have a greater potential for the diffusion of the proposed behavior within the community (Castro, Cota and Vega 1999; Ramirez, Villarreal and Chalela 1999). The concept of culture needs to be understood and deployed such that better services may be provided and better health interventions may be created. Culture serves as a resource that may be used to improve the efficiency of the healthcare system and to minimize the barriers that constrain the diffusion of the recommended health behavior.

The emphasis is on identifying the underlying values, beliefs and attitudes of the cultural community, so that a more effective health communication program may be developed. Let's take for instance a health campaign on family planning that seeks to promote the use of condoms among cultural members. Family planning campaigns are typically driven by the logic that smaller families ensure better allocation of resources per children and, hence, ensure better health. Now such a program is considered to be culturally sensitive when it conducts formative research with members of the cultural community to understand their beliefs, attitudes and behaviors and then responds to these underlying values, beliefs and attitudes in creating culturally sensitive messages that promote condom use. A culturally sensitive campaign might even go a step further and involve community members in the design and development of the message. In these instances, however, the campaign is supporting the status quo by conceptualizing family planning as the problem, while at the same tine ignoring other problem configurations such as lack of resources, unequal distribution of wealth in communities, and the broader global inequities that might underlie inaccess to resources.

Approaches to culture which emphasize social change focus on interrogating the power structures that marginalize cultural communities, and seek to alter these structures by engaging in health activism (Dutta-Bergman 2004a, 2004b, 2005a; Dutta and Basu 2007; Zoller 2005). Structure refers to the patterns of societal organization, institutional processes and practices, and patterns of resource distribution in society. In approaches that emphasize social change, cultural practices are examined in the context of their relationships with these societal structures. Concepts such as ideology and hegemony are activated in order for us to gain an understanding of the marginalizing practices of those in power. It is claimed that health experiences are embedded in the ways in which the privileged actors exercise their power and control through the widespread diffusion of the dominant ideology.

Ideology refers to the taken-for-granted assumptions, within the culture, which create conducive situations for the maintenance of the status quo, and hegemony reflects the unquestioned power held by a certain group of cultural members. By asking questions of ideology and hegemony, approaches of the social change type open up the material and discursive spaces of cultures to structural adjustments. They interrogate the assumptions of individual-level change, taken for granted in the biomedical model, and articulate the ways in which such efforts of individual-level change shift the emphasis away from those unhealthy structural inequities which are apparent in the marginalized sectors of the globe. The next section presents the overall categorization scheme generated by the combinations of these two distinct frameworks of categorizing cultures.

Box 3.2   The story of Louise

Louise is 42 years old and lives primarily on welfare because she has been rendered jobless with a disease called Multiple Chemical Sensitivity (MCS) that keeps her in bed most of the year. Louise is highly allergic to any chemicals in her environment and has to attempt to minimize the chemicals in her house so that she can prevent the attacks and frequent hospitalization. Louise developed this condition when she was 36 and has since gradually had to minimize the number of hours she puts in because she is unable to handle the chemicals at work, and feels more and more tired more often. Having been rendered jobless, Louise also can't afford health insurance and has gradually depleted most of her savings that she had from her years of work. Her husband left about two years back when her temper kept getting more and more difficult to handle and "he couldn't take it anymore." She doesn't know where to go to seek further help and is scared of the future that stands ahead of her three children. On most days, she can barely move around to take care of them.

How do we approach Louise's experience from a predictive standpoint? How would we approach Louise's experience from an "understanding-based" standpoint? How do we approach Louise's experience from a status quo framework? How would we approach Louise's experience from a social change framework?

Discussion point 3.2

- What are the advantages and drawbacks of the "status quo" approaches to culture in health communication?
- What are the advantages and drawbacks of the "social change" approaches to culture in health communication?
- Which of these approaches discussed here are you more likely to use in your work? Why?

Approaches to the Study of Culture

The combination of the two categorizing schemes, explaining versus understanding and status quo versus social change, provides the framework for locating the various ways of studying and applying culture in the context of health communication (see figure 3.1). The grid presented in figure 3.1 documents four different approaches to the study of culture in health communication. In the figure, the culture-centered approach is the combination of a perspective that centralizes understanding and a perspective that is directed at social change. Structural communication is directed at social change by quantitatively measuring and predicting the role of disparities on cultural variables and subsequent health outcomes, and by guiding us toward the gaps in policies and macro-level structures that promote health inequities. The cultural sensitivity approach, which regards culture as a barrier, focuses on explaining communication and health outcomes by quantifiable cultural factors and on applying these factors so as to minimize the barriers to effective health communication. Finally, the approach from the angle labeled cultural understanding seeks to provide the audience with a sense of understanding of the culture, its beliefs and values, and the communication practices around health. The emphasis of such an approach is on gaining an understanding of the meanings around health that circulate in the culture, without an implicit commitment to achieving social change.

As documented in chapter 1, the culture-centered approach provides the foundation for this book. According to the culture-centered approach, communication about health is culturally situated and is simultaneously tied with structural processes. In other words, the interactions between structure and culture is central to understanding the health experiences of cultural members. For instance, in his work with rural Haitians, Paul Farmer (1999) argued that the so-called cultural practices around health that were exoticized in published ethnographic accounts of Haiti systematically missed out the violence of the structural conditions that surrounded such practices, and the link between structure and culture in shaping such practices.

In contrast to the emphasis on the intersection between culture and structure articulated in the culture-centered approach, the structural approach to health communication seeks to examine the role of structure in explaining the health outcomes of individuals and communities.

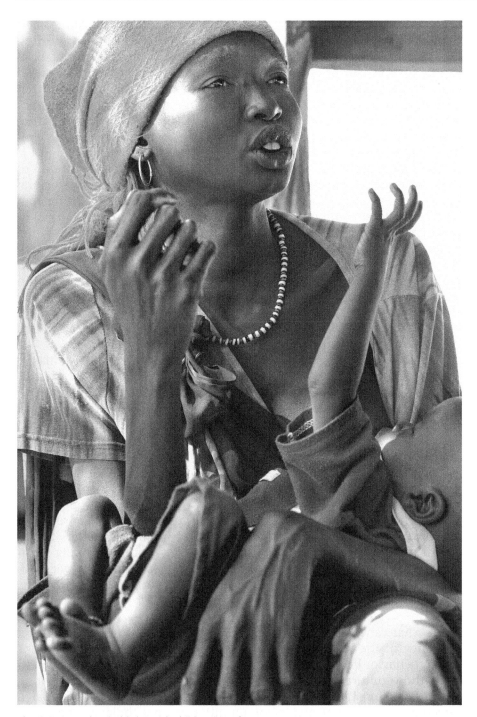

Fig. 3.2 A mother holds her sick child waiting for treatment
© Sven Torfinn @ Panos Pictures

Culture, in this context, is typically constructed as a variable that mediates or moderates the influence of structure on health outcomes and processes. An example of this approach is the growing body of research on social capital, published by public health scholars working on disparities (Kawachi, Kennedy and Wilkinson 1999). These scholars point out that economic inequalities in a community contribute to lower levels of community participation and trust (defined as social capital), which, in turn, contributes to the poor health outcomes in the community. Studies conducted under this approach are typically quantitative in nature and are based on large-scale surveys of communities that are compared in terms of their structural characteristics. The criticism offered against a structural approach to health is that it does not take into account the shifting contexts of the local communities within which health meanings come to be articulated. By extracting residual features of communities (such as the extent of community participation), such an approach omits the very meanings of health, constructed in the interactions between the cultural participants and the structures, and it also omits the local contexts within which health meanings, health behaviors and health experiences are constructed. Nevertheless, the structural approach provides a basis for social change by explaining the role of structure in health communication and by challenging structural inequities.

The culture-as-barrier approach to health communication is similar to the structural approach to the extent that it sees culture as a variable which could explain a communication phenomenon in the health context; the goal is to use culture for purposes of prediction. However, instead of emphasizing culture and its relationship to the structures that surround the health experiences of individuals, the culture-as-barrier approach conceptualizes culture as a barrier that prevents the enactment of the proposed health behavior, typically conceptualized under the biomedical model of health (Resnicow et al. 2002). This is also known as the cultural sensitivity approach, as it is couched under the broader framework of developing culturally relevant messages which are sensitive to the cultural mores while simultaneously minimizing barriers to the health behavior being promoted. In other words, being culturally sensitive is critical to the culture-as-barrier approach, so that the target audience of the intervention is drawn to the message and persuaded by it. The culture-as-barrier approach is the dominant approach in health communication, and is based on the notion that culture is a set of values and beliefs that can be quantified and taken into account to ensure greater efficiency of the system. These values and beliefs, in turn, explain the health behavior in question. The goal of the campaign planner is to minimize those cultural beliefs that act as barriers to the adoption of an individual behavior. Take for instance a hypothetical heart health campaign targeting immigrant Hispanic communities in rural Indiana. The objective of this campaign is to promote exercising in order to minimize the risks of heart attacks in this population, and campaign planners first conduct formative research in the community to determine the existing cultural beliefs that are barriers to exercising. Based on their research, the campaign planners identify that one of the barriers to action is the highly collectivistic character of the community: individual members do not want to take time away from their families to engage in exercising; they believe that exercising prevents them from spending time with their families. In responding to this cultural belief-based barrier, campaign planners design a message that addresses the issue of collective participation in leisure activities and presents the benefits of time spent exercising collectively. The message here addresses the barrier-belief that "exercising takes time away from collective time" and reframes it in a culturally sensitive manner. In this example, a culturally sensitive message simultaneously addresses a barrier in the culture and does it in a sensitive fashion.

Finally, the approach of cultural understanding is similar to the culture-centered approach in its emphasis on cultural meanings as articulated by people within the culture (Nichter and Nichter 1996). These meanings are contextually located and the emphasis here is on presenting this context, within which cultural members discuss their health experiences. In this approach, culture is dynamic, constituted through communication among cultural participants, and is embedded in the context within which meanings are articulated. Culture is seen as a lens which is articulated in the narratives of cultural members.

Although this approach of cultural understanding provides an invaluable alternative to the dominant biomedical model of health communication, which looks at culture as a barrier to health, it does not locate culture in the realm of the structural processes that surround it, and hence it does not provide an emancipatory space for health communication scholarship. The interpretations and meanings provide important insights about how health is culturally constructed, but they do not provide means for achieving social change by challenging the structures of marginalization which are integral to the experiences that these scholars talk about. By omitting structure, the approach of cultural understanding backgrounds questions of power, structural inequities and inaccess that are played out in the experiences of cultural members. Ultimately, the cultural understanding framework discusses the values, beliefs and practices of a culture as they are articulated in the meanings presented by the participants. All the approaches reviewed here share certain similarities, and yet they differ from each other in some fundamental ways. In the following section I will discuss the similarities and differences between them.

Similarities and Differences between Cultural Approaches

Similarities between various approaches to culture

Irrespective of their orientation, the approaches and theories of culture presented in this chapter share some common traits. They all draw upon a conceptualization of culture which belongs in a certain space, is built on the shared values and beliefs of the individuals living within that space, and is tied to certain shared practices that characterize the culture.

Space.   Culture is conceptualized in terms of a space that brings individuals together into a community. It is this space that typically offers the primary marker of the culture, because it is within this space that the values, beliefs, and practices of members are defined. It is also within this space that members communicate with each other; in other words, this space provides the platform for communicative exchange. It is also the site for the enactment of structural processes which define the fundamental characteristics of the space, such as its access to basic resources, its relationship with positions of power, its predominant communication avenues, and so on. As a material entity, it offers a defining framework for the articulation of cultural identities, beliefs, values and practices. The culture-centered approach, the structural approach, the culture-as-barrier approach, and the cultural understanding approach all draw upon the notion of space attached to culture.

At the most rudimentary level, scholars have defined cultures in terms of national boundaries. These cultures are referred to as national cultures. For instance, the work of Geert Hofstede compares national cultures on the four key dimensions of individualism–collectivism, power distance, uncertainty avoidance, and femininity–masculinity. Similarly, Airhihenbuwa's work with the PEN-3 model talks about African cultures that are tied to the geographic articulation of a space called Africa. Similarly, Farmer's work on the interactions of culture and structure in the realm of rural health focuses on the health of Haitians.

The rapid diffusion of technology, however, calls for more sophisticated understandings of culture that are constituted in technologically mediated communities and are not essentially linked to geographic locations. In other words, the spatial location of culture might also be articulated in terms of virtual spaces. For instance, a community of breast cancer survivors on the Internet might draw people from a variety of national cultures into a common space, where they exchange ideas and communicate with each other. In this instance, the online support community of breast cancer survivors becomes a cultural space. Worth noting is the presence of a platform for continuous exchanges of ideas, meanings, and values among cultural members.

Although space is conceptually linked with culture, some scholars have interrogated its monolithic construction in the context of globalization. For instance, the immigration of people from the colonized world to the centers of colonialism (the United States and United Kingdom) have fractured the notions of a first and a Third World. The increasing flow of people across the world challenges the geographically situated notion of culture, pointing out that cultures today are dislocated, constantly in flux and transition. Postcolonial scholars such as Homi Bhabha have suggested the notion of hybridity in order to articulate the multiple identities that

are continuously in play in postcolonial contexts. Irrespective of the frag-
mentation of the global landscape and of the realization of multiple identities, however, it needs to be pointed out that cultures inevitably are
attached to some sense of space. For instance, in the discussions of the
health experiences of immigrant Haitian cultures in the United States,
culture is conceptualized in terms of a space geographically located in
Haiti and a space geographically located in the United States.

Shared identities.   The shared spaces constituting cultures also provide the
basis for the articulation of cultural identities shared by the individuals
that inhabit these spaces. Identities refer to the ways in which individual
members of the culture view themselves and to the basic understandings
they have of what it means to belong to a culture. Individuals typically
draw on multiple identities at multiple levels. For instance, the identity of
a Hispanic immigrant in New Mexico is closely tied to his/her understandings of what it means to be Hispanic, what it means to be an immigrant, and what it means to be a Hispanic immigrant living in New
Mexico.

These identities are typically attached to the material characteristics of
the spaces, and evolve in relation to the structural processes that constitute such spaces. The communication between cultural members is based
on this shared identity, which defines what it means to be a member of
the culture. For both outsiders and insiders to the culture, the shared
identity provides the basis for articulating similarities and differences.
Cultural members are more similar to each other with respect to a certain
set of characteristics, in comparison with the members of other cultures;
also, with respect to these characteristics, they are different from outsiders. These similarities and differences constitute the demarcation of
cultural boundaries. For instance, Hofstede's work on national cultures
suggests that members of a national culture such as Egypt typically have
an interdependent self-construal, indicating that they think of their identities in terms of the groups they belong to, their kinship ties, their commitment to these ties and so on. Or take for instance a rural Bengali
culture. Identity here is typically constructed in terms of one's family
background; individuals first and foremost think of themselves as the son
or daughter of a particular family and are often asked about the family
they come from when meeting strangers within the community.

Cultural identities also commit individuals to relationships with the
culture to which they belong. Individuals who draw upon a cultural identity also have a certain public commitment to the culture. Membership in
a culture is attached to a set of implicit and explicit roles and obligations
with respect to that culture. For instance, being a member of the
American or British culture creates a certain set of expectations for cultural members. Patriotism is often an overt expression of this commitment to the culture, and is typically invoked when the culture is
threatened. In response to the attacks on the World Trade Center on 9/11,
the American public demonstrated their support for the nation by putting

up flags in front of their houses, by putting US flags on bumper stickers and the like.

Shared experiences.   Members of cultures are joined together by the commonality of their life experiences. Life experiences reflect what it means to be a member of the culture. They constitute the day-to-day activities of the cultural members. These life experiences are tied to the material conditions that embody the geographic space within which culture gets enacted, and they are integral to the identities of the cultural members. The shared experience of cultural members is intrinsically linked to the structural resources of the culture. For instance, the shared experience of the members of a Hmong community in California are connected with access to health resources, to mainstream communication platforms, to the jobs available to them, to health resources such as food, medical services, medical supplies, and so on. Members of a culture typically experience similar structural forces in their daily lives. The members of a rural Haitian community experience similar day-to-day struggles in finding daily jobs or in having access to transportation and communication channels, to hospitals and medical supplies, to sanitary systems and clean drinking water, and so on.

In addition, these shared experiences are also tied to the values and beliefs of the culture. Values refer to the culture's orientation toward important issues in life; beliefs refer to the thoughts of cultural members regarding these key issues. These values and beliefs provide the script for the cultural members' response to the structural processes surrounding the culture. They are also reflective of the traditions of the culture, pointing toward the conceptualizations of the sacred and profane within it. These traditions prescribe how cultural members will respond to a variety of health situations, and how they will interact with structural processes.

Shared values and beliefs.   Each of the approaches to the study of culture conceptualizes culture in terms of the values, beliefs, and practices that are common to the people who share the space. Values refer to the priorities of cultural members, reflecting the normative ideals of the culture. Beliefs refer to the underlying thoughts of the cultural members regarding the important issues in life. Beliefs represent the knowledge-base of the culture, reflecting what cultural members think of the issues under investigation. For instance, in Fadiman's study of the experience of a Hmong family with their daughter's epilepsy, the parents articulated the belief that the epileptic condition of their daughter was caused by the violent shutting of the door by their older daughter: here the beliefs provide an entry point into the culture.

Differences in the approach to culture

The approaches to the study of culture are characterized by four key differences: static versus dynamic concepts of culture; universals versus specifics; policies versus individual behaviors; and control versus agency.

Static and dynamic culture.   One of the ways in which culture theories differ is in how they refer to the concept of culture. The predictive models seek to extract from cultures certain residual characteristics in order to develop a categorization scheme. In this instance, the emphasis is on identifying stable characteristics on the basis of which cultures may be categorized and placed into different boxes. The emphasis in such an approach is on using culture to explain the variance in health outcomes. The interpretive models of culture conceive of culture as dynamic entities that are continuously shaped and reshaped through human action. For interpretive scholars working with the concept of culture, culture exists in the meanings that are created by cultural members and in turn, provides a script for the ways in which these meanings are created. Therefore culture is continually shifting, dynamic, and open to change.

Universals and specifics.   The universal approach to culture draws upon the notion of identifying universal characteristics that might be applied for the purposes of categorizing cultures on the basis of similarities and differences among them. At a broader level, the universal approach focuses on certain key variables that are applied across cultures, with the purpose of developing health communication practice based on them. The emphasis on cultural specifics focuses on the local context where meanings are created. In this approach, the best way to understand cultural meanings is in terms of the relationship of these meanings to the locally embedded contexts. These local contexts connect the macro-level structures and the day-to-day living experiences of cultural members.

Policies and individuals.   Individual-level approaches to the study of culture in health communication conceptualize the individual as the locus of change. The goal of these approaches is to modify the individual's beliefs, attitudes and behaviors. By contrast, the policy-based approaches to culture in health communication focus on identifying the unhealthy policies associated with the experiences of marginalization of certain cultures, and on changing these policies. Through engagement with members of the culture, they attempt to understand the opportunities for resisting the dominant power structures, which produce unhealthy conditions based on inequity.

Control and agency.   Whereas some of the cultural approaches described above deploy the concept of culture in such a way that the behaviors and outcomes of the cultural participants may be controlled by the funding agencies and campaign planners, other approaches to culture emphasize the co-construction of meanings. Control is linked to the positions of power; it is the means through which those in power exercise their impact on marginalized communities. It is also this relationship of control that ensures the privileged positions of powerful actors. The control-based perspective uses concepts such as cultural sensitivity to develop projects that would be better equipped to change the problematized behavior of the individual. On the contrary, approaches that highlight agency emphasize the ability of community members to define their goals and objectives and to engage actively in making sense of the structures that constrain their lives. Such an approach documents the many ways in which cultures resist dominant power structures and the other ways in which they work with such structures. The emphasis on agency brings forth both the transformative potential of agency and the constitutive role it plays. Agency offers the site of resisting the status quo by valuing the role of a dialogical space where cultural members might articulate the ways in which their health is threatened and suggest possibilities for social change.

Practices of Culture

The practices of culture in health communication are typically built around the predominant notions of culture as a barrier or culture as an enabler. These notions are in turn connected with the categorizing scheme presented earlier in this chapter. Although most studies of culture in health communication have emphasized the culture-as-barrier approach, a growing number of scholars in the area is calling for a shift that embodies the culture-centered approach to health communication (Dutta-Bergman 2004a, 2004b). Whereas the culture-as-barrier approach seeks to develop a predictive model of culture and to incorporate it in order to account for culture as a variable in behavior change interventions, the culture-centered approach calls for culturally based understandings of health meanings that would disrupt the traditional understandings and applications of health communication.

Culture as barrier

The approach to culture as a barrier has been extensively used in health communication scholarship and applications; it has also been referred to as the cultural sensitivity approach (Resnicow et al. 2002). In this approach, culture is conceptualized as a static entity, bounded by its geographic location and characterized by a set of well-defined factors. Also, the values, beliefs, attitudes and behaviors of the culture are quantifiable and allow the researcher to distinguish the culture from another culture. Take for instance the concept of locus of control. This concept refers to the extent of control individuals feel they have on their health outcomes. Cultures with external locus of control are typically considered fatalistic and hence must be changed so as to become able to achieve better health results. Once the defining characteristic of the culture has been identified, the health communication solution seeks to fix it, so that it may no longer be a barrier to achieving good health.

The culture-as-barrier approach attempts to extract residual characteristics from cultures such that a categorization scheme may be developed based on these traits. For instance, the locus of control research extracts the individual placement of responsibility on health behaviors and outcomes as a variable of interest. Based on this variable, it categorizes cultures into internal and external. Similarly, the research on family planning identifies barriers to the use of condoms in cultures and subsequently develops a campaign with the goal of removing these barriers. Health communication theories such as the theory of reasoned action, the health belief model and the extended parallel process model are based on this very notion of identifying underlying beliefs and circumventing the ones which prevent the adoption of the recommended behavior. Witte and Morrison (1995) describe a campaign where they used the extended parallel process model to identify the barriers regarding cultural beliefs about the effectiveness of condom use for family planning, and subsequently sought to realign cultural beliefs by pointing out that condoms were the most effective means for preventing pregnancies.

The culture-as-barrier approach has been criticized for imposing a set of alien values on a culture on the basis of the goals of the funding agency and of the campaign planner. Also, postcolonial scholars have questioned the neocolonial goals of health campaigns that seek to erase the local values of cultures by attempting to universalize Western values and beliefs. The family planning programs sponsored by the United States Agency for International Development (USAID) have been criticized for serving the agendas of the US by spreading a fundamentally value-based intervention to other cultural communities (Dutta 2006). In doing so, these programs have focused on the individual level and have assisted in propagating the agendas of population control as articulated by the transnational elite, simultaneously absolving existing power structures of the need to create accessible healthcare resources. Also, the individual-level focus shifts attention away from the need to change global unhealthy policies that might affect health adversely.

The culture-centered approach

The culture-centered approach is concerned with the ways in which the health experiences of the cultural members are marginalized, constructed as deviant or abnormal, and are accompanied by a minimal access to healthcare resources. Scholars working from this perspectve attempt to understand the health meanings of cultural members by engaging in dialogue with them.

The culture-centered approach formulates the importance of centralizing the voices of cultural members in the articulation of health with the goal of achieving structural changes that are meaningful to cultural members. This approach seeks to challenge the dominant structure fundamentally, by introducing alternative articulations of health and illness by means of engaging the voices of cultural members and simultaneously pointing toward the limits of the dominant structural system in generating conditions of better health for disenfranchised communities.

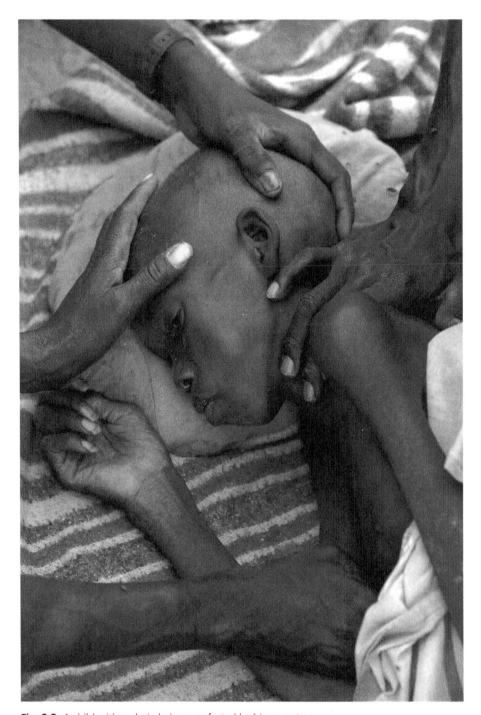

Fig. 3.3 A child with malaria being comforted by his parents
© Sven Torfinn @ Panos Pictures

As pointed out earlier, the culture-centered approach emphasizes cultural understanding. It accomplishes this by concerning itself with the voices of members of marginalized communities. On the one hand, it criticizes existing policies and practices in the context of the inclusion of the voices of cultural members. For instance, Airhihenbuwa provides a much needed criticism of existing theories of health communication with respect to the omission of the voices of African cultures. Similarly, in his work with Haitian communities, Farmer (1988a, 1992) documents the absence of Haitian voices in policy platforms and implementations which affect Haitian people directly.

The culture-centered approach also seeks to transform the status quo by questioning its practices. In this context, the culture-centered approach is fundamentally resistive. The resistance to the status quo is offered by way of examining the ideologies that serve the dominant paradigm. Ideologies refer to the taken-for-granted assumptions which retain the privileged position of the dominant paradigm and the power of those who practice it. For instance, scholars question the medicalizing ideology of the dominant paradigm that locates healing under the capitalist framework of modern society. Health in this realm is connected with the profit motives of the medical institutions, the HMOs, and the pharmaceutical industry. The individualizing ideology of health interventions, in addition, constructs health as an individual responsibility and therefore removes it from the realms of access, equity and transformation of structures.

Agency and context are two key elements of this approach. The approach engages in dialogue with community members to co-create their meanings of health and to understand the ways in which they see health problems. This dialogue is based on the understanding that cultural members are agents of change, who negotiate with the structural processes in their daily lives. Agency refers to the active participation of cultural members in the co-construction of meanings and in actions based on these meanings. Not only does agency draw upon culturally available meanings, but it also seeks to transform these meanings through the acts of individuals and collectives. Agency exists in a dialectical relationship with structure; the existence of the structural conditions constrains agency and enables it, and agency in turn creates, recreates and transforms structural conditions. The culture-centered approach also situates health meanings in the contexts in which they exist. These contexts act as references for the enunciation of communicative meanings.

Ultimately, the culture-centered approach questions the privileged positions of knowledge articulated in the dominant paradigm. It situates these positions of knowledge culturally and connects them to the capitalist interests of the cultural community of biomedical practitioners (physicians and patients), social scientists, and scientists of the Western world. It also provides a discursive space for rupturing the universal discourse of rationality that dominates the biomedical model by demonstrating its cultural roots and by articulating the irrationalities and inconsistencies inherent in the model. It questions the universal appeal of modernization that is central to much health communication work, and asks us to consider what we mean by modern and what we mean by primitive. Knowledge ultimately is culturally situated; how we know the world is intrinsically related to the culture in which we are born, the culture in which we grow up, and the culture in which we practice our scholarship. Culture therefore becomes the starting point for articulating knowledge; every knowledge is culturally based and is tied to the values of the culture. The culture-centered approach questions the taken-for-granted value of Western knowledge as the only way of looking at health, illness and its treatment. In doing so, it renders this universal knowledge position of the West as one out of multiple cultural possibilities for understanding health, illness and healing. It simultaneously opens up the discursive space of health communication to many other possibilities, based on other ways of knowing what health is, what illness is, and how best to treat it.

Discussion point 3.3

- What are the ways in which a culture-centered approach offers entry points for social change?
- How would you go about creating openings for social change through the culture-centered approach?

Conclusion

The goal of this chapter was to equip you with an understanding of the various approaches to the study of culture in health communication. With this goal in mind, the chapter began by offering two classification schemes for categorizing the study of culture in health communication: explaining versus understanding cultures, and status quo versus social change. The tendency to explain cultures emphasizes the operational definition of cultures, given on the basis of certain generalizable characteristics, and then studies the amount of variance in health results in the light of, or as explained by, these cultural factors. The tendency to understand cultures focuses on meaning-making, on developing a sense of understanding what it means to be healthy or unhealthy from the perspective of the cultural participants. The other classification scheme presented in this chapter focused on the relationship of the approach to the structural processes surrounding health. The status quo approaches focused on individual behaviors and sought to create support for those in power by removing health from questions of inequality. The social change approaches, however, question the uneven distribution of resources in the healthcare arena and seek to transform these inequities by understanding and explaining how they are associated with the health experiences of a culture.

The combination of the two classification schemes results in the culture-centered, structural, culture-as-barrier, and cultural understanding approaches to the study of culture in health communication. The culture-centered approach engages in dialogue with cultural members and seeks to generate an understanding of health meanings through this dialogue; ultimately, it seeks to transform the structures constraining the health experiences of cultures. The structural approach to health communication examines the predictive role of culture and its interaction with structure in the realm of the health experiences of community members. The culture-as-barrier approach attempts to explain the amount of variance in health results through cultural variables, and focuses on changing culture-based barriers to individual behavior modification efforts. The cultural understanding approach is similar to the culture-centered approach in its emphasis on understanding the health meanings of cultures, although it often operates within the status quo and does not really provide structural alternatives. Each of these approaches provides important entry points for looking at the role of culture in health communication.

4 Culture, Identity, and Health

Chapter objectives

In this chapter we will:

- study the role of identity in communication about health
- explore the relationship between culture and identity
- examine the role of narratives in health communication
- examine the relationship between narratives, culture, and structure

Identity refers to the ways in which we see ourselves, and is intrinsically connected to our understandings of health and illness, our relationships with others in healthcare settings, and the actions we engage in the context of health and illness (Bordo 1987; Shilling 1993). Identities are culturally situated, as the culture provides the contextual space within which individuals develop a sense of self, come to value certain aspects of the self, and come to enact this self-concept through their day-to-day actions. Cultural values and beliefs are played out in the realm of identity as they come to influence the ways in which the individual sees himself/herself, develops relationships with others and engages in day-to-day practices. As we will see throughout this chapter, *narratives* connect identity with cultural meanings; they provide both the ingredients and the recipes for meaning-making through which individuals construct stories about the self and the world, thus making sense of the world and acting in it. The ways in which the individual sees himself/herself are constituted through the stories shared in the cultural spaces; it is also through these stories that individuals shape the meanings and communications available to the broader culture. Healthcare narratives become the conduits through which individuals, groups, and communities come to understand who they are, comprehend the meanings of health and illness, and engage in their healthcare choices; it is also through these narratives that they shape the patterns and contents of communication and action in the broader culture. This intersection of identity, narratives and culture is the subject of this chapter.

The goal of this chapter is to equip you with an understanding of identity, what it is, and the ways in which it is tied with the health experiences of cultural members. In doing so, the chapter will first discuss the relationship between identity and health; in this section, attention will be paid to discussing the ways in which identity is tied to the meanings of health as understood by cultural members, and the health-related actions they engage in. The discussion of the relationship between identity and health will be followed by the exploration of the ways in which narratives serve as sites of enacting cultural identities and interrogating these identities in health contexts. These narratives offer insights into the meanings of health through the voices of the cultural members, and therefore connect the question of identity to the broader framework of the culture-centered approach.

Building upon the culture-centered approach, it will be argued that narratives are sites of contestation where cultural meanings are played out through dialogues among cultural participants. These dialogues demonstrate both the existing set of meanings that circulate within the culture, and the possibilities that might be presented in the interactions with the shifting contexts of health. In other words, narratives draw from existing cultural meanings and simultaneously offer opportunities for shifting these meanings based on the experiences of individuals, groups and communities. Finally, the chapter concludes by discussing the ways in which the interplay of identity, narratives and culture is enacted in the backdrop of the social structures within which individuals negotiate their daily health experiences. This discussion of structure emphasizes the ways in which the culture tells a dominant set of stories, and at the same time, omits other interpretations and possibilities of health and healing. Cultural narratives of health are juxtaposed in the backdrop of power, ideology and hegemony. This discussion of identity, narrative and structure provides a framework for examining the ways in which current health communication theory and application may be informed by the culture-centered approach, thus offering emancipatory possibilities for the practice of health communication.

Box 4.1   The story of Jake

Jake, a 45-year-old man, was recently diagnosed with prostate cancer. After this detection, Jake lost his sense of identity as a man. He felt that he could not perform sexually and could no longer have a meaningful relationship with his partner. This sense of loss profoundly affected Jake's life; these days he spends most of his time looking through the window. He also feels that he has failed in performing his duties, as he can no longer be for his family the provider he used to be.

As Jake's story shows, the ways in which he experienced his illness, sought out treatment options, and participated in the healthcare system as an individual were dependent upon how he saw himself as an individual, how he regarded his illness as being related to his identity, and how he navigated this identity in the backdrop of the broader social and cultural system and its normative ideals. For Jake, his identity as a man was threatened because of the impotence caused by prostate cancer. He could no longer have vaginal sex with his wife. In a culture where sexual identity (as a heterosexual man) is tied to the ability to have vaginal sex, identity is threatened by a disease such as prostate cancer. Identity therefore is the site where cultural meanings, values, and practices are negotiated on a daily basis. In the domain of the culture-centered approach, identity provides the theoretical entry point for understanding the ways in which culture plays out in the health experiences of individuals, relationships, groups, and communities. Culture, as conceptualized here, is both static and dynamic, providing a complex framework within which identity is negotiated and enacted. It is static because it supplies a set of values, beliefs and practices through which identity is constructed; it is dynamic because it offers a site for the contestation of these identities and for the negotiation of values, beliefs and practices of health.

Identity and Health

Jake's story elucidates that the ways in which members of a culture experience health and illness is intertwined with their identity; how they see themselves in the world and the ways in which they perceive their responses as members of the culture. Identity refers to the construction of self that is evoked in the day-to-day interactions of cultural participants, and provides the script for the ways in which participants construct meanings of health. Identity offers the conduit through which culture interacts with health experiences of individuals; it is the individual level manifestation of the cultural values, beliefs and mores. Therefore, identity of cultural members is related to the meanings they construct, the ways in which they communicate with others, and the ways in which they experience health and illness. Also, identity is central to the response of cultural participants to health messages, their adoption of preventive behaviors, the treatments they seek out, and the experiences they have with the healthcare systems. Identity, in essence, is central to the ways in which the participants respond to the healthcare system and what they do in response to the structural constraints within which they live their lives.

The identity of cultural members is responsive to the context and is dynamic in nature. In other words, different aspects of a patient's identity are evoked in different relationships and in different cultural contexts. For instance, Jake's sense of his identity as a husband and a sexual partner are evoked in his interactions with his wife, whereas his identity of having a successful career is evoked in his interactions with his colleagues. Although identity does have a stable component that draws upon the existing values, beliefs, and worldviews of the culture, it also has a dynamic component that shifts from context to context, and evolves in its interaction with the context. Identity is both a precursor of the interaction, and is determined by the nature of interaction. On one hand, it shapes the ways in which the participant responds to the context; on the other hand, it is shaped by the participant's response to the context. Take for instance the treatment choices enacted by Sarah, a breast cancer patient in a metropolitan US city in the Midwest. How Sarah responds to her breast cancer and the treatment she chooses are determined by her identity as a middle-class, Caucasian woman residing in a metropolitan

US city in the Midwest and working at a university. This identity is perhaps shaped by a variety of cultural factors along with the life experiences she has been through as a member of the culture. In addition, however, the treatment choice Sarah decides to go through and her experiences with the disease are also going to influence her identity, further influencing how she negotiates her health experiences in the future and how she talks about her health and illness. For instance, Sarah's journey with cancer might invoke discourses related to death and dying that might otherwise be inaccessible in the broader cultural space. As articulated earlier, identity is tied in with health through its interaction with meanings, relationships, health choices, and health experiences.

Identity is played out in the realm of meanings by shaping the ways in which individuals ascribe meanings to messages, and interact with them. For instance, the identity of a US teenager growing up in Chicago is quintessential to the meanings of sexual health he would construct in viewing a television program such as the "Real World." These meanings, in turn, would be quintessential to the actions the teenager chooses to take. Similarly, the identity of a middle-class Indian teenager growing up in New Delhi, India, would perhaps be intertwined with the meanings of "Real World" that he would interpret. These meanings once again would perhaps be very different from the meanings of "Real World" interpreted by a teenager in a small town in South India. These very different sets of meanings in turn would be quintessential to the response evoked by the message.

How an individual sees himself/herself in the world also influences the ways in which he/she interacts with others, the expectations he/she has from these relationships, and the role of these relationships in further shaping the individual's identity. In other words, identity is played out in the realm of relationships individuals participate in. It is after all based upon a sense of identity that individuals come to interact in the world through the interpretation and articulation of meanings in communication exchanges. Cultural values, beliefs and contexts influence the ways in which individuals perceive themselves and others in a relationship, and the ways in which they communicate with these others in relationships. For instance, the interactions with the healthcare system of a Hmong immigrant in Minneapolis would be different from the interactions of a middle-class Caucasian resident in the same city.

Identity influences health choices by being intertwined with the meanings and relationships individuals form with others. How an individual sees himself/herself is essential to the ways in which he/she approaches health. Take for instance, the interplay of identity and meanings in the realm of food choices. What an individual considers to be healthy is related to his/her cultural identity and the meanings associated with food. For Bengalis in Eastern India, being healthy is connected with eating rice. For African Americans in the Southern US, healthy eating is tied with eating green vegetables such as spinach and okra. The notion of healthiness of an upper middle-class yuppie in New York is tied to his/her choice of jogging around Central Park in the morning. Similarly, the types of choices individuals make in response to an illness are tied to their cultural identity. For example, individuals may seek out a variety of treatment options in response to an infection such as smallpox. Whereas in the Western medical community, the recommended treatment is one of antibiotics, in many communities in India, participants offer prayers to the goddess *Sitala* who is attributed the power of healing the illness.

Through its role in the context of health meanings and health discourses, identity also is central to the experiences of health and illness of cultural members. For instance, published research documents the different experiences of pain that vary with cultures. Whereas in some cultures, individuals report high levels of pain in response to a stimulus, individuals in other cultures report moderate or low levels of pain in response to the same stimulus. This experience of pain therefore is experienced through the markers of identity defined by the culture. In cultures where it is unacceptable for men to articulate their experiences of pain, men are less likely to report pain in response to illness experiences and are less likely to seek out health services. In other cultures, however, men feel comfortable articulating their illness and seeking out treatment options.

In summary, the ways in which identity is constructed ultimately shapes how health and illness is experienced. This experience of health and illness, in return, further influences the sense of identity of the cultural participant. The trajectory an individual chooses to take in response to an illness defines the ways in which he/she will think of himself/herself. For instance, a woman's choice to seek mastectomy will influence the ways in which she will construct herself. The interplay of identity with meanings, relationships, and health choices is enacted through the narratives shared by cultural participants. Identities at the individual level are manifestations of the interplay between values, beliefs, practices, and the shifting contexts within which these values, beliefs, and practices are played out.

Culture and identity

As a dynamic setting within which individuals experience health and illness, culture provides the backdrop against which identity is realized. It sets up the dynamic context within which meanings are negotiated in the articulation of identities. This is elucidated in Jake's story. How Jake thinks of himself as an individual is connected with the broader cultural meanings tied to sexuality, work-life, and the values of masculinity. It is within the foregrounded realm of cultural meanings related to questions of what it means to be a man that Jake experiences his prostate cancer. It is also in the realm of the broader cultural meanings that circulate around the responsibility of being a provider that Jake experiences a sense of having failed in performing his duties. Individuals think of themselves in the context of the meanings, symbols, values, and beliefs available to them within the culture, and these meanings, symbols,

values and beliefs, in turn, are impacted by the ways in which they negotiate their day-to-day lives. The combination of these meanings, symbols,
values, and beliefs constructs identities of individual members. How
these members see themselves is tied to the ways in which the culture
provides the backdrop for understanding the world, and the stories told
by the culture about the lived experiences of its members. In other
words, identity is negotiated in the arena of what it means to live life as
a member of the culture. Cultural members construct their identities and
act on the basis of these identities through their interpretations of what
it means to be a member of the culture. The values, beliefs and shared
meanings of the culture are implicit in the ways in which the individual
thinks of himself/herself. For instance, Harter et al. (2005) point out the
ways in which the cultural values of controlling and managing the body
play out in meanings of age-related infertility (ARI), connecting individual identity with broader cultural values. ARI-related individual identity
focusing on the right steps to manage one's body appropriately is shaped
by the broader US middle-class culture's emphasis on controlling one's
body. This is elucidated in the following reflection of Diana during an
Oprah Winfrey episode of ARI in 2002:

> I've always been one to take care of myself. I love to exercise. It's – It's a hobby.
> I began taking prenatal vitamins before I even got married. . . . I can't tell you
> the loss that you feel and how you wonder where you go from here and that
> you thought you were taking 10 steps forward just to find out you have to start
> over again (Harter et al. 2005: 6)

Diana's sense of loss is deeply embedded in her identity of having taken
the right steps to control her health, which in turn, is intertwined with
the broader cultural logic of control where "doing the right thing"
ensures that health is managed (ibid., p. 96).

Although they do draw from the possibilities of cultural meanings
made available to them, identities are also continuously in flux, and are
continuously negotiated by the members of the culture in their interactions with the daily contexts. Therefore identities are both static and
dynamic, building upon essential components of the culture, and yet
crafting new terrains in which health relationships and experiences may
be negotiated. Identities are connected with histories that tell stories of
the past, and simultaneously offer opportunities for carving out new
futures through the experiences of the present. For instance, the ways in
which women in the US construct their identities influence the types of
healthcare services they seek out during pregnancy. Whether a woman in
the US seeks out the services of a midwife depends upon how she sees
herself as a member of the culture and the ways in which she positions
herself in the context of the broader logic of the biomedical model that
privileges hospital births. This choice, in addition, provides the foundation for the sense of identity of the individual. The shifting context of
identities is elucidated in the reflections of health communication scholar
Kimberly Kline who discusses her personal struggles over the decision of

whether to have a midwife attend a home birth or to give birth in a hospital to her second child, reflects upon the birth of her first child by Cesarean section, and considers ways of engaging about this personal issue with her students in her health communication course (Babrow, Kline and Rawlins 2005: 42):

> With 10 years between pregnancies, Kim was poignantly aware of how time has altered her perspective on childbirth. Trying to make sense of her radically different concerns and desires during this pregnancy as compared to the last, Kim realized the difficulty of trying to tell someone 10 years younger (or 20 or 30 years younger) what a difference those years made in the way she understood the choices she made "back then." It didn't necessarily help her in making the choices she faced, but it did help explain the conundrum she confronted in justifying to herself and others the possibility of a home birth when her first child had been born using surgical procedures in a hospital. . .

Kline's dilemmas and tensions articulated in the realm of her choices of how to deliver her second child bring forth the shifting nature of cultural identities and the opportunities brought about by healthcare experiences for reconstituting these identities. In reflecting on how her story of the birth of her first child has taken a different turn, she wrote "Yes, the story has taken a different turn. . . is that so surprising given the different directions my life has taken?" It is in this realm of rewriting stories that new possibilities for health and illness are presented. Also, as articulated in Kline's narrative, the sharing of a story with others within the relational space offers further opportunities for shifting the broader cultural discourses around health and healing practices (the ways in which we think of midwifery in this case).

Identity and relationships

As articulated earlier in this chapter, relationships are built upon the identities of individual participants and their perceptions of the identity of the other in the relational *dyad*. The perceptions of self are integral to the meanings and interpretations drawn from messages, and the articulation of messages directed at the other participant in the relationship. The ways in which a Hispanic participant views himself/herself will fundamentally influence the ways in which he/she will communicate with the physician at an urban US clinic. Also, the nature of this interaction will depend upon the way in which the Hispanic participant perceives the physician, the way in which the physician perceives himself/herself, and the way in which the physician perceives the Hispanic participant. The relationship, therefore, is built upon the interactions between identities at multiple levels. Therefore, in the area of physician–patient relationship, the identities of the patient and the physician are integral to the ways in which the relationship is negotiated, expectations are laid out and communicated, and health outcomes are managed (see figure 4.1). Furthermore, the constructions of identity and expectations around

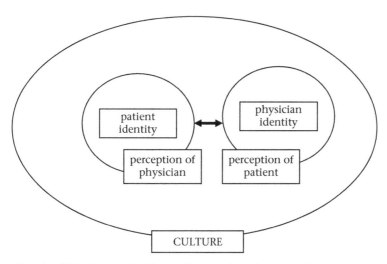

Fig. 4.1 The role of identities in physician–patient relationship negotiation

identity are located within the broader contextual spaces of cultures. In other words, cultural contexts, values, and meaning systems shape the ways in which identities are developed, and relational expectations are constructed and negotiated.

An example depicting the role of identity in the context of the physician–patient relationship is an article written by communication scholar Barbara Sharf (2005). In her essay, Sharf discusses the way in which she fired her surgeon in response to a problematic physician–patient relationship. Sharf writes:

> Dr Rigor and I were at ideological odds about our clinical relationship; he declined any attempts I initiated to negotiate with him. To remain as his patient would have meant conceding all control of decision making to him, the scenario that ostensibly provoked my dilemma. (pp. 340–1)

In this instance, the individual identity of the patient and her negotiation of this identity in the context of a healthcare interaction provide a starting point for interrogating the traditional doctor–patient relationship, and guided subsequent decisions. Her relationship with the physician then is built upon the ways in which she constructs her identity, and in turn, the relationship shapes how she negotiates her identity through the interaction with the physician.

Sharf's negotiation and renegotiation of her identity challenges the dominant discursive framing of physician–patient relationships by suggesting that patients play an active role in engaging with their illness experience and in the negotiation of decision-making between the physician and patient. Through the sharing of her story of firing her surgeon, Sharf opens up the discursive space to renegotiating the traditional power dynamic that places physicians at the center of the physician–patient relationship, and instead shifts control to the patient who ultimately chooses to fire the physician. Similarly, Rawlins (2005: 213) discusses the role of identity in the realm of the ways in which the physician partici- pates in relationships with his/her patients. In his example, Rawlins nar- rates the story of his father, Jack Rawlins, who was a physician. A reflective excerpt brings forth the relationship between identity and physician–patient relationship:

> My father's account provides several related lessons about a narrative stance toward practicing medicine. Committing oneself to understanding patients' health concerns and observable symptoms in and through the contexts of their own lived stories is foremost. Any person's health, disease, and treat- ment are thoroughly contextual and contingent experiences. Accordingly, familiarity with someone's unique personal history, habits, and values, where and how the patient lives, and the nature of his or her relationships with family and other persons is crucial for comprehending troubles and ills. I was impressed with dad's reference to house calls in this regard: ". . . going into somebody's house and seeing how they live just one time can make you a better physician for the next 10 or 15 years," as well as his well-versed uptake of one man's allusion to an elephant's foot in narrating his worrisome recent days.

In this instance, once again, the identity of the physician as a provider constitutes the relationships she/he experiences with her/his patients. How Jack Rawlins sees himself as a physician responding to a "calling" profoundly influences the ways in which he approaches his relationships with patients and the ways in which he goes about interacting with patients, listening to their own lived narratives, and treating them from a contextually located relational frame.

Identity and health choices

Identity not only influences how health meanings and relationships are negotiated, but also the ways in which cultural participants negoti- ate their health choices. As pointed out earlier in this chapter, the ways in which cultural members think of themselves intrinsically influence the types of preventive behaviors they engage in, the types of treat- ment options they seek out, and the ways in which they navigate the healthcare system. Health and medical choices are culturally situated practices and as symbols of the culture, they offer cultural members with opportunities for enacting their identities and relationships. The choices individuals make are reflective of their cultural values, beliefs and ten- sions, and these tensions are played out in the ways in which health decisions are made by individuals and their families. For instance, Kline's decision to choose the path of the hospital or the midwife for the delivery of her second child was located in the realm of her identity as a woman in a middle-class US context that unquestioningly celebrates the logic of biomedicine; this identity was further enacted within the broader realm of the culture, and the health choices it valued and fore- grounded.

Similarly, in her book on the experiences of a Hmong family with the US healthcare system, Fadiman (1998) demonstrates that the Hmong family's intrinsic Hmong identity was challenged by the dominant medical system that diagnosed the daughter of the family, Lia, as having epilepsy. In contrast, for Lia's parents, her condition was caused by her sister closing the door, which led her spirit to be caught. Based upon the illness explanation the participants believed in, two very different treatment options were put forth. Whereas in the narrative constructions of Lia's parents, Lia could be cured by burying a pot of ashes right beneath her bed, in the narrative constructions of Western biomedicine, Lia could only be cured through the appropriate implementation of medications. The two health treatments sought out in this case are fundamentally tied to worldviews and cultural identities. Whereas for the Western physician, his/her identity is located in the biomedical framework of modern science, Lia's parents' identities are located in their Hmong culture. The trajectories of health choices sought out in this instance are widely divergent depending upon the identities of the cultural members, and are connected to the broader logics of the cultures.

The relationship of health choices with culture is played out in the ways in which decisions are made in health crises. Within individualistic contexts, these decisions become the primary concern of the individual patient, with emphases placed on the privacy of the patient and how this privacy is negotiated in the healthcare decisions that are made by the individual. In contrast to the focus on the individual in decision-making situations in individualistic cultural contexts, collectivistic contexts provide greater room for the roles of family members in negotiating the decision–making process. In such situations, cultural members place greater emphasis on negotiating healthcare decision-making within families, and the responsibility of health is primarily placed on the family members who must negotiate the intricate web of relationships in reaching health decisions. The self-construal of cultural members as independent or interdependent serves as the conduit through which cultural values and beliefs come to shape the ways in which health choices are made. Cultures come to shape the identities and the choices of their members through the stories that circulate within them.

Identity and narratives

That cultural participants continuously construct identity through *narratives* is reflected in the writings of psychoanalyst Roy Schafer, who states: "We are forever telling stories about ourselves." Narratives, as suggested earlier, refer to a mode of reasoning through which cultural participants make sense of the world; they constitute the stories that cultural members share with each other and the processes through which these stories are shared. It is through stories that individuals come to understand who they are, and communicate this sense of understanding to others. Referring to this link between the self and narratives, Frank (1995: 53) writes: "Stories do not simply describe the self, they are the self's medium of being." In other words, the self comes to exist in the realm of the stories that are constructed and shared with others.

In the context of illness, these stories offer ways for the self to come to an understanding of itself. Frank suggests that becoming seriously ill brings forth occasions of storytelling as ill people seek to repair the damage that the illness has done to their sense of where they are in life and where they may be going, and communicate with others about the illness. Discussing his own illness experience with cancer and the medical tests and surgeries he went through, Frank points out that he had to tell and repeat versions of his story to family members, work colleagues, and medical workers, each with their different communicative requirements for the stories. Schafer refers to these stories as "self-stories" (p. 31), and suggests that self-stories are simultaneously told to others and to oneself; relationships with others are reaffirmed (as suggested in the section on identity and relationships) through these stories that are shared and the self is reaffirmed in its existence after the disruption caused by the illness. In other words, through the self-story the ill person reaffirms that "he is still there as an audience for himself" (p. 56).

Frank suggests that illness begins as a disruption and entails the condition of living with "perpetual interruption" (ibid.). He shares the story of Nancy Mairs (1993: 122), whose meditations about God in reconciling with the indignities of living with multiple sclerosis is interrupted by the spilling of diet coke onto the floor that she is too disabled to clean. She interrupts her story about her belief in God as she notes that she will "have to continue working on this passage with my feet in a sticky brown puddle". Mairs's story is an interrupted story that is wrought with ambivalences. Illness stories, therefore, break away from the norms of conventional narratives and require a new kind of storytelling that is responsive to these continuous interruptions that divert the stories from tidy ends. The untidy ends give the illness narratives their inconsistent quality that physicians find uncomfortable in patient's stories. Frank suggests that it is precisely because of this uncomfortable quality that the illness stories need to be told so as not to silence the interrupted voices. He points out that the ill person as a patient has been interrupted by the disease, and is now, "infinitely interruptible in speech, schedule, solvency, and anything else" (p. 57). The presence and roles of the medical staff and the protocols of medical treatment are set in the realm of these interruptions in the life of the patient, with the goal of achieving medical control over the body of the patient. Medical sociologist Waitzkin writes that illness narratives are continuously interrupted because "the patient's story may not contribute to the doctor's cognitive process of reaching a diagnosis; the patient's version of the story may be confusing or inconsistent; telling the story may take more time than is perceived to be available; or parts of the story may create feelings that are uncomfortable to the doctor, the patient or both" (Waitzkin 1991: 28). In order to create legitimate spaces for the voices of patients, our understandings of narratives styles need to open up to the continuously interrupted and ambivalent stories of patients. By interrogating the taken-for-granted assumption underlying the privilege of the biomedical model and its practices and by emphasizing the necessity of listening to culturally situated narratives, the culture-centered approach offers an entry point for the telling of alternative stories that challenge the conventional practices of storytelling.

The disruptions in illness narratives are also disruptions in memory as the connections with the past and the future need to be reconstituted. A coherent sense of life's sequence is disrupted by the illness and the illness story serves as a way of connecting the past to the future, mediated through the presence of the illness experience, thus bringing about the possibility of coherence in the illness narrative articulated through the experience of the patient. Spence (1982: 31) refers to the idea of narrative truth that reconfigures the past in terms of what was foregrounded and backgrounded in order to create a sense of "continuity and closure". Sharing the illness story with others becomes a way of constituting memory as the process of creating the story also "creates the memory structure" (Schank 1990: 115). The self comes to be constituted through the process of narrating the story and brings about discursive openings for learning about illness and the meanings of illness. The responsibility of the self, in this context, is to rise to the occasion by narrating a good story that discovers the narrative truth in it and shares the truth with others. Telling the truth, as Frank points out, "involves recognizing that your life has not turned out as you wanted. What went wrong must be acknowledged and examined; mourning will attend this examination" (Frank 1995: 63). By refusing denial and coming face to face with the pain of suffering, the good story refuses to fit into the dominant conventions of storytelling. The good story is often uncomfortable for the dominant biomedical model as it defies the logic of control embedded in the model, and therefore is often silenced when physicians become uncomfortable with the story, thus limiting the possibilities of what might become truth as articulated through the experiences of the storyteller.

Frank suggests that what makes an illness story good is the act of witnessing that draws upon the experiences of the ill person who states "I will tell you not what you want to hear but what I know to be true because I have lived it. This truth will trouble you, but in the end, you cannot be free without it, because you know it already; your body knows it already" (ibid.). In rising to the occasion by narrating a story truthfully, the ill person bears the responsibility of memory as she/he becomes a witness and reaches out to the consciousness of the culture in narrating what needs to be learned from illness experiences. The ill person as witness challenges the dominant underpinnings of the biomedical model as she/he draws upon her experiences as someone who has been through the illness and hence has legitimacy to talk about the illness to the greater community, thus offering points of departure for exploring truths about questions of body, mind, and soul that often lie outside the realm of the biomedical model. Pointing out the narrative truth embodied in the self-story of Cathy Hainer, a journalist whose reflections on her journey with cancer were published in the *USA Today* in the late 1990s, Beck (2005) draws our attention to the capacity of the narrative to engage with alternative meanings and explore new languages for talking about illness experiences. The following excerpt from Hainer's column of April 20, 1999 is particularly instructive of the role of illness narratives in the realm of the collective consciousness.

> Whether I was accepting my possible demise or denying it, I wanted very much to talk about it. I wanted to be keenly aware of what was happening to me, what death might mean, how it would feel. I didn't want to be cheated out of the experience because the subject was taboo. Of course, it was nearly impossible to discuss such an unknowable subject in any rational way. But I demanded that my family and friends engage me on this matter. (p. 1D)

Hainer's quest for narrative identity constituted through discourse creates discursive openings for the ways in which we think and talk about death and dying, and the meanings of death that become available to us through our experiences, opening up opportunities for new language that is otherwise unavailable to us in everyday discourse. By going into the realm of discursive practices that are conventionally unacceptable, Hainer engages her readers with questions that typically stay beyond the realm of the dominant discourse. Along with her readers, she creates a public discourse about the lived reality of cancer embodied in "our story" (Beck 2005: 77).

The dominant biomedical framework that constitutes the discourse of illness not only interrupts the stories of patients but essentially takes away their voice through its continued emphasis on the cure of the body; therefore, one of the key goals of the self-story is to reclaim the self from the diagnostic identity imposed by biomedicine (Frank 1995). Through the self-story, the patient creates a new language for articulating illness experience, a language that runs counter to the language of biomedicine that leaves a limited number of options for action (Waitzkin 1991). The feminist writer Audre Lorde writes about this necessity to reclaim oneself by making the self available after her mastectomy: "In order to keep me available to myself, and be able to concentrate my energies upon the challenges of those worlds through which I move, I must consider what my body means to me" (Lorde 1980: 65). Through her story, Lorde seeks to find a language that allows her to speak as a one-breasted woman, thus not only connecting with her self but with other women who have experienced mastectomy. Making oneself available to oneself not only means reconnecting with the body after the illness experience, but also of finding a connection with others who share the condition. It is through the sharing of the self-story that the patient struggles for a coherence, and it is through this struggle that she/he connects with the truth of the story. Hainer's story encouraged her readers to co-construct their life stories and connect with their personal experiences with cancer, thus becoming "our story" (Beck 2005: 66). This connection of the self-story with the collective consciousness as an opportunity for learning is articulated in the following excerpt from Russel Shaw:

> Cathy had spoken so eloquently and beautifully – not only for those who have or have had cancer, but also as a teacher for those who love someone with cancer. . . There are many who have learned from Cathy's words. The world is a better place because she lived and wrote. Because her words live on, she will, too. (*USA Today*, December 17, 1999, p. 30A)

Cathy's story became a window into a world that is inaccessible in the discursive realms of biomedicine, thus creating new language and new opportunities for engaging with questions of disease and illness. It is precisely this ability of the self-story to open up new discursive spaces for the collective that gives it its political character.

The sharing of the story demonstrates the political context of narratives as they open up the possibilities for exploring questions of being and ways of knowing situated beyond the realm of the biomedical model. This is evident in Hainer's narrative discussed earlier as she struggles with meanings of death and dying in the context of her cancer. Illness narratives, in this sense, open up the discursive space to alternative articulations of knowledge by bringing into question that which we know and the ways in which we know it through the struggles and challenges of the ill. Frank writes, "The good story ends in wonder, and the capacity for wonder is reclaimed from the bureaucratic rationalizations of institutional medicine. Being available to yourself ultimately means having the ability to wonder at all the self can be" (Frank 1995: 68). The capacity to wonder is once again richly elucidated in Hainer's quest for understanding the meaning of death discussed earlier in this section.

Narratives are intrinsically connected to the culture as they are stories told by the members of a culture, drawing upon the repertoires of meaning available to cultural members. These are stories of the culture, about what it means to live as a member of the culture. It is through these stories that a culture passes on its traditions, values and beliefs. It is also through these stories that cultures find transformative spaces for forging new paths. For cultural participants, these stories become conduits for understanding, interpreting and meaning making in the world. It is through this process of understanding, interpreting and meaning-making that cultural participants provide a glimpse of who they are. Exploring the narratives of health and healing opens up the discursive space to culturally situating health and illness experiences, and locating health experiences in local contexts.

The culture-centered approach suggests that cultural participants enact their identities through the stories they tell about their lives, their health, and their illnesses. Through these narratives, cultural members co-construct their identity; they tell us who they are, how they see the world, and the ways in which they interpret meanings of health in the world. As stories of the culture, health and illness narratives provide insights about the culture, its values, beliefs and hallowed practices. It is also through these stories that cultural members find avenues for enacting change, articulating openings for creating new identities through which they see the world and reaching out to other members in the cultural community. This was exemplified in the self-story of Cathy Hainer who reached out to the broader cultural consciousness around illness and dying through the sharing of her personal experiences. Therefore, narratives are contested spaces; they are spaces within which cultural meanings are articulated and played out. Whereas some of these meanings are foregrounded, yet others are backgrounded in the discursive space. They simultaneously offer opportunities to connect with the stable dimension of culture, and introduce new interpretations and meanings that circulate in the culture. Narratives in other words are both connective and transformative.

Narratives of Health

Narratives are stories told by the members of a culture. It is through these stories that cultures maintain the traditions. Yet, it is also through these stories that cultures create openings for social change. Therefore the stories are related to culture in a complex and transformative fashion such that stories both reinforce the culture and offer avenues for cultural change. These continuous and transformative aspects of narratives are embodied in the example of Kline and her discussions of childbirth practices. Whereas on one hand, Kline draws on the cultural mores of biomedicine that privilege hospitalization of pregnant women for delivery, her sharing of the story regarding the choice to have a midwife help deliver at home creates a new storyline, thus offering an opportunity for challenging the dominant biomedical framework and creating new openings for articulating meanings of health and healing. Fundamentally, narratives provide a framework for making sense of illness experiences. They offer a window into the illness, the impact it has on those affected by it, the ways in which treatment is negotiated, and the ways in which the illness has shaped the life course of the individual affected by it.

The power of stories

Individuals make sense of their life experiences, their experiences of health and illness, their experiences with the curing and healing of the illness through the sharing of stories. These stories are the threads through which meanings are articulated. As markers of sense making, stories provide participants with a framework for understanding and interpreting their own health experiences. Stories are powerful because they offer the conduit through which individuals make sense of their lives.

Box 4.2 The story of Cecilia

In their essay on the healing power of narratives, Cecilia Bosticco and Teresa Thompson (2005) offer the story of the loss of Cecilia's daughter, Teresa. Cecilia was in her second semester of graduate work when Teresa was diagnosed with cancer. Cecilia narrates how she attempted to find a sense of coherence in her life once she returned to school ten months after her daughter's death. She needed to understand what had happened to her, and every class she took and paper she wrote became vehicles for explaining this. It is through this experience of exploring the meaning of her loss that Cecilia discussed the power of sharing stories with others in the process of grief. She writes that the sharing of her story became a way for her to understand herself and her decisions, continuously opening possibilities for revisiting the interpretations and for re-explaining the same events on the basis of changes in meanings and experiences. She refers to this process as "re-storying," i.e. the rethinking and retelling of stories in new ways, until they become believable explanations.

What purpose does storytelling serve in the realm of bereavement? In the instance of Cecilia, what are the ways in which storytelling helped her heal? What do you think are the functions of re-storying? How does re-storying connect the individual to his/her relational network and community?

Furthermore, the story of Cecilia suggests that stories of loss are situated in the realm of the broader culture. The symbols and the meanings that cultural participants draw upon in narrating their stories are intrinsically linked with the values and the mores of the culture, and are very much situated in the realm of the culture. What are the cultural norms within which stories of bereavement are shared within the US? What are the ways in which these culturally situated stories of bereavement might be challenged?

Health communication scholars discuss the healing power of stories (Sunwolf, Frey and Keranen 2005). Stories heal by providing closure to health and illness experiences and a way for making sense of these experiences. Stories also offer the patient an avenue for expressing himself/herself and connecting with others. They form the foundation for communities of individuals who have been through similar experiences. For instance, the stories shared by an asthma support group (on Yahoo) connect the group members to the shared experiences of illness. They offer a mechanism for coping with these and serve as exemplars for the members of the culture. In other words, a culture teaches the values of health, illness and its treatment through stories which pass from one generation to the next and through stories which circulate among cultural members. Stories constitute the culture, at once connecting what is transmitted across generations with what is dynamic in the culture. Stories also offer opportunities for cultural shifts, as they serve as sites for negotiating and renegotiating identities and relationships among cultural participants.

Meanings of health

Stories communicate both general and particular meanings of health. At a general level, they demonstrate what it means to be healthy and what

Box 4.3   The story of Amy

Amy is 42 and a successfully tenured Professor of Communication at a major US university. Amy has had a productive academic career, and in the first few years of her tenure as assistant professor she worked really hard at being productive. Between teaching and publishing her research, Amy kept herself immersed in her work. When Amy took up her job as an assistant professor after finishing her PhD, she and her husband Scott had decided to wait until Amy got tenure to think about having a child. This was a difficult decision, as, a year into their marriage, Amy and Scott started feeling pressure from their family members about when they were going to conceive.

Now that Amy feels secure in her career, she wants to start thinking about having a child. In the past few months, Amy and Scott have, however, experienced difficulties in conceiving. Although each of them independently remembers having read stories about age-related infertility (ARI), they were optimistic, as Amy worked hard at maintaining her health and at taking preventive measures. These days, Amy catches herself feeling guilt, feeling as though she has let her family members down by prioritizing her career. Amy remembers how her mother used to say: "The time will pass before you know it." This image of her mother has been recurring the past few months, as Amy has struggled with the decisions she had made.

What are the dominant stories that circulate in your culture around ARI? What are the cultural functions served by these stories? How do you respond to Amy's story presented above? How does your response to Amy's story connect with the cultural discourses within which you are located? In this chapter, we have learned about the role of stories in challenging cultural discourses. What are the opportunities for Amy's story to rewrite the cultural texts around ARI? How would you rewrite such a story?

it means to be ill; at a more specific level, they communicate particular ways in which health meanings may be negotiated and treatment options may be sought out. Through their plots, stories communicate to their readers the nature of the culture, the conventions and mores of the culture, the ways in which it understands health and illness, and the constructions of healing and curing built around the experiences of illness.

Health meanings are continuously negotiated through the sharing of the stories. The narration of stories of health experiences of individuals, groups, and communities provides important lessons and markers concerning the ways in which the members of the culture ought to negotiate their experiences of health. These stories also offer openings for cultural change, as they provide interesting entry points for renegotiating identities and relationships.

Ultimately, the health experiences of the cultural participants are built upon the meanings of health they construct. These meanings are both dynamic and complex; they are deeply intertwined in layers. The way cultural members understand health and the way they come to understand the treatment of illness are intertwined with the values, beliefs and meanings that circulate within the culture. It is through their understandings of health choices and treatment options that individuals come to make decisions about the prevention and treatment of illness. Therefore interrogating the meanings of health and illness helps us to understand better the ways in which individuals and communities make health and treatment choices in their day-to-day lives. These health meanings are understood through dialogues with cultural members.

The dialogical turn

As pointed out in the introduction to this chapter, the culture-centered approach is built upon a commitment to dialogue (Dutta-Bergman 2004a). Dialogue, in turn, is built upon foregrounding the voices of the cultural participants. These voices become the starting points for understanding what health is, what the health problems faced by the community are, and the ways in which such health problems might be dealt with. Dialogue, in other words, is the starting point for the identification of problems and solutions in the context of emancipatory approaches to health communication.

The dialogical approach provides a space for presenting alternative viewpoints and for contesting the dominant framings of health. By respecting the agency of the subaltern participant, the dialogic approach acknowledges the limits of the dominant paradigm. It simultaneously points toward possibilities for change. The subaltern participation in the discursive space challenges the dominant paradigm by its very presence, because the dominant paradigm has been traditionally built upon telling target audiences what to do. In this paradigm, messages flow from the center to the periphery; the persuasive agenda of such messages is to change and influence the target audience such that the proposed behavior will be diffused into the population. The dialogical approach challenges the dominant paradigm through its very focus on engaging with subaltern participants, who have typically been silenced in the dominant health communication discourse. It becomes a site of engagement where multiple meanings are at play, forming a complex and intertwined web of dynamic cultural meanings around health issues.

Narrative, Culture and Structure

Narratives not only provide the framework for understanding cultures, but they also suggest possibilities of social change through the circulation of stories of oppression and resistance (see chapter 9 for further discussion of the resistive aspect of storytelling). When narratives are located in the realm of structure, participants discuss the ways in which their lives and possibilities are constricted by the surrounding structure. This sharing of the stories of structure and of the ways in which it constrains the possibilities of health for cultural members opens up new possibilities of social change in the healthcare context.

Narratives as culturally situated entities

Every narrative of health is understood within the context in which it is played out (Dutta-Bergman 2004a, 2004b, 2005a, 2005b; Garro 2000). Garro suggests that culturally situated knowledge about illness and its causation is a resource that guides the interpretation of the illness experience and the stories constructed around it. The narrative becomes meaningful in its relationship with the cultural context. In her research project on the meanings of diabetes in an Anishinaabe community located in Manitoba, Canada, Garro documented the culturally situated meanings of diabetes as a "new illness" or a "White man's sickness," brought by the Europeans to North America and caused by a move in the economy, from the Anishinaabe subsistence activities of the past that produced healthy and fortifying foods, toward store-bought foods. This culturally situated narrative of diabetes is reflected in the following excerpt from Garro's conversation with Mrs Spence, a 50-eight-year-old woman who presented herself as no longer having diabetes and described how her experience with it led to significant changes in the way she and her family ate (Garro 2000: 78):

> This is why I think someone has sugar today because of the foods someone eats now. I also did quit eating the foods I used to eat before. I quit food or meat from the can. Another thing, canned milk was never used before – no canned milk in earlier days. Now I never use that milk. That canned milk.

This excerpt brings to the fore the ways in which the experiences of diabetes in the Anishinaabe community are located in the broader realm of eating practices and lifestyles connected with the modern economy. The explanation of diabetes offered by the cultural participant is situated within the local context of food practices and lifestyle choices, connecting the story of diabetes not simply to a personal history, but to a community history, on the basis of the shared experience of the community (Good 1994). Here's another excerpt from the conversations with Mrs Spence, which elucidates the location of the illness in the context of the community history even further:

> What I think is because of the foods. I was working at [name of business located off the reserve] at the time. I never ate right. We always ate "Klik" or "Spork" [these refer to canned meat products], anything at all, so that is where I think it came from. I was always busy and I had no time to cook a proper meal. (ibid.)

Here, once again, the narrative of diabetes is connected to the cultural context of the lived experiences of community members. Diabetes is contextually situated within the realms of being able to eat right and finding the time to cook a proper meal, both of which are in turn situated in the realm of the work-lives of community members.

The individual experience of Mrs Spence thus gets connected to a broader community experience of diabetes; the "White man's sickness" is everywhere in the community, since a substantial number of persons is affected by it. The relatively recent emergence of this ubiquitous sickness is connected with busy work-lives, dependence on convenience foods, and the chemicals that are consistently sprayed on crops and used in processing canned foods.

The context is much like a dictionary, which helps us decipher the story and its moral. Narratives are played out in the culture through the meanings attributed to the cultural rituals built around health-related issues; these rituals are formalized and habitual actions are performed by cultural members. Therefore, in the health context, narratives are enacted in the realm of health-related cultural rituals. It is through these rituals that cultures dramatize stories of health, and provide plots around which health meanings are articulated. For instance, consider the ritual of the operation theater. In this ritual, the doctors and nurses walk in wearing clean clothes and masks, the patient is anesthetized, his/her bodily parts are cut open, the operation is conducted like a coordinated drill, the patient is sewn up, and the ritual ends with the patient being wheeled out to another room. Now an operating room story narrated by a doctor, a nurse or a relative of the patient would make sense when the ritual components are incorporated into the story. The ability of the audience to understand the story would depend upon a meaningful incorporation of the rituals into the story structure. The rituals gain meaning through the shared understanding of what they are, what their value is, how to perform the rituals, and how such rituals work.

Narratives also present the taken-for-granted assumptions of the culture about health and the ways in which it ought to be treated. For instance, the narrative of a cancer patient in Chicago discusses the experience of the patient with the surgeries and the chemotherapies. In this narrative, the cultural value of curing is embodied in the *medicalizing* ideology that underlies the narrative. Here the assumption is that the only plausible narrative is one of medicalization, which simultaneously eliminates from the discourse other possibilities such as healing or spirituality. In other instances, narratives of treatment often focus on the public sphere of health and illness, simultaneously limiting the private nature of health and illness. The articulation of health and illness in the public sphere present the sick body as a public site to be acted upon, as a publicly presented body to be acted upon by the medicalizing ideology and the agents of the medical structure; the sick person becomes a site to be acted upon by the medicalizing logic in order to be restituted to his/her normal role as a productive citizen. In this sense, the medical ideology functions to support the logic of efficiency of the broader capitalist structure within which it is situated, ensuring the adequate supply of labor and the efficient treatment of sick persons.

Thus narratives demonstrate the values and beliefs of the culture not only by looking at what is present, but also by looking at those elements that are absent or backgrounded. The absences are just as critical as the presences. Such cultural narratives provide insights regarding questions of power, ideology and hegemony within the culture. As shared by the status quo, they communicate understandable ways of looking at the world, they make sense of this world for the audience, and build a meaningful framework. The next section situates narratives of health in the realm of the broader structures within which they are constituted; attending to these structures sensitizes us to the political agendas of narratives.

Discussion point 4.1

- What does the narrative of the Anishinaabe community on diabetes as the "White man's sickness" communicate about the location of diabetes within the broader context of the community?
- Compare the narrative of "White man's sickness" with the narrative of the "biomedical model" in the explanation of diabetes. Which one of these narratives seems more acceptable to you? Why? In discussing your choice of a particular narrative, reflect upon the cultural location of the narrative which is more likely to appeal to you.
- Think of the last time you visited a physician's office. Write down a few key things that you can remember from your interaction with the physician. How do you think the ways in which you communicated with the physician were tied to your identity? How do you think your concept of the physician's identity influenced the nature of your interaction?

Narratives, structures and politics

Narratives are inherently political because they embody a certain interpretation of health processes, experiences, and healthcare systems (Mattingly and Garro 2000). The narratives that are circulated in the dominant culture are, typically, the narratives of the power structure, those which support the status quo and propagate its control on the subaltern classes. These are stories told by those in power and often involve individual-level actions of prevention that lead to better health. For instance, the stories told by dominant public health actors in the United States (such as the United States Department of Health and Human Services, National Institutes of Health, Centers for Disease Control and Prevention) explain cancer in terms of failure to consume at least five servings of fruits and vegetables daily, thus emphasizing individual choice in its prevention and reducing the role of unhealthy structures in its aetiology. Similarly, in their analysis of USAID-funded health promotion campaigns which promote contraception, Dutta and Basnyat (in press) point out that these narratives focus on population control as a solution to poverty in the South and shift attention away from questions of resource inequities and structural adjustment as solutions to poverty. In doing so, such narratives serve the status quo by maintaining the configurations of power, and shifting the onus onto the underserved communities of the South.

The political role of such narratives is to foreground the emphasis on the individual and his/her choices and, the same time, to background the role of the surrounding structure in limiting healthcare access. The broader agenda here is to define health problems as problems of the individual, thereby absolving the status quo of its responsibility to contribute to change initiatives by adjusting the structures and redistributing the resources. The individual enactment of these narratives throws light on how individual identity is constructed around health issues. Therefore, in the dominant narrative, the individual sees his/her identity as that of someone who engages in, or does not engage in, a certain lifestyle rather than seeing himself/herself in relationship with the structure that constrains his/her life.

Those who have access to power also determine the stories that circulate within the discursive space of the culture. *Ideology* refers to the taken-for-granted assumptions which resonate in the cultural practices and cultural stories, and *hegemony* refers to the act of maintaining control without the use of coercive forces. Power is maintained through the exercise of the ideological devices in the stories that circulate in the culture. The medicalizing ideology is one such ideology, which is continuously in circulation in the dominant culture; it suggests that the capitalist consumption of medical technologies and services is the elixir to the health problems of individuals. In the realm of health, narratives serve the status quo by foregrounding certain aspects of their stories and simultaneously backgrounding other core elements. Hence the act of interrogating the stories told in a culture draws our attention to the mechanisms by which power and control are maintained within that culture.

Discussion point 4.2

- Select a health issue that is currently salient to you. What are the current cultural narratives around this health issue? How do these narratives serve the power structure?
- What are the cultural narratives of smoking prevention campaigns which encourage adolescents to not smoke? How do these narratives serve the status quo? What are the possibilities of alternatives to these dominant cultural narratives of smoking prevention?
- Refer back to a time when you and/or a close family member suffered from an illness. How did you talk about this illness? How did your family members and friends talk about it? What stories around the illness did you share with others? What purpose did these stories serve?

Resistance through narratives

Cultural members *resist* the power structure through the re-creation of alternative narratives (this resistance is further theorized in chapter 10). Such alternative narratives are ways of redoing the script; they retell the story, thus providing new beginnings for experiencing health and its treatment. They are alternative writings of health communication, with alternative ways of looking at how health is experienced in the world. They challenge the dominant paradigm by presenting a different picture of health. The story is told differently, the actors are presented in a different light, and the ending is different. The overall message of the story takes on new beginnings and suggests new ending points. It sees different problems altogether and therefore suggests different starting points for solving them. For instance, in the narratives of diabetes discussed earlier, the community history locates diabetes in the realm of the ongoing contamination of the environment and food supplies, thus resisting the dominant biomedical framework in its explanation of diabetes:

> That's because of those bombs they're testing. . .That's going to settle down. You'll even get it from the milk, you'll get it from the crop. . .That's why people are going to get weaker and weaker. . . I believe that now. . . (Garro 2000: 82)

This narrative of health constructs it in the realm of the environment and challenges the very modernist project within which biomedicine is situated. Disease and illness are constituted as negative outcomes of the project of modernity, and therefore modernity is resisted through the articulations of the violence that is intertwined with it.

Similarly, in research conducted in the Santali communities of rural India, peasant members of marginalized communities which have minimal access to resources discuss the ways in which structural constraints impede their health choices, and they narrate stories about this inaccess as one of the key markers of their lived experience:

> I say this, have a full stomach and live a happy life. We don't need much you know. Just enough *panta* [referring to rice soaked in water] for the day and this body is happy. It is fed and it is happy. But even that is hard to come by. (Dutta-Bergman 2004b: 1112)

Thus, the narratives of health articulated by the participants draw attention away from the dominant stories, which construct health as a matter of individual choice, and locate it instead in the context of structural constraints and economic resources. Health is conceptualized as intrinsically connected to the economic condition and, in formulating it this way, the narrative offered by community members challenges the agendas of dominant policy organizations and health promoting agencies, which focus on individual-level prevention. This is further articulated in the following narrative shared by Ram, who points out the corruption in the healthcare system which fundamentally impedes the realization of health in subaltern communities:

> I can't read the paper. I only tell you what I see and hear. They get medicines, all the expensive ones. But then, they channel them out through the back-doors and sell them to the dispensary across the road at a cheaper price. (Dutta-Bergman 2004a: 256)

In this instance, the sharing of the story of limited structural access is, in and of itself, a narrative of resistance; it foregrounds the oppressive nature of structural inaccess in a discursive space that has typically omitted structure and has focused instead on change in individual behavior, induced through the dissemination of prevention messages.

Furthermore, members of subaltern communities share stories of change, where they articulate their hope for a different world, where they would have access to resources, and discuss participating in community platforms to change the structural constraints. They say:

> You just can't sit and watch it happen [referring to poverty]. . . I went to the meeting and they asked me to come every two weeks. I talk about my problems, and they all work with me. We all help each other out. They also help me out with money when I need it. . . I participate in processions and meetings. (Dutta-Bergman 2004a: 258)

This hope for a world with greater access introduces new possibilities, which have otherwise been silenced. Such stories also become ways of presenting the voices of cultural participants and thus enacting their agency.

Yet another example of an alternative narrative is the example of Minoti and Balaram in chapter 2 (see Box 2.1). Instead of deciphering the choices of these subaltern participants as reflective of an intrinsic lack of agency, I suggested the relevance of attending to the structural components of the story. These components are typically absent in the dominant framing of the story, which would typically discuss the choices of Minoti and Balaram without presenting the context within which they experience their health.

In addition to introducing different interpretations and meanings, narratives in structural contexts also serve as tools for *mobilization*. The mutual sharing of stories creates a sense of community around an issue. For instance, the telling of the story of shop-floor pollution at a steel mill becomes the organizing point for bringing together the workers, who protest at the poor working conditions. The sharing of stories among sex workers about non-compliant clients who would not use condoms serves as a mobilizing point for sex-worker solidarity, so that the use of condoms among clients becomes mandatory. This sharing of stories creates greater awareness and a sense of belonging to a larger collective. The story connects the individual to the collective, and it is through this collective that the individual resists the status quo.

Resistance is enacted through the retelling of story in new ways. This retelling or re-narrating of the story breaks the conventions of the dominant cultural narrative and violates the normative expectations of the culture imposed on the narrative. This is exemplified in the retelling of the story of diabetes as a "White man's sickness." By breaking the conventional patterns and by pulling away from the conventional expectations of the moral of the story, the retelling opens us to new possibilities of social change. Once again, the example provided by Sharf (2005) documents the ways in which alternative narratives resist the dominant medicalization discourse. In this example, by firing her physician, Sharf narrated an alternative story of power where the patient is not simply the target of the medical system to be acted upon as a passive recipient. Instead, her firing of the physician positioned power in the realm of the patient, thus providing an alternative to the dominant reading of physician–patient interactions.

Discussion point 4.3

- What are the ways in which resistance is enacted through narratives in health settings?
- What is the relevance of resistance in the domain of health communication in marginalized settings? As health communication students and scholars, why should we study resistance? What are the possible health communication applications that might be developed on the basis of narratives of resistance?

Conclusion

In summary, the culture-centered approach provides a dialogical space for enacting social change in healthcare contexts, through the performance of narratives of health which disrupt the ideological framings of health solutions under the dominant paradigm. Through its articulation of identities, the culture-centered approach provides an opening for locating health experiences in the domain of individual identities. These identities, in turn, are connected with the health meanings, health choices and health experiences of cultural members. By presenting the culturally situated identities in healthcare contexts, the culture-centered approach directs us toward understanding the ways in which health meanings are constructed and negotiated.

The culture-centered approach articulated in this chapter connects the individual-level identities present in relationships and health choices to cultural processes at the macro-level. Narratives provide the channels through which identities are presented and negotiated in the culture, and therefore are reflective of these identities. They show us the ways in which individual members of the culture make sense of cultural practices, and come to understand their health experiences. They also demonstrate how individuals negotiate their health choices and how these choices relate to the broader values of the culture. They provide publicly presented platforms for enacting mutually meaningful cultural identities, and offer opportunities for rewriting these identities.

One important contribution of the culture-centered approach is the theorization of narratives in the realm of the structures that surround the health experiences of marginalized communities. Much of the existing research on narratives and culture undertheorizes the role of structure and hence, in most instances, fits into the cultural sensitivity framework suggested in chapter 2. By contrast, the culture-centered approach suggests that narratives are enacted within structural processes, and hence provide openings for interrogating and resisting these structural processes. Narratives are ideological devices which serve the status quo and which might also provide entry points for challenging the status quo through the telling of alternative stories, built around a different plot.

5 Pathways of Curing and Healing

Chapter objectives

In this chapter, we will:

• study the cultural location of the biomedical model
• examine the cultural roots of the different pathways of curing and healing
• introduce the polymorphic approach to health communication

As outlined in the introduction of the book, the culture-centered approach calls for dialogue that opens up spaces for those voices that have historically been marginalized (Dutta-Bergman 2004a, 2004b, 2005). Furthermore, the culture-centered approach criticizes both the dominant models of cognitive behavioral approaches, which underlie much of the current health communication theorizing and applications, and the biomedical approach, which informs the ways in which health and illness are constructed as modernist projects. So far we have examined the cognitive behavioral theories and models of health communication. In this chapter we will examine the culturally situated nature of the biomedical model and explore alternative pathways of healing and curing, which have traditionally been silenced by the modernist project of biomedicine (Lupton 1994). It is worth noting that the classification of these approaches as alternatives is tied to the politics of knowledge which backgrounds the culturally situated nature of the biomedical model and offers it as such, as a universal solution to questions of health and illness. Therefore much of the discussion of this chapter focuses on the politics of knowledge production, which privileges certain forms of knowing and simultaneously downplays other ways of approaching health and illness.

Drawing upon the culture-centered approach, this chapter discusses the ways in which culture influences the way disease and illness are understood by its members and the way community members approach the matter of healing and curing disease and illness. As outlined in chapter 3, in the culture-centered approach culture is not simply a finite set of values and beliefs enclosed within a box that remains static throughout human interactions. Rather, culture is dynamic, and is continuously realized as its members navigate through life experiences; in other words, these life experiences and the actions of individual members influence the values

Box 5.1   The story of Basanti

Basanti is 62 years old and works as a maid-servant to eight families in the village of Rampur in West Bengal, India. Basanti barely makes her living and depends upon her ability to secure daily work to ensure that she and her children have enough food for the day. In her discussion of health, Basanti presents a complex web of healing and curing. In some instances, when she considers the illness to be serious, she goes to the state-sponsored subsidized hospital, which has limited resources of doctors and hospital supplies. In the case of persistent fevers of her children, she takes them to the local allopathic doctor and pays the exorbitant visitation fees to get the child treated. In yet other instances, she points out that she visits the local homeopathic doctor, whose medicine is much more affordable to her compared to the allopathic doctor at the clinic. Basanti also visits the *kobiraj* (Ayurvedic practitioner). Ultimately, says Basanti, although allopathic medicine can provide temporary relief, it cannot really heal the condition the patient faces. For healing to occur, the underlying causes have to be dealt with, and, for Basanti, these underlying causes are connected with divine forces. Therefore she explains that she offers *manat* at the temple of the Goddess *Kali* so that she will be appeased.

and beliefs of the culture, which are continuously in flux (Dutta-Bergman 2004a, 2004b). Also, culture seamlessly interacts with structure and agency in constituting the meanings of health and illness and in defining pathways for action (Dutta-Bergman 2004a, 2004b, 2005).

The purpose of this chapter is to elucidate how culture is played out in the domains of health, illness, curing, and healing. The perception of illness and the response to it from the cultural participants are the products of their lived experiences and, in turn, shape these experiences, together with what the culture sanctions as knowledge, the values it puts on it, and the uses it makes of it as a resource in the daily lives of the cultural members. Thus, as we shall see in these pages, it is through the lived experiences of its members that we come to understand a culture and its approaches to illness, curing and healing.

The example of Basanti illustrates the centrality of culture in the way one perceives illness. The fact that she locates the ultimate cause of illness in the realm of the divine (with the Goddess *Kali*) is informed by her cultural notion of health and illness, which, in turn, is further informed by her life experiences in seeking out health. The structural condition of being deprived of resources informs the options that are sought out by cultural participants. In addition, the notion of a divine origin of health and illness is influenced by other models of health, illness, curing and healing, available to the patient beyond the biomedical model – models which define the complex terrain of the cultural space within which health, illness, healing and curing are negotiated.

This chapter will begin by presenting the biomedical model as culturally constituted, interrogating its universal logic on the basis of the culture-centered approach, and examining the link between culture and illness. The following section will present alternative ways of healing and curing, located outside the biomedical model. Finally, the chapter will conclude with the presentation of the *polymorphic* approach to health and illness that foregrounds the multiplicity of approaches to illness and its treatment.

The Dominant Framework: Biomedical Knowledge

The biomedical model is presented to us as the only viable model, one which is scientifically based and therefore is perhaps the only legitimate resource for dealing with issues of health and illness within the modernist project (Comaroff 1982; Good 1994; Hahn 1983). The prevalence of the biomedical model is tied to the taken-for-granted assumptions around what constitutes knowledge in the realm of health and which techniques and technologies are legitimately equipped to generate such knowledge (Baer, Singer and Susser 2003). The assumption underlying much of the medical and allied sciences is that the biomedical model provides a truthful account of reality when compared to more primitive forms of healing and curing practices, which are not empirically based and hence are irrational. The widespread diffusion of the modernist paradigm of development and the expansion of the global market economy played key roles in popularizing biomedicine as the pre-eminent medical system in the world (ibid.).

At the onset, it is vital to recognize the relevance of the biomedical model in delivering effective solutions in certain instances. Indeed, the problem faced in resource-deprived parts of the world is often one of inaccess to the basic resources of the biomedical system. Having said that, the goal of this chapter is to establish that the biomedical model is one among many ways of approaching health, illness, and well-being; and that the legitimacy of the biomedical model is constituted within a contested space, which is always open to new meanings and new possibilities. This notion of contested spaces of negotiating health and illness draws upon complementarities among the different approaches to health and illness, as well as upon tensions between them. This contestation, I would argue, becomes particularly relevant in the realm of marginalized communities, who struggle with their limited structural resources in order to find healthcare solutions that fit their needs (Dutta-Bergman 2004a, 2004b).

Discussion point 5.1

- What do you understand by the biomedical model? What, according to you, are the basic features of the biomedical model?
- What are your gut responses to the biomedical model? Where do you think these gut responses come from?
- What are the culturally circulated stories about the biomedical model? What purposes do these stories serve?

Conceptual framework

The conceptual framework of illness in the biomedical model is that illness is caused by the malfunctioning of a specific bodily part, and that the part in question needs to be treated so that the illness may be removed. The emphasis is on curing the diseased bodily part. This conceptual framework is located within the broader notion of control through empirical observation, and is driven by evidence found from controlled experiments or studies. Biomedicine specifically focuses on patho-physiology, depending on a type of physical reductionism that radically separates the body from the non-body (Hahn 1983).

Good (1994) argues that the language of clinical medicine takes a natural science approach to the relationship between language, biology, and experience. The biomedical model treats diseases as "universal biological or psychophysiological entities" (p. 8) which result from "somatic lesions or dysfunctions." These dysfunctions manifest themselves in signs which are measurable physiological characteristics, and symptoms, which consist in communications regarding one's experience of distress associated with the sign. Note that, under this model, the signs and symptoms are intrinsically related, and the validity of a symptom is predicated upon the existence of a sign. "Real pathology" in this context is a reflection of disordered physiology, and the objective knowledge of such pathology is provided by contemporary technical medicine through its physical findings, laboratory results, and the visual markers of reality generated by contemporary imaging techniques. Hence the biomedical model emphasizes technologies that are created and fine-tuned for the purposes of detecting the signs of distress.

The primary tasks of the physician are diagnosis, that is, the identification of an appropriate underlying disease entity, and rational treatment, which seeks to intervene in the disease mechanism. In this framework, diseases are "biological, universal, and ultimately transcend social and cultural context" (ibid.). The legitimacy of a patient's complaint therefore depends upon its connection with a clearly identified underlying physiological condition which is identifiable by the tools created by the model. To the extent that such a condition cannot be tracked down, the complaint is seen as reflecting subjective opinions and experiences, and not grounded in objective reality. In other words, the existence of an illness is ultimately predicated upon the ability of the technology to detect the signs of illness, demonstrating the culturally situated West-centric emphasis on technology.

Baer et al. (2003) point out that within the US context, biomedicine incorporates certain core cultural values, beliefs and metaphors that are continually communicated to patients. These values and beliefs reflect broader cultural beliefs such as self-reliance, independence, rugged individualism, pragmatism, empiricism, atomism, militarism, profit-making, emotional minimalism, and a mechanical concept of the body and the way it is repaired (Stein 1990). An example cited in the work of Baer and his collaborators is that of the war on cancer: popular and scientific portrayals of cancer depict a prolonged war against a deadly and evil internal growth that is led by a competent oncologist with sophisticated tools and carried out by a courageous, stoic and obedient soldier, the patient. Erwin (1987) refers to this process as "medical militarization." The emphasis, in biomedicine, on individualistic values deeply connected with aggression, critical medical anthropologists argue, is related to the location of biomedicine within a broader culture which values individualism and aggression as ways of solving problems.

The cultural location of biomedicine is particularly evident in Payer's comparison of medicine in France, Germany, Britain, and the United States (1988). He reports that French medicine results in significantly longer doctor visits when compared to German medicine, because of its strong orientation toward abstract thought. Whereas French biomedicine locates the liver as the locus of numerous diseases, including complications such as migraine, headaches, general fatigue, and painful menstruation, German biomedicine regards poor blood circulation as being at the root of a variety of ailments such as hypertension, tired legs, and varicose veins. Both German and French biomedicine rely heavily on the capacity of the immunological system to resist disease, and therefore they de-emphasize the use of antibiotics. On the other hand, US biomedicine tends to rely much more heavily on invasive forms of therapy such as Cesarean sections, hysterectomies, breast cancer screenings, and high dosages of psychotropic drugs. Baer et al. (2003: 13) note:

> US biomedicine manifests a pattern of aggression that seems in keeping with the strong emphasis in American society on violence as a means of solving problems – a pattern undoubtedly rooted in the frontier mentality that continues to live on in what has for the most part become a highly urbanized, postindustrial society. In this sense, the war on cancer and the war on drugs are symbolic cultural continuations of the war against Native Americans that cleared the frontier for White settlement.

Economic interests

The ascendancy of biomedicine to a dominant position in the West coincides with the rise in industrial capitalism and is entrenched within the assistance from the capitalist class, whose interests it serves (Baer et al. 2003). Contextually locating the history of biomedicine in the realm of capitalism, Brown articulated that the project of "scientific medicine" funded by the Rockefeller and Carnegie foundations placed heavy emphasis on the germ theory of disease, and only those medical schools and research institutions were funded which reflected this broader agenda. The germ theory of disease was an ideology that legitimized the capitalist interests by drawing attention to discrete external agents rather than to social structural and environmental factors, and "was compatible with the worldview of, and politically and economically useful, to the capitalist class and the emerging managerial and professional stratum"

(Brown 1979: 12). Biomedicine further served the economic interests of the capitalist class, with its emphasis on creating a healthy and productive workforce that would contribute to economic productivity and profit. This notion of profit and economic productivity is evident in much of the dominant discourse of biomedicine, which talks about disease states in terms of lost productivity. In order to create a productive labor force, biomedicine focuses on treating the body as a machine that requires periodic repairs so that it may perform assigned productive tasks that contribute to the economy. For instance, in discussing the control over the reproductive space exerted by biomedicine, Martin (1987: 146) discusses that "birth is seen as the control of laborers (women) and their machines (their uteruses) by managers (doctors), often using other machines to help".

The increasing popularity of biomedicine globally has brought its greater control over various aspects of the lives of individuals and communities, globally (Baer et al. 2003). This has led to a process of ever-widening the net of biomedicine, with greater segments of social lives and human behaviors being brought under its control through the continuous extension of medical pathological terminology to cover new conditions and behaviors. This increasing coverage of human life under the purview of biomedicine is referred to as medicalization. The medicalization process has become pervasive in social life, as health clinics, health maintenance organizations, and other medical providers offer classes on managing stress, controlling obesity, overcoming sexual impotence, alcoholism and drug addiction, and promoting smoking cessation (ibid.). Medicalization is deeply connected with the profit to be made through the discovery of new diseases and the development of new treatments. It contributes to the increasing social control held by physicians and health insurance institutions over behavior, and transforms a structural problem into a problem of individual behavior that can be controlled (Waitzkin 1983). The culture-centered approach suggests a discursive space for interrogating the universal logic underlying medicalization and for interpreting the biomedical model in the realm of structure, power, and control.

Discussion point 5.2

- How does biomedicine serve the interests of the capitalist classes?
- What role does the medicalizing ideology play in the context of managing dissent in the laboring classes? How?

The Culture-Centered Critique of the Biomedical Model

Why do we need a critique of the biomedical model? In answering this question, let's pay closer attention to the story of Basanti. In this story, we learn that Basanti relies on a variety of treatments to deal with the illnesses faced by her and her family. She traverses the different worlds of treatments, shifting from one to the other, depending upon the nature of the illness, the location of the patient in the family structure (children have the highest priority over the resources), the price of the treatment, and the other resources (such as time and the price of transportation) needed to secure the treatment. These treatments are intertwined and integrated into a complex web of meaning-making which is juxtaposed in the backdrop of the structural resources available to the patient and his/her family members. Listening to the story of Basanti opens up the possibility of a variety of approaches to healing and curing that lie outside the biomedical model, and yet engage with it. Furthermore, Basanti's experiences help her with her life choices and, in turn, consti-tute discursive spaces for her health and illness, thus making it possible to value the stories and lived experiences of individuals, groups and communities and to reject the dominant practice of simply taking for granted the tools of biomedicine and the arguments of scientific ration-ality, as if they were the only legitimate entry points for knowing about health and illness.

Basanti's story, through its very embodiment of a complex life that continuously enacts agency at the intersections of social structures and cultural meanings, challenges the privilege of biomedicine, which we typically take for granted in our work as health communicators. When evaluated through the lens of the biomedical model, Basanti's choices are quickly identified and discarded as "primitive" or "magical." In order to create a meaningful discursive space for understanding the health choices of cultural community members such as Basanti who survive within very limited structural resources, we need to disrupt the univer-salistic and exclusive logic of the biomedical model. In doing so, we need to focus our attention on the ways in which the constitution of the bio-medical model marginalizes underserved sectors of the population, not only by denying them access to the basic infrastructures of biomedicine, but also by marking the choices of the community as "primitive" on the basis of its own scientific–rational standards. It is this discursive marking of the subaltern as primitive that legitimizes the unequal power struc-tures and the privilege enjoyed by the status quo and further reified by biomedicine.

Basanti's story suggests that the decision-making cues used by parti-cipants are located at the intersections of culture and structure (Dutta-Bergman 2004a, 2004b, 2005), reflecting the ways in which locally contextualized values and beliefs interact with the social structures that sur-round the lived experiences of individuals and their families. In a global-ized context, these pathways of curing and healing are multi-dimensional and geographically dispersed, albeit located within the intricacies of structures of modernity, where they are formed. The culture-centered app-roach responds to this complexity by locating health choices within the local contexts in which they are constituted and at the intersections of structures and cultures articulated through the voices of people and com-munities. Also, the culture-centered approach provides an entry point for interrogating the complex relationship between health, illness, healing and curing. It provides a vantage point for understanding the multiplicity of perspectives on illness and its treatment, and the culturally situated nature of these perspectives. In doing so, it regards the biomedical system as one of the many culturally determined approaches to illness and treatment, and therefore problematizes the universalized notions of truth and reality in health and illness embodied in the biomedical model. This act of making visible the values underlying the biomedical model is both a discursive and a political stance.

Thus the culture-centered approach interrogates the rationality of the scientific discourse of the biomedical model, and understands it in the context of projects of modernizing the world. This ruptures the scientific notion of biomedicine as "an objective body of scientific knowledge external to culture" based on the notion of science as antithetical to culture (Lupton 2003: 19). By understanding the biomedical model from a cultural perspective, the culture-centered approach opens up the space for understanding other ways of conceptualizing health, illness, and healing. The questioning of the universalizing tendencies and rational claims of the biomedical model brings forth issues of power, ideology and hegemony, which underlie the tendencies to construct the biomedical model as the only viable option and as the only point of access to truth in the realm of health and illness.

Box 5.2   The story of Jennifer

At the age of 43, Jennifer was diagnosed with breast cancer. She still remembers the trip to the doctor's office, when the doctor shared with her the report of her biopsy. Having worked as a medical administrator, Jennifer was familiar with the hospital system and had a good network of physicians, nurses and administrators among her friends. She decided to start looking at the various treatment options on the very first day of her trip back from the doctor's office. In addition to going through the medical literature, she also received a lot of feedback and input from her friends. The most common response that she heard was: "Just take it out." She operated on this mind-frame for a while, and even set an appointment to have surgery. However, as the date of the surgery approached, she was more and more unsure. As the days passed by, she read more and more materials which questioned the efficacy of surgery and suggested a variety of alternatives. These alternatives ranged from Yoga to meditation and guided imagery. Jennifer wondered whether she should go for the surgery or whether these other alternatives might be more meaningful for her. Her friends told her that she was losing precious time, but Jennifer was not so sure about surgery as she was within the first few days of receiving the news.

What do we learn from the story of Jennifer about the health decisions and choices we make and the ways in which we go about navigating the medical system? As one of Jennifer's friends, what would you suggest to her? How does your suggestion connect with the scripts of health, illness, healing and curing in your culture?

Hegemony of the biomedical model

The culture-centered approach draws our attention to the inequitable access to structures that create conditions for legitimizing certain values and certain ways of knowing as acceptable and commonsensical, simultaneously de-legitimizing other values and ways of knowing as unacceptable or impossible. In the widely circulated biomedical model, which is the dominant model of health, knowledge claims and bodies of knowledge are evaluated in the backdrop of their ability to correspond to an external reality. What this reality is and what tools are used to verify it, however, depends upon the socio-cultural system within which this body of knowledge is proposed. Therefore the culture-centered approach draws our attention to power and interrogates its role in pushing a certain social construction of reality as superior, or as a better form of knowing. The technologies of biomedicine are located within the cultural realm of Western science, and are accorded a privileged position on the basis of access to power and to the economic system of capitalist societies, which operate on the logic of efficiency and productivity (Lupton 1995a, 1995b). This access to the positions of power in modern society from which knowledge claims may be evaluated underlies the universalization of biomedicine (Dutta-Bergman 2004a, 2004b).

Alternative ways of knowing have been undermined because of their limited access to the positions of power within which knowledge is articulated and circulated in the global order (Dutta-Bergman 2005a; Lupton 1995a, 1995b). They have been discarded as primitive or unscientific, which thus maintains the privileged position of the biomedical community and the unquestioned social control enjoyed by the biomedical model. An American Medical Association (AMA) report on alternative medicine demonstrates this intrinsic bias against alternatives and the attempts of the medicalizing ideology to locate alternative forms of healing and curing in the realm of the supernatural and the unscientific.

> Buckman points out that reports of success for many of the therapies being embraced by the public may be explained in several ways. The "cures" may have come from misdiagnosis, and when the anecdotes of healing are traced to the original sources, no data can be found. Patients may not have had the diagnosis for which they were "cured" or the data may have been falsified or misinterpreted by the healer. They may have experienced self-limiting or fluctuating illnesses, remission of which was wrongly attributed to the alternative treatment. After therapy, patients may not have been followed long enough to accurately assess cure or observe relapses. Concurrent conventional therapy is often being taken by patients who undergo alternative treatments, with inappropriate credit given to the unconventional method. Finally, misinterpretation of information by patients who believe themselves miraculously cured is often at the core of their success story. However, he points out that some of the clinical trials examining different areas of alternative therapy have raised enough questions to make further investigation of these methods desirable, in order to help answer the essential question in this debate: do these methods merely make one *feel* better, or do they really help one *get* better? (http://www.ama-assn.org/ama/pub/category/13638.html)

Notice the privileging of the dominant discourses of biomedicine to explain away possibilities of curing and healing located outside its own realm. The stance of the AMA toward alternative forms of healing and curing as elucidated in the above excerpt also demonstrates the privileging of "getting better" over "merely making one feel better." Intrinsic to this statement is the comparison between "really" getting better, as determined by physiological measures that can be tracked down through the modernist technologies of biomedicine, and the patient's experience of feeling better. What is real is that which can be measured by the technologies of biomedicine. The notion that the reality of curing can only be measured through physiologically observable characteristics helps maintain the privilege of biomedicine and its technologies, simultaneously erasing forms of healing and curing and patient experiences that draw from other ontological and epistemological roots. To the extent that these alternative forms of healing and curing seek legitimacy in the realm of the hegemonic configurations of biomedicine, they do so by subjecting themselves to scrutiny under the methods and tools of biomedicine. Note in this excerpt the ways in which alternative forms of healing are discounted through the offering of several other, non-scientific explanations for their workings.

The same report further elucidates the discursive uses of the language of rationality to legitimize the control of biomedicine and simultaneously devalue other ways of knowing.

> Some of the interest in alternative medicine may be due to an "outbreak of irrationalism" that includes New Age interest in "channeling" and astrology. Television talk shows and the proliferation of books and tapes on alternative therapies are gobbled up by an uncritical public that does not understand how to sort quack theories from what might be reasonable. Carl Sagan has recently lamented the phenomenon of our increasing scientific illiteracy and the rise of pseudoscience and superstition, noting that "baloney, bamboozles, careless thinking, and wishes disguised as fact . . . ripple through mainstream political, social, religious, and economic issues in every nation."

The growth of alternative medicine in the US is connected to the outbreak of irrationalism and scientific illiteracy. In this context, the scientific claim of biomedicine serves an important political role in maintaining its privileged status, the privileged position of the medical experts, and the privileged position of the medical industry, which depends upon this discourse of authority to maintain its legitimacy and to ensure a growing market for its goods and services (Baer et al. 2003; Waitzkin 1983).

This privileging of biomedicine as scientific, and hence modern and progressive by comparison with the retrogressive tendencies of alternative forms of healing, is further elucidated in the following excerpt:

> In an essay in the *New York Times*, two university scientists who discuss the OAM conclude, 'Should there be an Office of Alternative Medicine to evaluate unconventional practices? Not one that elevates magical notions to matters of serious scientific debate. . . . It is important to distinguish these experiences [such as kindness or sunsets] from claims that ignore natural law.'

Once again, the serious scientific debates of science are set up in the backdrop of experiences such as of kindness and of sunsets, demonstrating the taken-for-granted assumptions underlying what is valued and what is not valued as ways of knowing. Whereas science is certainly considered to be a serious enterprise, what is also hidden in the statement is the implication of frivolousness in the unscientific tendencies of alternative medicine. The excerpt reveals the hegemony of scientific discourse in discursively constructing what is knowledge and what is not; unconventional practices are quickly relegated to the realm of magic, which does not deserve scientific attention.

Furthermore, to the extent that alternative forms of healing enter into the discursive spaces of modernity, they do so through their uses of modernist marketing techniques (as witnessed in the rise of Yoga-marketing in the US, or in the formation of the Office of Alternative Medicine at the National Institutes of Health), or through their legitimization by the biomedical enterprise (as reflected in the formation of the OAM, the attempts to develop controlled trials for certain alternative treatments, and the development of "new" disciplines of medicine such as mind–body medicine). To the extent that the discourse of science gives its blessings to these alternative therapies, they acquire legitimacy. In this process, specific techniques or processes are extracted from their epistemological and ontological roots and are imbibed (hence co-opted) within the scientific discourse for purposes of application.

Some scholars argue that present-day biomedicine can no longer be squarely placed in the realm of the West, because well-established medical research organizations and research bodies today are widely distributed across the globe, in countries like China, India, and Japan. Although this is indeed an important argument, it is also critical to point out that much

Box 5.3   The story of Vanessa

Vanessa has grown up as a doctor's daughter. He father was a well-known medical practitioner as well as a medical anthropologist who studied Chinese ways of healing. Vanessa herself has studied medicine and went on to practice in a Native American reservation in South Dakota. Her patients, she realizes, have a very different value system from hers in approaching their health. Although, as a doctor trained in biomedicine, she feels many a times that she knows what the best options are for her patients, she is also uncertain, as she doesn't really know the appropriateness of her knowledge. For instance, at certain times, although she is quite sure that surgery is the best option for her patients, she is also aware of the profound ways in which surgery violates the epistemological framework of Native American healing. At times she struggles, caught in the tension between these two very different worldviews that she has come to respect and admire.

How would you suggest Vanessa approach her job? Is it possible for her to resolve the tensions between the different approaches? What suggestions would you have for Vanessa as a culture-centered health communication scholar?

of the current biomedical knowledge continues to be articulated and debated within the Western geographic realm, is historically situated in the context of the Enlightenment project, and is used as an argument for Western chauvinism, tied to the origins of the rational scientific enterprise in the scientific revolution of Europe.

In summary, the biomedical model of health is closely aligned with the modernization project, being pushed globally as the only viable and rational model of health, illness, and treatment. Other models, typically discussed in the backdrop of this model, are considered to be ancient or primitive, lacking a sophisticated theoretical system or empirical basis for meaningful generalizations, and therefore lacking in their scientific capabilities. In this section we will understand the cultural bases of the biomedical model and present its limitations as a culturally configured model, developed in the West and linked with the industrial revolution and its objectives. Even in the critique of the biomedical model as an entry point for discussing alternative models of health and illness, it is important to recognize its effectiveness in dealing with certain conditions, the large-scale need for the solutions it provides, and the scarcity of some of the basic resources of the biomedical model in the marginalized sectors of the world.

The West-centric roots of the biomedical model

The biomedical model is located within the period of Enlightenment, between the late seventeenth and the late eighteenth centuries, drawing much of its discourses and practices from the Enlightenment project, which privileged developments in science and technology as essential elements of human progress. A medicine based on science and technology was seen as providing the solutions for problems of disease and illness throughout the European Enlightenment. Emphasis was placed on the power of reason as critical to the development of human understanding, and on the rejection of superstition and religion (Lupton 2003). This emphasis on scientific principles and the celebration of rationality was accompanied by the professionalization of medicine and by greater control over the licensing of medical practitioners (Jewson 1976).

Also referred to as the cosmopolitan system, scientific system or Western system, this medical system originated from the Greek tradition. As Charles Leslie (1976) points out, the Greek tradition, however, is only one out of the three great medical traditions, Chinese, Greek and Indian, which were independent, maintained a clearly defined social organization and were based upon generic physiological and cosmological concepts. In spite of this diversity of traditions, as explained earlier, the biomedical model has enjoyed special position in the modern period owing to its associations with the scientific process and the efficacy of the technologies developed within the model. In other words, what has propagated such widespread acceptance of the biomedical model was its commitment to technology and its widespread use, which provides efficacious answers to health problems.

The biomedical model is based upon a conceptual framework that addresses the treatment of illness through surgical and pharmacological options, and primarily draws from germ theory. The invention of the microscope was a key marker in the history of biomedicine, as it facilitated the movement toward technological innovation, scientific prowess and laboratory-based knowledge, away from knowledge based on bedside interactions (Rosenberg 1988). The emphasis on rigorous and objective modern scientific knowledge in biomedicine puts tremendous powers in the hands of the practitioner and simultaneously minimizes the power of the patient to navigate his/her choices, reducing him/her to a passive and uncritical role in the consultative relationship (Lupton 2003). Furthermore, the domain of medicine extended from the hospital to communities, as the modern European states of the seventeenth and eighteenth centuries became more concerned about the welfare of the population and the maintenance of its growth in the context of industrialization, free market economy and increasing urbanization.

Good (1994) argues that the predominant view of scientific language as transparent to the natural world has dominated the medical behavioral sciences; it is a cultural language linked to a specialized version of reality and a system of social relations that is linked to culturally located values. In this approach to knowing, the effectiveness of a system depends upon its ability to capture clearly the one reality that exists in the external world. Therefore the emphasis is on finding one-to-one correspondences between the concepts within the model and an external reality that it seeks to explain. One of the central cultural values driving the model is built upon the notion that observation provides the only point of access to ascertaining the reality of the material world. Yet another value embedded in the model is that the material world provides the only point of access to reality. Furthermore, it is assumed that empirical observations would provide the needed explanations for understanding health, illness, and dying.

It is also interesting to observe that individualism as a cultural value lies at the core of the biomedical model; the individual patient is seen as the site of the disease, and biomedical technologies are deployed with the goal of curing the patient (Lupton 2003; Stein 1990). The lens is further narrowed, to focus on a diseased bodily part or condition that needs to be treated and/or removed (Comaroff 1982; Gordon 1988). In doing so, the biomedical model de-contextualizes the illness from the whole body, from the multiple relationships of the patient with other family members, from the location of the patients within the social system, from the cultures within which the patient lives, from the structures surrounding him/her, and from the environment that surrounds his/her day-to-day life. Biomedicine demonstrates much of the same values of contemporary Western culture and its roots in the Enlightenment project, particularly in the realm of valuing naturalism, autonomy, independence, and mind–body dichotomy (Lupton 2003). Gordon (1988: 40) notes that biomedicine constitutes an "image of the modern self, capable of nearly absolute freedom from social determinacy, able to disengage in order to reach a higher level of truth." Furthermore, rugged individualism and independence become the key values recommended for patients within the biomedical model: patients are urged to co-participate in the war against disease through the use of aggressive technologies (Baer et al. 2003). In the next section we will examine how the biomedical model (a) exerts its power over other ways of knowing, in the context of the project of modernization, and (b) maintains power in the hands of the providers, thus creating an unequal terrain in which medical knowledge is played out and put into practice.

Discussion point 5.3

- In the section on cultural values in biomedicine, we discussed the ways in which the biomedical discourse reflects individualistic values. What other values do you see reflected in the biomedical system today?
- What do these values say about the current role of biomedicine in human society?

Relationships of power and the biomedical model

Exactly which out of the many models of healing and curing gets adopted and widely circulated in society depends upon questions of access to power (Dutta-Bergman 2005; Lupton 2003). Power refers to the force exerted by a particular system within a social order based on its access to the discursive and material spaces. The culture-centered approach suggests that power is situated in the realm of the social structures, and it is through its access to these structures that power exerts its control over the socio-cultural spaces. The power enjoyed by the biomedical model through its support by the state and civil societies in the context of modernity is central to the valorization of biomedicine and to the monopoly it enjoys.

Take for instance the power of doctors in the biomedical system. Cultural analysis of the physician–patient relationship suggests that physicians exert a great deal of power in the framing of an illness, in categorizing it and giving it a name, in choosing a treatment regimen, in monitoring the regimen, and in evaluating its effectiveness (Freidson 1970; Willis 1989). Physicians draw this power from their authority over knowledge; the discourse of scientific rationality places this authority in the hands of the physician (Starr 1982). The power of the medical profession is tied to the objective and scientific value of biomedicine, and is further supported by the state through its emphasis on the professionalization and licensing of medicine (Freidson 1970). By strictly controlling the entry into the medical profession and the knowledge and practice of medicine, and by controlling the number of doctors through quotas placed upon entry to medical schools and through strict restriction laws, the state accords the medical profession the "right to its monopoly over expert knowledge and practice" (Lupton 2003: 116). Political economists argue that there is also a socio-economic gap between doctors and their patients, who continue to preserve this unequal power relationship. Furthermore, regulatory organizations such as the Federal Drug Agency (FDA) further participate in supporting the dominant power structure through their regulation of the types of healing and curing choices that become available to patients within capitalist societies, and by creating an infrastructure that supports the dominance of major pharmaceutical corporations.

The implicit power exerted by biomedicine serves not only the medical profession, but also capitalist interests, by drawing attention away from socio-structural roots of health problems to the individual-level aspects of health (Waitzkin 1984). Through their dominance over patients, doctors reinforce the messages of capitalism; to patients suffering from depression or stress, they recommend to exercise, do Yoga, meditate, or take mood-altering medications; they direct patient behavior to non-threatening channels, thus shifting attention away from the socio-economic factors that cause the conditions. Medicine "helps to legitimize and reproduce social class structure and the economic system. It thereby maintains the position of dominant interests, and in the process, achieves power for its members" (Lupton 2003: 116). Capitalism is further reinforced by biomedicine, with its focus on using health products manufactured by large-scale corporations as solutions to health problems. This power is extended through medicalization, as more and more aspects of human life are brought under the purview of biomedicine with the invention of new diseases and the deployment of new solutions, thus creating whole new markets for new medical products.

The widespread power of the biomedical model is exemplified in the notion that we accept it as the standard model for understanding the human body, human health, illness, and treatment. This discursive framing of health and illness simultaneously influences the policies that are created to govern and regulate the different approaches to health and illness, the options available to patients and their families, and the ways in which resources are allocated.

Spaces for dialogue

The dialogical stance in the culture-centered approach creates communicative spaces for conversation, opening up avenues for a two-way flow of communication and knowledge. It enables us not only to look at the cultural bases of the different pathways of curing and healing, but also to adopt a stance of respect in our interactions with various cultural systems and the ways in which they approach disease and illness. In doing so, the dialogical stance foregrounds the mutually interdependent flow of communication among the different approaches to health, illness, healing and curing, thus creating spaces for the exchange of meanings. Rather than attempting to change the participants into a receiving culture, on the basis of inherent positions of power enjoyed by the biomedical model, the dialogical approach places emphasis on meanings and new possibilities.

The need for alternatives: locating culture

Why do we need alternatives to the biomedical model? One of the basic answers to this question is that these alternatives already exist, have existed long before the biomedical model and have robustly co-existed with it. As the medical anthropologist Charles Leslie eloquently argues in his introductory essay to the seminal text, *Asian Medical Systems*, the singular acknowledgement, in historical accounts of medicine, of the Greek tradition, which was the precursor to Western medical science, and the simultaneous omission of the Indian and Chinese medical systems served to maintain Western hegemony through a monopoly over the claim to scientific knowledge. It also maintained an intrinsic power differential, through the position of superiority automatically assumed by the Western cosmopolitan centers of modernity as the primary locales of scientific work. This ethnocentrism of the scientific claim is evident in the following introduction by Wilson (1971: xiii) to a collection of essays by anthropologists and philosophers on the nature of rationality: "Only in advanced western societies is the detached and systematic approach to social (and perhaps also to natural) phenomena at all commonly adopted – or adoptable. It is in this society that the dilemma of how to understand the world arises as an intellectual problem . . ."

Criticizing this exclusive claim to science from the biomedical model, scholars of Indian and Chinese medical systems point out that these systems of medicine are scientific in their "rational use of naturalistic theories to organize and interpret systematic empirical observations" (Leslie 1976: 7). Needham goes on to argue that some fields of knowledge in Chinese traditions were significantly more sophisticated and advanced than those of Greece, and that modern science borrowed the Hindu–Arabic notation, trigonometry and other knowledge from Asian civilizations. What lies at the heart of the spatio-temporal claim of the scientific monopoly of Western medicine is a specious argument that privileges a certain set of culturally derived practices over another set of culturally derived practices, on the basis of having access to power and determining the terrain of the knowledge networks.

Health communication scholarship has unfortunately continued this ethnocentrism by taking for granted the biomedical model as a primary site of investigation and by basing its investigations on the model's assumptions of scientific rationality. In fact, almost all of the introductory texts of health communication, and the *Handbook of Health Communication*, focus on the biomedical model alone. Much of the discussion of health communication is carried under the rubric of the biomedical model and ignores the issues of communication that are played out in these alternative spheres. It is within the biomedical system that healthcare organizations, relationships and identities are examined. Similarly, much of the work on health communication campaigns operates on the presumptions of the biomedical model, and the targets of prevention interventions are identified on the basis of their biomedical roots.

This ethnocentric bias is also evident in yet another system of categorization, which is used to separate the biomedical from the other models. In this system, the biomedical model is presented under the name of modern medicine, whereas the other medical systems are presented as traditional systems. Inherent in the discursive construction of tradition versus modernity is the openness and flexibility to change of the modern system, compared to the conservativeness of the traditional system, which is closed to change and hence irrational. As Leslie (1976) and others working on Asian medical systems point out, this categorization is highly problematic because both Indian and Chinese systems of medicine demonstrate openness to change; they have in fact survived the onslaught of cosmopolitan medicine because of this very openness. Leslie's line of thinking has been continued by an emerging body of scholarship that demonstrates the ways in which practitioners of Chinese and Indian medicine often adapt and incorporate elements of the biomedical model into their practice.

Simply reducing the study of health, and our communication about it, to the biomedical model vastly ignores other bodies of knowledge, which provide meaningful and viable ways of understanding health and illness. Also, limiting the study of health and illness to the biomedical model limits the knowledge of health communication to a culturally determined system, that of the West, and closes off ways of knowing practiced elsewhere in the world. Although much of the theory and practice of the biomedical model is based upon the blind assumption that the model has the best answers for health, illness and treatment, careful examination demonstrates otherwise. Although, as noted earlier, the model does provide valuable and efficacious solutions to certain illnesses, there are domains in which the model clearly seems to falter and not to have clearly defined answers. For instance, the ways in which the model approaches rare order diseases such as multiple chemical sensitivity (MCS) and fibromyalgia demonstrate the limits of the explanations it can provide and treatments it can offer; its incomplete approach to diseases such as those of the thyroid, or diabetes and asthma, and its lack of clearly defined answers to the treatment of these diseases, further point toward its limitations; and so does its inability to have well-defined and non-contradictory answers, based on logical empiricism, to the prevention and treatment of illnesses such as cancer, diabetes, or heart disease. The model's emphasis on surgical and pharmacological options to illness produces side effects that might do more harm than good, and the comparisons offered between the risks versus efficacy of widely used treatments are limited. As discussed earlier, the model takes a narrow approach to health and illness, focusing on one bodily part, which needs to be removed or treated with medicine or surgery, rather than understanding the health of the complete individual. In doing so, the model prescribes treatments based on a narrowly defined approach to

---

Box 5.4   The story of Meina

Meina came to the US from China in 1998, as a graduate student in physics. Having been trained as a physicist, she is fairly familiar with the scientific way of doing things. Having grown up in China, she is also familiar with the Chinese system of healing and is in the habit of using a variety of ways for approaching disease and illness. However, since coming to the US, Meina has limited access to the options available to her back in China. She is sometimes at a loss, because she feels her options in the US are fairly limited. She also feels it would be silly to ask someone about possible options.

What do you think underlies the vastly different experiences that Meina had in China and in the US? How would the healthcare system respond to the needs of individuals such as Meina? How would the culture-centered approach equip you to approach Meina's limited choices?

---

illness and does not take into account the interconnections between the various components of the body, the relationship between the body and the mind, the relationship between the human being and his/her surroundings, and so on. Finally, it is worth noting that, in various parts of the world, the biomedical model co-exists with other models such as the Chinese and Indian systems, and this is more and more the case in the Western centers of the globe, where the biomedical model used to be the predominant model. In the next section, we will examine some of the most widely circulated pathways of curing and healing which exist outside the biomedical model and yet engage with it in the possibilities they create in the current healthcare landscape. At the onset, it is important to point out that this chapter only provides a starting point for discussions about alternative ways of knowing about health and illness. Detailed discussions of these ways of knowing are beyond the scope of this book, and need to be taken up in future scholarship.

Spirituality and Health

Spirituality is the organization of human consciousness, flowing from the basic questions of human existence such as "Who am I?" "Where am I going?" "What do I know?" "What must I do?" and "For what can I hope?" (Morgan 2002). For Becker (1975: 3), spirituality is "an expression of the will to live, the burning desire of the creature to count, to make a difference on the planet because he has lived, has emerged on it, has worked, suffered, and died" (p. 3). Spirituality is intrinsically tied to health because it asks the fundamental questions of life and death, and provides entry points for understanding the meaning of suffering. Offering a window into the nature of human existence and its fundamental basis, spirituality provides a framework for understanding human health, illness, pain and suffering. The introspective nature of spirituality opens up possibilities for self-reflection in connection with the nature of health, illness, death and dying. It transcends the realm of the immediate

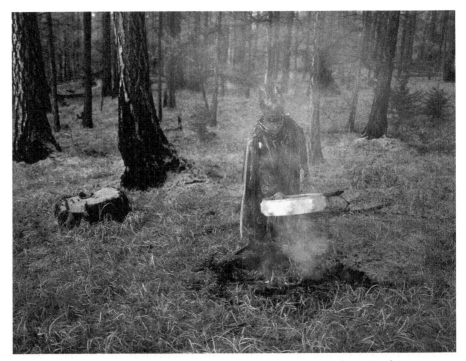

Fig. 5.1 A shamanic ritual in the taiga near Shadan, connecting with the spirit of the trees and of nature
© Yann Mingad @ Panos Pictures

into a sense of the universal, defined in terms of "oneness with respect to many" (Reese 1980: 597).

Morgan (2002) suggests that all conscious human activity is a form of spirituality, to the extent to which it is connected to the state of being. Above and beyond this conscious human activity, current discussions of spirituality typically focus on a level of self-awareness where this process becomes the unique center of knowledge and valuation, being tied with an awareness that we are self-creations. This self-aware spirituality is, on the one hand, a reminder of our loneliness as it bestows upon us the responsibility for our actions, yet on the other hand it connects us to other persons, to the environment, and to our sense of God, as our ego boundaries become permeable. Spirituality makes us aware of "a higher order of the universe, a meaning in the universe, in which we participate but which we do not control" (p. 61). Spirituality opens the doors to coping with illness, pain, suffering and death by providing a sense of changelessness in the midst of change, by transforming the tragic events of life through hope and love, and by connecting the human being with a deeper sensitivity of the spirit, higher aspirations of service, and a greater understanding of the cosmic purpose as creative goodness. Faith offers courage and direction in the midst of grief and pain; it offers a sense of purpose in the midst of suffering, health and illness. Each of the major religious worldviews provides systems of spiritual meaning-making which guide the interpretations of life and death.

Christianity and health

Healing is integral to the Christian way of life. In Roman Catholicism, Jesus was the manifestation of God's love and healed people physically, mentally, and spiritually, in his faith encounter with them. In Jesus' ministry of healing, sin and sickness were deeply connected; not only did he heal the skin but also the soul wherein the disease resided (Constantelos 1991). This healing mission of Christ is embodied in the mission of the church to reach out to the homeless, poor, sick, elderly and dying. In the Roman Catholic faith, the pastoral care of the sick is signified by the signing of the cross, which signifies the life, death and resurrection of Christ; the healing community of the church and the rituals that manifest this healing action; the healing guidance of the chaplain or the spiritual caregiver who facilitates the communication of emotional and spiritual care for the patient and their family; and the sacraments of healing, rituals which include the laying on of hands (praying for the sick person), anointing the sick person with oil which is blessed by the bishop during the Easter Vigil on Holy Saturday; and a prayer that corresponds with the condition of the sick person.

Judaism and health

Jewish spirituality is based on the foundation that all life is sacred and deeply interconnected in profound ways (Silberman 2005). According to the Jewish tradition, life is drained by worry, travel and sin, and is enriched by beautiful sights, sounds, and smells. One way of healing in the Jewish tradition is through connection with religious texts such as the Talmud (the primary body of Jewish legal opinions), the Shulhan Aruch (the codification of Jewish law), and the Jewish prayer book, offering insights about the soul, the presence of God, and the act of healing. The Jewish community and the rabbinical counselor offer the support and care for the patient through the communal responsibility of visiting the sick, known as Bikur Cholim. Prayer is one of the most accessible resources for the Jew during the illness experience. In addition, illness interrupts the normal flow of events and offers an opportunity for observance of the holy time, also referred to as Shabbat.

Hinduism and health

Hindu spirituality is founded on the quest for the Brahman or the ultimate external reality; this notion of an ultimate external reality is built on the foundation that the reality that is perceptible to the senses is not, perhaps, the ultimate reality, and that there is something that exists beyond the realm of the senses. Brahman is defined as "that which makes great" and is characterized as inaudible, invisible, unsmellable, indestructible, and without beginning or end (Koller and Koller 1991). The nature of Brahman is mysterious, elusive, and beyond the realms of the empirical world and thought.

This quest for the ultimate external reality is coupled with a quest for the ultimate Self referred to as Atman, the Self that exists as total consciousness, beyond the material constructions of the body and its need for food, the life of the food that feeds the body, the sensory perceptions, and the intellectual activities. The Self cannot be known as an object because, to the extent that it becomes an 'it,' it is no longer the ultimate knowing subject. It can be realized in direct self-awareness, through immediate experience, where it is illuminated by its own light. This impermeability of the Self, as an object, to sensory perceptions is further elucidated in the following excerpt from *Brihadaranyaka Upanisad*: "You cannot see the seer of seeing, you cannot hear the hearer of hearing, you cannot think the thinker of thinking, you cannot understand the understander of understanding. He is your Self which is in all things." (III.4.2, as cited in Koller and Koller 1991: 25). Thus the Self exists much beyond the realm of the body, in the context of health and healing. Hinduism draws upon this profound realization of the Self, which is indestructible and without any beginning or end. As opposed to the biomedical model, which is focused specifically on the body as the site of the disease and treatment, Hindu thought conceptualizes the body as an illusion or *maya*.

Furthermore, the Upanisads go on to elucidate the realization that the Brahman was identical with the Atman and that the same Self exists within all beings. Therefore by knowing the Atman, all is known, embodied in the famous teaching "Tat Tvan asi": "That which is the subtle essence, this whole world has for its Self ("Atman"). That is the true. That is the Atman. That art thou" (ibid.). Atman must be known through direct self-experience and, therefore, cannot be made publicly available to others through the demonstration of evidence, as it is only through direct experience that the Atman can be known. This emphasis on direct experience as the only legitimate entry point for self-realization contrasts with that of the biomedical model, which emphasizes the development of sophisticated tools and technologies of empirical observation that can detect the problem and treat it. As opposed to the biomedical model's emphasis on empirical observation as the tool for knowledge, Hinduism begins with the knowledge that observations perceived through the senses are ultimately an illusion, and suggests the need to transcend these material perceptions of reality to truly know the Atman and the Brahman.

Also, drawing upon the indestructible nature of the Self, Hinduism articulates the notion of Samsara, connected to the cycles of life, death and rebirth; Samsara not only denotes the wandering of the individual from life to life, but also the continuous flux in the world processes (Iyengar 1996, 2005). Hindu spirituality fundamentally contradicts some of the basic tenets of biomedicine because it emphasizes mind–body union and suggests that the separation of mind and body is an illusion.

One of the ways in which Hinduism directly addresses questions of health is Yoga. Yoga is concerned with the basic question of practicing a discipline that leads to self-awareness and to the attainment of wisdom. The *Purusa* or pure subject realizes that it is simply the spectator of *Prakriti* and not actually a part of it or connected to it. Suffering results from ignorance and the inability to separate the *Purusa* from the *Prakriti*, from the lack of the ultimate realization that the suffering self is merely an illusion. In other words, *Purusa* is really free from suffering, but this realization is prevented through ignorance (Koller and Koller 1991).

Thus Yoga is a disciplined method for removing this ignorance; it is prescribed as a form of self-discipline designed to overcome ignorance, laid out in Patanjali's *Yoga Sutra* (Iyengar 1996). Sage Patanjali describes Yoga as the restraint of *citta*, consciousness – which consists of mind (*manas*), intelligence (*buddhi*), and ego (*ahamkara*). *Sadhana* is established as a methodical, sequential means for the seeker to accomplish his/her four aims in life: right duty (*karma*), rightful purpose and means (*artha*), right inclinations (*kama*), and emancipation (*moksa*). The Yogic disciplines that channel the energies of the organs of action and the senses of perception in the right direction are *yama* (restraint) and *niyama* (practice).

The discipline of postures is referred to as *asana*, and it makes us knowledgeable about our bodies and capable to distinguish between motion and action. The combination of effort, concentration and balance in *asana* channels us to live in the present moment, "physically in the rejection of disease, mentally, by ridding our mind of stagnated thoughts or prejudices; and on a very high level where perception and action become one, by teaching us instantaneous correct action; that is to say, action which does not produce reaction" (p. 32). *Asanas* involve the positioning of the body as a whole with the involvement of both the body and the mind, and they act as bridges that connect the body and the mind, and the mind and the soul (ibid.). Iyengar further writes that "the body is the temple of the soul. It can truly become so if it is kept in health, clean and pure through the practice of asana" (ibid.).

The regulation of breath with attention is referred to as *pranayama*. *Pranayama* is the control of the breath which results in the expansion of the life force (ibid.). The practice of *pranayama* prepares the mind to meditate for the vision of the soul by removing the veil of ignorance covering the light of intelligence. It has three elements: inhalation, exhalation and retention of breath. These elements are carefully learned and controlled by elongating the breath and prolonging the retentive period, and by directing the precision of movements. By controlling the senses and the mind through the *asanas* and *pranayama*, the *citta* is drawn towards its source, the *atman*. This drawing inwards of the perception, mind, and intelligence is referred to as *pratyahara*. *Pratyahara* releases the seeker from the world of the senses so that she/he can embark on the journey of the soul; the senses take a reverse turn, now being guided by consciousness toward its own desire for self-realization. Complementing the five elements of *yama*, *niyama*, *asana*, *pranayama*, and *pratyahara*, the internal quest of Yoga comprises of concentration (*dharana*), meditation (*dhyana*), and total absorption (*Samadhi*). *Dharana* develops and sharpens intelligence, *dhyana* cleanses consciousness, and *samadhi* leads consciousness toward the soul. In the realm of Yoga, then, the ultimate quest is total absorption and the spiritual journey is interwoven with the cleansing of the bodily organs, of the senses of perception, of energy, and of the mind. Questions about the health and healing of the bodily organs are interwoven with processes of spiritual enlightenment and with the ultimate vision of the Atman.

Islam and health

In Islam, health is a valuable resource that must be maintained in order to serve God (Islamic Medicine). Cleanliness and personal hygiene are emphasized as important elements of preparing for prayer, five times a day, with bodies and clothes that are spotlessly clean (Abouleish and Athar at http://www.islam-usa.com/im3.html; Qur'an, 4: 43 and 5: 7). The human body is seen as existing in unison with the spirit, and therefore the spiritual pursuit of Islam is intrinsically tied to taking care of the body. *Salaat*, which roughly translates as "prayer," consists in washing all the exposed parts of the body, including hands, feet, face, mouth, nostrils, and so on five times a day, and in the recitation of the Qur'an – both of which have preventive and healing effects on the body. The association between prayer and healing is laid out in the Qur'an (10: 57): "O Mankind: There has come to you a direction from your Lord and a healing for the (disease) in your hearts – and for those who believe in guidance and mercy." Islamic fasting is seen as a way of disciplining the mind and body and training in self-restraint. Proper nutrition is considered integral to Islam, as the following verses reiterate: "O you mankind: Eat of what is lawful and good on earth" (2: 168); "Eat of the things which God has provided for you lawful and good, but fear God in whom you believe," "Forbidden to us are dead meat, blood and flesh of swine" (5: 4) and intoxicants (5: 93 and 2: 219). Furthermore, moderation is emphasized in verses such as: "But waste not by excess for God loves not the wasters," (7: 31) and "Eat of the good things we have provided for your sustenance, but commit no excess therein, lest my wrath should justly descend on you, and those whom descends my wrath do perish indeed" (20: 81).

Emphasizing the relevance of engaging in healthful and preventive actions, Prophet Mohammed (PBUH) states, "Everything good that happens to you (O Man) is from God, everything bad that happens to you is from your own actions." Illness brings human beings closer to God by making them aware of their own weaknesses and by making the patient aware of God through suffering. Accepting disease as the will of God and asking him to remove the affliction is recommended in the Qur'an: "If God touches thee with affliction, none can remove it – but He; if He touches thee with happiness He has power over all things" (6: 17). Islamic medicine starts with physiotherapy and diet, followed by the prescription

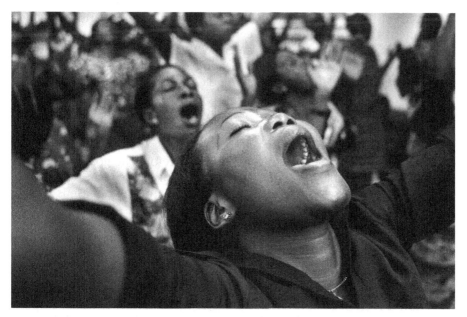

Fig. 5.2 Healing session in the Mama Olangi hospital. The medical staff use a mix of medication and prayers to treat their patients
© Dieter Telemans @ Panos Pictures

of drugs; it resorts to surgery only if all else fails. It has had a long development as a systematic tradition of healing.

A growing body of research on religiosity suggests that religion is positively associated with a greater sense of well-being, stronger self-esteem and better personal adjustment (Chamberlain and Hall 2001). For instance, in his comparison of the degree of religious involvement among one hundred mentally ill persons with one hundred similarly matched controlled persons, Stark (1971) observed that the mentally ill were significantly less likely to be religious as compared to the control group.

Discussion point 5.4

- How would you engage with ideas of spirituality from a biomedical framework?
- How would you engage with biomedicine from a spiritual framework?
- Are their possibilities of dialogue between biomedicine and spirituality without one co-opting the other? If so, how?

Alternative Systems

The Indian medical system

The Indian medical system addressed in this chapter is called Ayurveda. Ayurveda is a medical tradition that focuses on the prevention and treatment of illness; it is built on a theoretical component and an applied component that inform its practice. The epistemological and ontological foundations of Ayurveda are located within the realm of Hinduism, because Ayurveda as a system of healing developed within the philosophical realm of Hinduism. Ayurveda means knowledge of life or longevity. As a naturalistic healing system, Ayurvedic theory states that the body goes through changes that are necessary in order to purify and liberate the essences within the body. This purification and liberation of the essences happens naturally when the flow of life within the body is orderly and unobstructed (Trawick 1992). Therefore the goal is to ensure that the channels of flow remain open, clear, and free. The rightness of material life processes is the focus of Ayurveda and the disease is treated by facilitating these processes.

According to the Ayurvedic model, each person, and the cosmos, are made up of two components: *Prakriti*, a female–physical component, and *Purusa*, a male–spiritual component (ibid.). *Purusa* is the soul, which is indivisible, atomic, and immutable, while *Prakriti* is made up of several components and is subject to change. An individual's bodily construction is his/her *Prakriti* and consists of three *dosas* which are responsible for all good and bad bodily processes, *vata* (wind), *pitta* (bile), and *kapha* (phlegm). *Vata* drives all movement in the body, including breath and bowels; *pitta* is the essence of all health and light, for instance fever and healthy glow of eyes and skin; and *kapha* stabilizes and facilitates cohesion.

The word *dosa* also refers to fault, illness and suffering, suggesting that the body is primarily a site of pain. The body, a *Prakriti*, is the site of change, and hence is the locus of death. Any change from the normal state causes sickness and is seen as leading to death and destruction. The locus of change may vary, from between season, diet, or place to a person's temperament and habits. According to the Ayurvedic texts, *Susruta* and *Caraka*, time itself is change and leads all life forms to death. Also, life is change and, as such, is called "the flux." Change is inherently painful as it leads to death, and yet it also leads to the liberation of the soul.

The functioning of the body depends upon the flow of substances through the bodily channels and upon the transformations of these substances into one another. Each substance flows through its own channel and the goal of Ayurveda is to keep the physiological processes going, such that the substances may not flow over into alien channels. Sickness is caused when a channel is blocked and the substance normally flowing through that channel spills over into another. Therefore the goal of Ayurvedic practice is to ensure that the channels are unblocked. This unblocking is mostly achieved by seeking to bring the body to its natural state.

Take, for instance, the case of an Ayurvedic doctor treating a patient who has multiple blocked processes such as improperly functioning heart, dim eyes, blocked ears, numb feet, and what he considers as severed connection between the skin of the feet and the flesh (Trawick 1992). On the basis of his diagnosis, the physician prescribes orderly food directed toward quickening the body of the patient. He suggests that the patient should avoid eating tamarind because it is believed to cause dullness, and that she should avoid heavy food, which would keep feeling from flowing into her nerves. In summary, the Ayurvedic medical system connects mind and body in understanding the meanings of health and illness, and in approaching the treatment of illness.

The Chinese medical system

Porkert (1976) pointed out that traditional Chinese medicine follows an inductive and synthetic pathway to knowing, and is interested in function rather than in substratum. The emphasis of this system is not on determining causal pathways, but rather on developing empirical techniques for observing functions. With its reliance on the inductive and synthetic method, traditional Chinese medicine has developed organic energetics such as orbisiconography, sinarteriology, pharmaco-dynamics, and phase energetics. The primary task of inductive science is to determine the relationships between different functions, which are defined in qualitative statements tied to conventional standards of value.

The basic standards of value governing Chinese medicine are the polar combination of *yin/yang* and the cycle of Five Evolutive Phases (*wu-hsing*). Defined as polar aspects of interrelated phenomena, *yang* taps into the active, competitive, negative, centrifugal, aggressive and expansive components whereas *yin* taps into all that is contractive, positive, centripetal, structive, conservative, and substantive. The classification of all phenomena as *yin* and *yang* provides a comprehensive picture of effects which complete one another and effects which are neutral toward one another. The *yin* and *yang* classification is combined with the cycle of the Five Evolutive Phases. Four of these Five Evolutive Phases constitute critical phases in any evolutive activity, namely potential activity (Wood), actual activity (Fire), potential structivity (Metal) and actual structivity (Water). The Fifth Element is Earth and is considered to stand in neutral indifferentiation (Porkert 1976).

The traditional Chinese medical system, therefore, focuses on establishing systems of technical correspondence in terms of the basic quality standards. Orbisiconography describes the interactions of the functional orbs of the organism, sinarteriology describes the relationships among the physiological signs, pathological symptoms, and therapeutic measures, phase energetics suggests criteria for examining the influence of cosmic (i.e. meteorological and immunological) functions on those of the organism. These systems of technical correspondences provide the theoretical framework for the applied disciplines of Chinese medicine such as pharmacotherapy, the use of drugs derived from animals, plants, and minerals, and acu-moxi-therapy, which focuses on the use of needles or cauters to sensitive spots at the body surface.

Placing the focus on functions, the Chinese physician uses four diagnostic methods to achieve a complete appraisal of the functional situation of the patient: inspection, interrogation, olfaction, and palpation (Porkert 1976). In his comparison of Chinese and Western medicine, Porkert points out that the former can offer specific therapy that is keyed to the functions and thus responsive to the differentiated symptoms, as compared to Western medicine, which can often offer only an unspecific treatment because no specific organic disorder can be diagnosed. Chinese medicine offers diagnosis and treatment for so-called chronodemic diseases, which typically flare up over vast territories and, according to Western medicine, are probably caused by virus. In Chinese medicine, these diseases are explained in terms of deficiencies or redundancies of energy in certain orbs that are conditioned by current immunological condition. Finally, Porkert points out that Chinese medicine offers early diagnosis and prevention of organic diseases such as cardiac failure, diabetes or cancer, which are preceded by stages of growing functional disorders. In Chinese medicine, if patients are given an early diagnosis and specific treatment that corresponds to it, they can be prevented from entering an advanced stage of the disease.

The paradigm of systematic correspondence in the traditional Chinese system of healing focuses on the entire human organism, including its mental and physical states, and its relationship with the greater whole of the social and natural environment of the human being (Unschuld 1992). What is important in this systematic correspondence is the link between the individual and his/her environment. It is understood that individual health exists in relationship with the environment. Geomancy is a practical application of a system of correspondence, and is one way of conceptualizing the relationship between humans and their environment, seeking to channel or alter natural processes for the purposes of curing illness and achieving the well-being of the individual (Seaman 1992).

The macrocosm–microcosm analogy drives much of Chinese geomancy, such that physiological and pathological processes are interdependent with cyclic astronomical, meteorological, climatic and epidemiological factors. The macrocosm–microcosm analogy plays out in the relationship between human health and the rhythms of the earth. Therefore, the alterations of the earth bring repercussions upon the health of individual human beings Seaman 1992). Geomancy typically involves experts at two levels: (a) the professor who uses the theoretical models of Chinese geomancy to understand the relationship between space, time, and energetic forces; and (b) the craftsman who applies the principles of geomancy to the common problems of individuals and actually exhumes the bones during the secondary burial.

Recent ethnographic accounts demonstrate the adaptive nature of the Chinese medical system, documenting ways in which it has adapted so as to incorporate elements of the biomedical model. This line of research also documents the current popularity of the Chinese medical system not only in China, Taiwan, Hong Kong and Singapore, where this form of medicine has been traditionally practiced, but also, and increasingly, in other parts of the world, including the US, Canada, UK, where the bio-medical model seems to dominate. Therefore health communication scholarship ought to examine the interplay of culture and structure in the use of the Chinese medical system, in its relationship with the biomedical model, and in the role it enjoys in the realm of global politics.

Native American systems of healing

For the Native American systems of healing, the traditional healer was the shaman, a qualified person who has the knowledge to deal with illness in the realm of the sacred. The shaman is singled out from childhood for special religious training about the sacred ways of the native American. The purpose of the shaman's life is to find the cause of an illness and treat it; and he is typically knowledgeable about earth, humans and nature, seeking to determine the spiritual causes of the illness, above and beyond the physical causes. Holistic medicine allows the shaman to look at, and treat, the multiple causes of the illness; she may rely for instance on a dream or a vision. Because the illness is typically brought about by an imbalance, the shaman administers both physical and spiritual medicine that attempts to restore the balance. In this worldview, death cannot be averted by the shaman if one is meant to die. Such unnecessary efforts at averting death may be seen as ways of affronting nature; death is not to be feared, but one is meant to appreciate life and the loved ones. Natural medicine is a major component of the healing arts of native Americans and the basis of the healing lies in nature and natural processes. The herb medicines used in healing are natural, are usually picked through natural processes, and are distributed and administered via rituals. The specific beliefs, steps and processes used by the shaman in healing vary from tribe to tribe.

Socio-Structural Contexts of Healing and Curing

The alternative ways of healing and curing discussed in this section are located within a socio-structural context that engages with the modernist paradigm; although the epistemologies these systems draw upon indeed predate the Enlightenment project, our accessibility to these epistemologies is very much located in the realm of the modernist framework (Baer, Singer and Susser 2003). In other words, the popularity of these various forms of healing and curing is embedded within the politics of capitalism in late modernity. Spirituality in this sense also has a price and can be purchased in the global economy. To the extent that you can shell out the money, you can go to a weekend retreat, immerse yourself in spirituality and come back refreshed to participate in the global economy and con-tribute to its effectiveness as a productive worker.

The logic of capitalism that constitutes the discursive space suggests that spirituality is the luxury of the rich and upper middle-class corporate citizens of the global economy who can shell out the exorbitant sums of money required to purchase it. Yoga and Ayurveda have been reduced to techniques for the rich to give them moments of peace in the New Age culture, accompanied by the widespread use of Yoga and meditation, in the form of workplace fitness programs which seek to balance the over-worked employee. In this context, the locus of the problem is shifted, from the structural imbalances and unhealthy workplace demands, to the management of the self through spiritually accessible technologies and techniques. Spirituality has become the next "in thing," much like a fashion statement that can be work by those who have the purchasing power to get it.

For instance, consider the popularity of Deepak Chopra in the United States. The website of the Chopra center for healing opens with a link that connects you to the Chopra store. As you browse through the Chopra store, you can buy candles at $70.00 a set, the Chopra relaxation CDs at $285.00, and the Chopra audio kit at $55.00. As you think of this "New Age" social class, you wonder where they get the purchasing power to buy these instruments for achieving a mind–body balance. As you browse through the website further, you get your answer to this question. You realize that many of the Chopra well-being courses are targeted toward celebrities and corporate executives, and to the upper and upper middle classes, who can afford to buy this packaged commodity of New Age living.

Also, consider the accessibility of Yoga and the structural inequities attached to this accessibility. As we hear celebratory stories about the rising popularity of Yoga in Hollywood studios and in the boardrooms of multinational organizations, subaltern communities in India, the socio-cultural point of origin of Yoga, have minimal access to the epistem-ologies, ontologies, tools and techniques of Yoga, as these have been systematically backgrounded from the discursive space through tools of science and rationality. Furthermore, epistemologies of Indian and Chinese systems have been systematically erased as techniques from these traditions have been extracted and incorporated into the biomedical model. The establishment of the complementary medicine division of the National Institute of Health is one such move, which seeks to co-opt the techniques of other healing systems under the dominant scientific frame-work and study them under this framework (Baer, Singer and Susser 2003). Furthermore, creating a centralized structure within the National Institutes of Health becomes a device for monitoring and managing these other ways of knowing by the larger biomedical and scientific–technical industries. The development of clinical trials to test the effectiveness of meditation, for instance, removes meditation from its epistemological roots and does violence to it by placing it within the parameters of the scientific enterprise; epistemologically, it co-opts meditation by funda-mentally denying its roots and interjecting it into a dominant scientific language. In this sort of approach that is prevalent today, the biomedical model continues to enjoy and retain its privilege, while other techniques such as acupuncture and meditation are incorporated into its system under the name of holistic medicine; but their epistemological roots are obliterated and erased from the discursive space. In the next section we look at an alternative framework for conceptualizing healing and health that is not based on co-opting, but on the possibilities of engaging with many voices and simultaneously respecting the epistemological roots of these different alternatives and opening up to the possibilities of their co-existence. We look at polymorphism as a way of approaching parallel and meaningful healing and curing systems.

Discussion point 5.5

- How would you locate yourself with respect to the different systems of healing and curing?
- What are your responses to these different ways of approaching health?
- What does your response to these systems of healing and curing tell you about yourself and your values?

Polymorphism

Polymorphism focuses on the many realities that co-exist in the experience of the world, engaging with these realities in understanding the world and acting in it. In other words, polymorphism articulates that there are many truths in this world, and that these truths often co-exist in complementary relationships rather than in dichotomous either/or categories (Dutta-Bergman and Doyle 2001). The thrust of polymorphism, therefore, is spaces of harmonious co-existence rather than antagonistic battles based on the either/or categories. Resisting the notion of polar opposites such that the existence of one precludes the existence of the other, polymorphism touches upon multiplicity and explores the possibilities of dialogue. Mikhail Bakhtin (1981) sensitized us to this concept of multiple possibilities and interpretations in any social situation in his discussion of *heteroglossia*.

The way we see the world depends on how we approach it; the lens used by the researcher in locating and describing the practices of the world is fundamental to the way the world is constructed (Bakhtin 1981; Cheney 2000; Dutta-Bergman and Doyle 2001). A polymorphic approach to health communication is based on the understanding that the various systems of healing that are available to human beings work in harmonious and complementary ways. Unlike the dominant view of health and healing that foregrounds the biomedical model, simultaneously ruling out other models and approaches, the polymorphic approach highlights spaces of multiple existences that tend to overlap. For instance, in the example of Basanti presented in the introduction, the seeking out of various types of treatments to the various conditions reflects a polymorphic worldview where the type of treatment sought is contextually

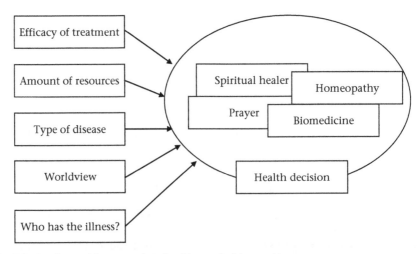

Fig. 5.3 A polymorphic approach to healthcare decision-making

defined, and various types of treatments are simultaneously sought out by the diseased individual, depending upon the type of disease, the amount of resources available, the efficacy of the treatment, the worldview of the individual, and who in the family is ill. In other words, various systems of healing and curing become part of a complex web of meanings.

The meanings and interpretations of these systems of healing are inter-dependent, drawing upon their contextual location with respect to the individual. In making sense of this complex system, the polymorphic approach provides openings for dialogue. It is, after all, in this dialogical space that patients seek out varieties of treatments, and providers con-tinually flow from one system to another and work with each other in delivering a meaningful experience to the patient. At the crux of the poly-morphic approach lies the interrogation of the dominant biomedical framework as a monolithic way of knowing the world and existing in it. This also suggests that, although the singular dominance of the biomed-ical model is challenged, it should also be acknowledged for the solutions it does provide for the patient. The relevance of this dialogical space in engaging different worldviews on health and healing is reflected in the following excerpt from Lori Alford's book *The Scalpel and the Silver Bear*, where she discusses her journeys as a Navajo tribe member in the world of biomedicine, as a surgeon (2000: 144–5):

> I could see both sides of the story. One side – the trained medical practitioner, who fathoms the body's mysteries as a detective directs a beam of light into a dark room to look for clues about the source of physical disharmony – said, *Roll her into the OR now!* But the Navajo part of me, who had once been a little girl, could see the inappropriateness of interfering. Navajo eyes warned: The beauty of the body would be disturbed. A surgical knife would defile an intact, minia-ture universe, with rules and systems that evolved naturally over millennia. I could see the sacredness of that body, how all its many parts are one harmonic system.

In her journey through the biomedical system as a member of the Navajo community, Dr Alford presents to us reflexive moments where she goes back and forth between the worldviews and engages them in dialogue. On the one hand, she is trained as a medical practitioner who sees the relevance of invasive surgical procedures, and on the other hand, she sees through her Navajo eyes the violence of the knife, which defiles the sacredness of the body. It is in this space that Dr Alford discusses the possibilities of dialogue:

> My Western medical training told me that the eight-year-old girl could die if we did not remove her appendix right away. But her grandmother's fears and objections were just as real and true. The two worlds were colliding. The solution lay somewhere in the uncharted territory between them. (p. 144)

A polymorphic approach to health communication theorizing and application development focuses on locating and harnessing the multiplicities of communication, on integrating the rich body of communication theories, and simultaneously retaining their diversity (Dutta-Bergman 2004a). As articulated in the previous sections, no one level of analysis (intrapersonal, interpersonal, small group, organizational, or mass-mediated) and no one paradigmatic approach is adequately positioned to capture the complexity of communication; for the study of health communication processes to be meaningful, multiple levels of communication from multiple perspectives engaging multiple contexts of healing and curing need to be simultaneously activated. In this polymorphic approach, health communication is a complex web of interrelated treatments and worldviews that continually interact with each other, enriching and metamorphosing each other, and offering continuous opportunities for growth through dialogue.

Discussion point 5.6

- How does the polymorphic worldview enmesh with your view of health, healing and curing? Please locate your response in the realm of the broader cultural norms and practices which constitute you.
- How would you put into place a polymorphic approach to health communication in looking at the healing and curing of disease? More specifically, what steps would you take in order to create and sustain a polymorphic approach?

Conclusion

This chapter demonstrates the relevance of the culture-centered approach to our understanding of health and illness and to the approaches we take to them. Medical systems are culturally situated, and are intrinsically tied in with values, embedded in certain ways of looking at the world. A polymorphic approach to health communication opens up the dialogical space, and encourages the exploration of the intersections of the varying systems, the overlaps between them, and those intertwined spaces of medical theorizing and practice where these systems co-exist in meaningful ways. Ultimately, the chapter provides an entry point for the consideration of alternative models of health, illness, curing and healing that lie outside the rubric of the traditional physician–patient relationship, which has been at the center of much work within the field. For instance, how does the relationship between the Ayurvedic practitioner and his/her patient differ from the traditional doctor–patient relationship conceptualized in the literature? How do patients in polymorphic contexts negotiate the multiple relationships with biomedical practitioners, Ayurvedic practitioners and acupuncturists? These questions may be answered once we start exploring the complexity of health communication experiences and treatments available to patients and used by them.

6 Culture and Marginalization

Chapter objectives

In this chapter, we will:

- understand the nature of marginalization
- describe the key characteristics of marginalization
- examine the link between culture, structure, and marginalization

One of the key elements of the culture-centered approach is its emphasis on marginalized contexts (Dutta-Bergman 2004a, 2004b; Dutta and Basu 2007). Marginalized contexts refer to those cultural settings that are typically rendered voiceless and invisible in mainstream discourse and are structurally deprived of material resources. The culture-centered approach challenges the grand narrative of the dominant paradigm of health communication and examines the ways in which these dominant articulations of health serve the status quo and silence the voices of marginalized communities. It argues that communication is central to the experience of marginalization of certain communities; economic marginalization typically goes hand in hand with communicative marginalization such that communities without access to material resources are also rendered voiceless through their inaccess to communication platforms where policies are debated, implemented, and evaluated. In other words, the culture-centered approach argues that the ways in which we communicate about issues of health in mainstream discourse further contributes to marginalization by reinforcing certain dominant messages about the marginalized communities and by restricting the resources available to them.

We will first discuss the experiences of marginalization and identify common features of the state of being marginalized. This exercise will help us understand the question: What does it mean to be marginalized? The discussion of the experiences of marginalization will be connected to the health outcomes experienced in marginalized communities and to the ways in which cultures are marginalized. We have already seen marginalization at the cultural level in the previous chapter, where the dominance of the biomedical model is placed in the backdrop of the subordination of alternative ways of healing and curing, such as the Chinese and Indian medical systems. In our discussion of culture, we will examine how culture continues to play an important role in determining who gets to say what to whom and how the control over the discursive space is connected with issues of power. The symbolic constitutions of discursive spaces are situated in the realm of the material bases of such spaces.

The chapter will argue that marginalization is played out both structurally and communicatively. The communicative enactment of marginalization will be discussed both in relation to communicative processes and in relation to the messages that circulate in social systems. The discussion of power and structure will touch upon social inequalities in healthcare and the ways in which these social inequalities are maintained by the healthcare system. We will discuss issues of access and inaccess to healthcare resources and examine the nature of structural violence in marginalized communities. The last section of the chapter will present the ways in which marginalization is communicatively enacted. In this section, those communicative messages and processes will be discussed that are inherently linked with marginalization.

Marginalization

What is marginalization? Marginalization refers to being at the periphery of a dominant system (Abraham 1993; Dutta-Bergman 2004a, 2004b; Farmer 1992, 1999; Kleinman 1980; Kleinman, Das and Lock 1997). Therefore being marginalized implies a status of inaccess to the dominant healthcare system. Individuals and groups who are marginalized in the healthcare system are unable to secure health resources and typically have a minimal say in the designing and implementation of healthcare policy. Marginalization occurs both at the individual and community levels. In most instances, individuals experiencing marginalization at the individual level typically reside in communities that are marginalized.

Box 6.1   The story of Roberto

As a migrant worker in El Paso, Texas, Roberto works in a farm from 8 am in the morning to about 7 pm at night. During the day, he hardly ever gets a break from his busy work schedule. He is not conversant in English and is not aware of any health resources available to him in town. In his conversations about his health, Roberto states that he is worried because he does not know where to go if something was to happen to him; he cannot really speak English or find his way around the area. He also says that he saves up almost all his money to take it back home and can barely make ends meet. His wife and children live back in Mexico and have limited access to healthcare. Roberto cannot read the local newspapers or the pamphlets that are handed out by the healthcare workers.

What does Roberto's story tell us about the nature of marginalization? What do we learn from this story about the ways in which individuals, groups, and communities are marginalized and about what it means to be marginalized? What roles can we, as health communicators, play in addressing issues of marginalization?

Roberto's health and the health of his family are intrinsically tied with his ability to find work. As a migrant farm worker, he is unaware of any health resources available to him. He states that he sometimes feels anxious at the thought of not knowing what to do in situations of health emergency. Roberto's situation may be classified as one of being marginalized within the US healthcare system, marked by the absence of health resources that are integral to survival. Note that this condition is also marked by lack of access to information and to communication resources that are considered to be the basic elements of health capacity. Not only does Roberto have minimal access to healthcare resources, but he is also far removed from his community and not aware of the availability of support and resources in it. His condition is one of informational marginalization.

Marginalization is embodied in the position of being under, of being silenced, of being without a voice and of being without resources. This positionality of not having a voice is epitomized in the following articulation of a marginalized community member from Panama, "the community has no voice; here there are no leaders" (Narayan et al. 2000: 107). In the realm of health communication, marginalization refers primarily to the condition of inaccess to health resources, to the organizations which implement the distribution of health resources and to those policy platforms which determine the allocation of these resources. Consider the experiences of an unemployed man from Ivanovo, Russia: "Before, medical treatment was free, now one has to pay for everything" (Narayan et al. 2000: 102). This excerpt reflects the fundamental lack of access to basic health resources. The condition of marginalization is also marked by exclusion from those processes which determine how health policies are evaluated and critiqued, an exclusion manifested in the limited access of the marginalized actors to the discursive space of health policies.

Communicatively, marginalization refers to the condition of being unseen and unheard; it is the condition of not having a voice in the state of affairs that affect the individual, his/her social group, and/or his/her community (Dutta-Bergman 2004a, 2004b). In other words, it reflects a state of existence in which an individual or a group does not have communicative presence within the mainstream discursive space and within those policy platforms that regulate the distribution of health resources. This lack of communicative presence is accompanied by the lack of access to those basic health resources that are required for survival. In the context of healthcare, marginalization is therefore indicative of the inaccess to basic health care resources such as basic medical supplies, preventive resources, and hospital staff. It is this inaccess that influences the health outcomes of the marginalized. Worth noting here is the complementary relationship between health resource marginalization and communicative infrastructure marginalization, both of which are typically clustered within certain demographic indicators such as social class, racial identity, gender, nationality, and so on. For instance, the working poor in the US have limited healthcare resources, and also have limited access to communication platforms where policies are debated and discussed. Similarly, the digital divide research suggests that Hispanic communities with minimal access to healthcare resources within the US also face the problems of the digital divide, where they have limited access to communication technologies that might equip them with health information and knowledge about vital health resources (Dutta-Bergman 2006).

In addition to having minimal resources, marginalized sectors of the globe typically have minimal say in the development and deployment of healthcare policies that affect their lives. As members of resource-starved sectors, marginalized people are typically placed at the peripheries of democratic processes and denied access to those channels of communication that are critical to the functioning of democracies. So-called participatory channels in democracies serve the agendas of those with access to resources and to the communicative platforms that can shape local, national and transnational agendas. This is reflected in the following observation of a Guatemalan participant: "these community organizations do not listen at the local level, only help the better off" (Narayan et al. 2000: 154). Typically, being marginalized is indicative of this basic lack of access to the resources of mainstream civil societies that impact and monitor the local, national and transnational agendas, including agendas related to health. Sekovici, a rural participant in the Narayan project, states: "nobody asks the people anything" (p. 182). This sense of being silenced is further reflected in the following excerpt: "sometimes they do not even let you talk. They say that they already know the problem and that they will solve it" (p. 190). The interpenetration of communicative and health-resource marginalization is further evident in Dutta-Bergman's dialogues with Santali communities of Bengal (2004a: 256): "where do we have anything babu? Where do Santal's [sic] get to say anything?" The experience of not having anything goes hand in hand with the experience of not getting to say anything.

The agency of the marginalized is backgrounded in the dominant healthcare discourse in such a way that the individuals in question who are marginalized do not feel as though they have a say in the communication of health to them. According to a rural participant from Zawyet Sultan, Egypt in the Narayan project, this feeling of being silenced is reflected in the notion that "only God listens to us" (Narayan et al. 2000: 182). As pointed out in the previous paragraph, the marginalized are typically constructed to exist in a position of being communicated to, rather than being engaged as active participants in the discursive space. Health campaigns, for instance, address marginalized communities as target audiences of health campaigns developed by outside experts (Dutta-Bergman 2005a, 2005b; Dutta 2006). For instance, in an article discussing multicultural health campaigns, Witte and Morrison (1995: 240) suggest that "fatalism is an important variable to consider in health communication campaigns because people who believe they have no control over their health will have not motivation to engage in health promotion or disease prevention activities." In this instance, the fatalism of the target audience is categorized as the variable that needs to be addressed in order to carry out the health promotion effort. Furthermore, Witte and Morrison go on to portray East Asian cultural beliefs in the following terms, "reluctant to disagree or contradict those with high status. May say 'yes' even when they do not understand. Multidrug therapy is common and they like colored medication. Injections are popular" (p. 232). The "other" in this context is portrayed in childlike terms, unlikely to disagree and likely to prefer colored medications.

This exhumation of agency in the dominant discourse serves the hegemonic control of dominant actors over the discursive and material spaces; in other words, the political economy of health campaigns is justified by the portrayals of the marginalized populations as being without agency and hence in need for interventions manufactured by the experts. As a result, much of the health communication that does take place in the context of marginalized populations is top-down, flowing from the discursive spaces at the center to the marginalized locales of underserved societies; health campaigns are manufactured by experts located in the US or UK, in collaboration with the national elite. The construction of the marginalized in terms of passivity is used as rationale for the deployment of communicative strategies directed at the marginalized. In this context, the subject position of the marginalized serves as the target audience of top-down messages to be acted upon, to be targeted through communication strategies, and to be altered through one-way messages. Such messages are directed at the marginalized, attempting to change their individual behaviors which are typically treated as causes of poor health. This is exemplified in the articulations of Witte and Morrison (1995) discussed earlier, where the authors talk about developing communication strategies to modify the unhealthy behaviors of the target public.

Discussion point 6.1

- In your experience, what are the ways in which we communicate about hunger?
- What are your perceptions about the causes of hunger? Where do you think these perceptions come from?
- What is the role of communication in the context of hunger?
- What roles do you think we can play as health communicators in addressing questions of hunger?

The experiences of marginalization

Marginalized individuals and groups share certain common experiences that distinctly identify their state of being marginalized. One of the key experiences in marginalized communities is lack of access. This lack of access is played out in a variety of ways, each one demonstrating inequities in the distribution of basic resources of health. In other words, marginalization becomes evident in the form of inequity – where the access of an individual or community to a set of resources is starkly different from the access enjoyed by some other individual or community (Atkinson and Micklewright 1992; Kawachi et al. 1994; Kennedy, Kawachi and Prothrow-Stith 1996; Wilkinson 1994; also, both studies conducted by Kawachi in 1999). Some economic theorists argue that conditions of utmost marginalization such as famines are often caused by human acts of marginalizing rather than by the absence or depletion of natural resources (Sen 1999). In other words, basic structural deprivations are created and sustained by structural inequities and unequal distributions of resources, created and sustained by unhealthy policies which are, in turn, created and sustained by those in positions of power (Sen 1999). In his book, *Famines in India*, Bhatia equates famines with poverty, arguing that during the colonial rule of India the frequency of famines increased substantively because people were rendered poor by the land taxes imposed on them to raise money for the financing of the Indian Army, and by the introduction of a market system which made grain available at a price they could not afford.

One of the fundamental characteristics of marginalization is the lack of access to food. Members of marginalized communities often discuss the lack of access to basic food supplies that are central to maintaining good health; the experience of going to bed hungry and of being unable to feed one's children are quintessential to the narrative of marginalization. The following excerpt from a woman in Macedonia (Narayan et al. 2000: 44) narrates this:

> Up to a few years ago, I didn't even ask myself the question: What shall I cook? Today there are times I do not have anything to put on the stove and this is very difficult for a mother [crying]

This lack of food and the pain that comes with hunger is articulated in the following excerpt from Dutta-Bergman's journey in the spaces of rural Bengal (2004b: 1112):

> How can I stand their pain? How can I see them go hungry? I am the father. I gave them birth. They look at me, they think I will take care of them. But I can't. I can't even offer them food. I think about this. I think. But then, what do I do?

Here a father discusses his experiencing the pain of not being able to feed his children. For him, health is fundamentally the ability to provide food for his children, and it is this basic capacity that he does not have because of the inequities in the system. This pain of not being able to feed one's child is further elucidated in the narrative of a mother: "often she has to decide who will eat, she or her son" (p. 35). According to a participant from Senegal, "your hunger is never satisfied, your thirst is never quenched; you can never sleep until you are no longer tired" (Narayan et al. 2000: 35). Similarly, according to a participant from Vietnam, the experience of going to bed hungry is a frequent occurrence: "In the mornings, eat sweet potatoes, work. At lunch, go without. In the evenings, eat

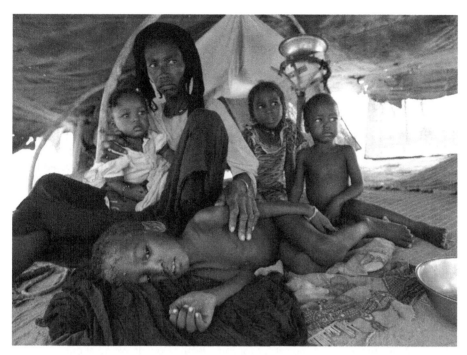

Fig. 6.1 Hunger in Kalahandi, India

sweet potatoes, sleep" (ibid.). Note the juxtaposition of hunger in the backdrop of the work of marginalized community members and of their ability to find work. News reports in India often discuss hunger-related deaths in resource-starved areas (http://ndtv.com/template/template.asp?template=Starvation&slug=Food+elusive+for+%5C).

Communities face inaccess in terms of the sheer availability of food resources in community spaces. For participants in marginalized spaces, food has become a commodity that has to be purchased at a price, and it is their very poverty that marks their inability to find food. For Nimai, a rural participant in my work (Dutta-Bergman 2004b: 1113):

> Fruits like bananas and apples are important for them [referring to his children]. I know I should feed them an apple or a banana. I walk by the fruit stall every day, you know, when I go to work. Money. But where do I get the money? . . . I have to get work every day so they are not hungry. Especially, during slow time, there isn't any work.

Although Nimai knows that it is important to feed fruits to his children, he points out that he really can't do this, as the fruits that grow naturally in the region have to be purchased at a price at the local markets. Notice that the ability to secure food as a commodity in the marketplace is intrinsically connected to the ability to secure work; health, therefore, has become a commodity that can be purchased in the modern economy by workers who supply their labor to the economy. However,

Box 6.2   The story of Fan Wang

In August 2006, the Associated Press carried a story on Fan Wang, a mother from Hangzhou province in China who had poisoned her four children and then killed herself after having gone hungry for about two months. The story discussed how Fan sold her blood to the local blood banks, which operated illegally, in order to make ends meet and feed her children. Then, one day, she felt weak and started having fevers. She no longer could muster the energy to walk the six or so miles to the blood bank to sell her blood. A few weeks went by and she managed to scrape up whatever food she had stored through the year. But then she was out of food and didn't really have the ability to walk or move around. The social worker who visited the village every few months heard about Fan from other villagers who visited the clinic and went to pay her a visit. At her very first visit, she speculated that Fan probably was infected with HIV/AIDS, like many other members of the village who were selling their blood at the illegal blood banks. The social worker knew that the rainy season was approaching and a few more weeks would pass before she could get any help for Fan. She assured Fan that she would be back with further assistance. In late October, when the social worker was finally able to arrange a visit to the village, she heard the story of how Fan had fed rat poison to her four children and then poisoned herself.

What do we learn from Fan's story about our roles as health communicators? What do you think are the underlying causes for Fan's death? How do we go about addressing these causes?

in resource-starved contexts, work is difficult to come by, and therefore food becomes an inaccessible commodity.

Although in a marginal yet growing body of work in health communication this lack of food has been articulated as one of the fundamental health capacities that are absent in marginalized communities in the global healthcare system, much of the dominant discussions of health communication look at individual behaviors as roots of health problems and background these issues of structural inaccess (Dutta-Bergman 2004a, 2005a). My own review of the health communication literature demonstrates that most health campaigns focus on individual behaviors as roots of health problems, and shift attention away from issues of structural inequities (Dutta-Bergman 2005a). Although, when asked about their health, members of marginalized communities often primarily talk about the experience of hunger, much of the dominant health communication framework does not really address this issue in conceptualizing health and in discussing health communication interventions. In summary, discourses that emerge from marginalized contexts suggest that, for members of many marginalized communities, the health of the individual, family or group is fundamentally tied to this ability to secure basic food supplies; this fundamental articulation of hunger challenges the dominant discourses of what it means to be healthy.

Discussion point 6.2

• Think about a marginalized community in the US. What are the ways in which this particular community is marginalized? What are the messages in mainstream discourse which marginalize this community? How?
• Imagine that you were to develop a health communication project which challenges the marginalization of this particular community. How would you go about developing a communication program which addresses the marginalization in mainstream discourse?

In other instances, members of marginalized spaces point out that they have minimal access to hospitals, physicians, and basic medical supplies. The following heart-rending story about the death of a small boy in a poverty-stricken area of Ghana expresses this lack of basic health resources (Narayan et al. 2000: 45):

> Take the death of this small boy this morning, for example. The boy died of measles. We all know he could have been cured at the hospital. But the parents had no money and so the boy died a slow and painful death, not of measles, but of poverty.

In this instance, the death of the small boy is directly related to lack of access to a hospital; he died because his parents could not afford the costs of taking him to the hospital. In her research with the homeless in Ohio, Harter draws our attention to the basic supplies of healthcare, which are unavailable to the homeless. Similarly, Basu et al. demonstrate that the homeless members of a small community in Indiana face problems in accessing the mental health system. In his work with the members of a marginalized community in rural India, Dutta-Bergman (2004a, 2004b) demonstrates that community members face healthcare inaccess in the form of unavailability of doctors, unavailability of necessary vaccinations, and unavailability of necessary medical supplies. Reba, member of an impoverished Santali community in rural Bengal, states that:

> I don't even think of going to the state hospital. I went many times, waited in long lines, lost a whole day. . .What's the use if I have to pay Rs. 40 to get the medicine after waiting in long line to see the doctor, and losing Rs. 15 because I missed the day's work? (Dutta-Bergman, 2004b: 256)

In this case, although free medicines are promised, most of these medicines are beyond the economic reach of the marginalized community members. This is articulated in the following narrative of corruption at the local hospitals: "They get medicine, all the expensive one. But then they channel them out through the backdoors and sell them to the dispensary across the road at a cheaper price" (Dutta-Bergman 2004b: 256). Although policy discourse talks about making health resources accessible, the reality about health resources is far removed from the policy talk. Corrupt elite practices limit the basic health resources available to community members.

Given that much of healthcare in the capitalist social order is tied to the ability of individuals to find work, marginalization is also experienced in the inability of individuals to find work that would provide them with the economic resources to access healthcare. Healthcare as a resource needs to be purchased, and is tied in with the productivity of the worker in the social system. In other words, those at the margins are doubly limited – by their inability to access healthcare resources and by their inability find access to those economic resources that might provide them access to such healthcare. Furthermore, the cycle of poverty gets perpetuated as individuals find themselves in positions of minimal access to those economic resources that are quintessential to securing the competencies and skills necessary to find jobs in the global economy. The absence of jobs and the absence of resources such as educational ones, which would facilitate the ability to find work, limit the overall healthcare access of individuals in marginalized communities.

Marginalization is also experienced in the realm of access to the political processes that influence the fate of the marginalized. Members of marginalized communities often discuss the ways in which the key international and national political actors serve elite interests and are dismissive of the interests and needs of the marginalized. Legislative and judiciary systems operate in a discursive space which is typically inaccessible to the marginalized. Political platforms on key issues in the global system typically operate through bureaucratic processes that limit opportunities for participation and use communicative tools that are only accessible to the elite actors. This elite bias is also reflected in the widespread growth of civil society platforms in capitalist societies that typically continue to reflect the agendas of the elite rather than serving as conduits for expressing the concerns of the marginalized. For instance, multiple non-governmental organizations operating in the South continue to reflect the agendas of dominant global agencies such as World Health Organization and the United States Agency for International Development (USAID) rather than offering participatory platforms for expressing the voices of the marginalized. In his work on civil society, Dutta-Bergman (2005b) argues that mainstream civil society platforms operate as hegemonic devices that co-opt the participatory power of the marginalized rather than offering opportunities for participation directed at affecting tangible social change in the communities.

Ultimately, the experience of marginalization is marked by the absence of a voice in policy platforms and in academic work that reflects the current state of knowledge about the marginalized sectors of the world. Marginalization is marked by erasure from spaces where policies are articulated, debated and evaluated. Policies are often constructed for the marginalized without creating opportunities for their participation, and are often justified by the argument that the marginalized need to be represented by dominant social actors. For instance, in the US, policies regarding the homeless are passed and implemented without the participation of the homeless themselves to such policy platforms. Similarly, the academic literature in health communication targeting marginalized sectors of the globe typically takes a top-down approach and presents discourses that continue to portray the marginalized actors as being passive and in need of interventions dictated by the elite actors (see for instance Witte and Morrison 1995).

Elite actors at the center first decide the key objectives for messages targeting the marginalized. Based on these predetermined conceptions about the nature of the problem, top-down communication is sent out to the marginalized spaces. Therefore the positions of the sender and of the receiver get fixed within the discursive space, being intertwined with access to power. Marginalized populations exist to be written about, to be spoken to, and to be worked on by the elite actors at the center, who typically have the power or have access to the discursive sites of power. The goal, ultimately, is to find ways to control the outcomes in marginalized spaces; the targeted outcomes are those desired by the privileged actors at the center. As a consequence, much of the communication that occurs in the context of the marginalized sectors of the globe focuses on serving elite interests and biases, at the same time further marginalizing the marginalized through the use of the discursive space to construct the target audience as undesirable, as lacking in something, as marked by an absence of agency. To the extent that the marginalized can be portrayed in terms of absences, these absences serve as discursive tools that justify the inequities. In the colonial context, for example, to the extent that the colonies could be portrayed as primitive spaces that needed the message of enlightenment, imperial presence in these colonies could be justified.

Discussion point 6.3

- What role does health communication play in promoting health inequalities? How do health campaign efforts promote health inequalities?
- What role do you suggest health communicators play in addressing structural inequalities? Please outline specific steps that health communicators might undertake in addressing structural inequities.

Health outcomes

Structural and communicative marginalization work in unison to create conditions of overall inaccess to health resources within the community (Farmer 1996, 1999). It is within this climate of overall inaccess that community members experience poorer access to preventive resources, support resources, and treatment resources. The combination between minimal access to health prevention and to health treatment generates conditions of overall health depletion; the individual faces a variety of health problems which ultimately influence his/her health negatively. Extant research also documents that individuals living in marginalized communities experience greater levels of stress as they struggle with the minimal resources that are available to them on a daily basis (Wilkinson 1994; both studies conducted by Kawachi, with various collaborators, in 1999). The day-to-day struggle for basic resources, embodied in the conditions of poverty, influences the emotional and spiritual health of community members, which, in turn, influences a variety of other health results.

A growing body of work on the *epidemiology* of health documents the ways in which income inequities in communities influence the health problems of these communities (Atkinson and Micklewright 1992; Kawachi et al. 1994; Kennedy et al. 1996; Wilkinson 1994; both studies conducted under Kawachi in 1999). These scholars suggest that greater income inequities contribute to lower levels of social cohesiveness, interpersonal trust and community ties within these very communities, and these indicators of poor community social capital, in turn, directly exhaust the health of community members, so that they become more likely to suffer from a variety of chronic health conditions. In this line of research, therefore, community members experience greater levels of marginalization within communities which have greater disparities.

The marginalization of culture

The marginalization of underserved communities is further accomplished through the communicative portrayal of these communities in terms of absences, often framed within an individualized context and articulated in terms of drawbacks of the culture (Dutta-Bergman 2005a; Dutta 2007). In the dominant approach, culture is defined as static, as a set of values and beliefs that are typically constructed as barriers to the health interventions being proposed for the community. For instance, Witte and Morrison (1995) discuss the relevance of the extended parallel process model in multicultural health campaigns, so that cultural barriers can be identified and addressed through campaign messages. Cultures are marginalized through the discursive framing of values and beliefs within the dominant framework, which continues to present the concept of culture in terms of an exotic "other" that needs to be transformed through the value-free and rational efforts of the dominant system. This conceptualization of culture as a static entity offers the impetus for efforts to change, led by the dominant power structures. This notion of the "other," depicted in dominant discourses of development, supports the economics of a whole body of knowledge, and, further, the logic of imperialism on the basis of the notion that imperial entries into cultures are attempts to help modernize primitive cultural spaces. This is nicely captured in the following writing of Arturo Escobar on the economics of development (1995: 103–4):

> To be blunt, one could say that the body of the malnourished – the starving "African" portrayed on so many covers of Western magazines, or the lethargic

South American child to be "adopted" for $16 a month portrayed in the adver-
tisements of the same magazines – is the most striking symbol of the first world
over the Third. A whole economy of discourse and unequal power relations is
encoded in that body . . . it all becomes, for Western science and media, help-
less and formless (dark) masses, items to be counted and measured by demog-
raphers and nutritionists.

Culture, therefore, serves as a conceptual framework that feeds into
the marginalization of peoples and communities by offering conceptual
vessels that justify the prevalence of the dominant paradigm. For instance,
family planning programs targeting the southern nations of the world
often portray these cultures of the South as rapidly producing masses of
progeny who ought to be taught the benefits of the modern family; hence
the focus is on teaching the modern values of development, which begin
with an emphasis on the smaller family (Dutta and Basnyat, in press). For
instance, the Radio Communication Project in Nepal, a campaign sponsored by the USAID, juxtaposes the primitiveness of the culture, implicit
in desiring too many children, in the backdrop of the modernist tools of
family planning gifted by development projects:

> Health Worker: Is it God's will that we have too many children or is it God's
> will that we take advantage of modern medical science to be able to control the
> size and spacing of our family? The well-planned family these days has only
> two children. Health Worker: Happily today, modern medical science has
> provided us with safe and reliable contraceptives so that we can all plan our
> families well. We should remember that a well-planned family is the basis of
> the clean and safe environment. (Johns Hopkins University/Center for
> Communication Programs 1998: 135)

Note that the traditional values of the culture, expressed in the notion of
having "too many" children, is positioned in the backdrop of the boons of
modern medical technology. What is constructed as a target of the health
interventions is the traditional value of the culture, and the intervention
seeks to demonstrate how a modern lifestyle can provide the panacea to
the limited resources faced by the communities. The absence of resources
is typically framed in the realm of passivity or the lack of agency of community members, and is tied to cultural values defined in terms of variables such as self-efficacy, locus of control, and fatalism. These values are
constructed as barriers that need to be worked upon and therefore
changed by the campaign planner, in order for the community to achieve
development and contribute to the global economy. In other words, the
discursive construction of underdevelopment is intrinsically linked to the
economic interests of the status quo. For instance, much of the USAID-
funded health communication programs typically focus on the problem of
population control as the key problem underlying underdevelopment and
poverty, thus locating the problem in the realm of deeply rooted primitive
cultural values that need to be changed; it shifts attention away from questions of resource redistribution and social equity (Dutta 2006; Farmer and
Bertrand 2000).

By placing the blame on primitive cultural practices, questions of structural violence are backgrounded and the need for campaigns targeted at transforming cultural behaviors is foregrounded; nations which control their population problem, it is argued, will be better able to manage their resources and to participate effectively in the global economy. This economic agenda of health communication efforts is expressed in the following excerpt from Madeleine Albright:

> International family planning also serves important US foreign policy interests; elevating the status of women, reducing the flow of refugees, protecting the global environment, and promoting sustainable development which leads to economic growth and trade opportunities for businesses. (http://usinfo. state.gov/journals/itgic/0998/ijge/gj-14.htm)

The individual and the community are constructed in terms of broader cultural stereotypes which portray the community as devoid of the basic human agency to seek and achieve change, and the impetus for change comes from the sources of power that define the problems of development and articulate the accompanying solutions – which, according to these sources, are about to bring about development in the community. Metaphors used to describe the community are, typically, metaphors that depict the underdevelopment of the community and its so-called lack of progress by attributing them to individual-level characteristics of the community members (Dutta and Basnyat, in press). For instance, the RCP (Radio Communication Project, an entertainment education program launched in Nepal) drama script addresses the "problem" of overpopulation in the following manner:

> It's the problem of family size. As you know, traditionally people in Nepal have had many children . . . too many . . . well, certainly nowadays we cannot go on having such large families. The country cannot support them for one thing. For another thing, modern medical science has proved to us that it is extremely unhealthy and dangerous for a woman to have a lot of children (JHU/CCP 1998: 135)

Note the placement of the traditional Nepalese value of having too many children in the backdrop of the modern technology that allows people to have well-planned families. The contrasting of tradition in the face of modernization further uses the discourse of modernity to paint the so-called traditional practices as dangerous and unhealthy. In this context, the marginalization of the community is played out in the realm of the communicative construction of the community as primitive, savage, and unable to take care of itself. It is through this process of marginalization that actors at the center define their legitimacy in exerting power and control over the positions at the periphery.

Power and Structure

At the heart of marginalization are the concepts of power and structure. Power refers to the hold that certain sets of actors within or outside the community have over other actors within or outside the community; it reflects the differential in the ways in which communication flows from one predetermined location to another (Dutta 2007). Power is typically predicated upon the resources available to the actors within the system, and upon the ways in which these resources determine access to communicative and material avenues. Those with power typically have greater access to resources and hence are able to define the agendas that ought to be pursued, whereas those without power or with limited access to it have limited access both to communication and to material resources. These agendas, in turn, shape the ways in which social structures are experienced by members of the communities.

Structure refers to the material entities within and outside the community that are constitutive of the life experiences of the individual and of the community. It typically consists of organizations, resources, and networks within and outside the community, and the access to these organizations, resources and networks determines the ways in which community members live their lives. Individuals, groups, and community members experience structures in the ways in which they navigate the healthcare system. Structure both enables and constrains human agency, on one hand offering opportunities for its enactment, on the other hand presenting barriers that minimize the ways in which agency is enacted within the community. The extent to which structure enables and constrains human agency depends upon the ways in which it interacts with the distribution of power within the social system. The interconnected web of power and social structure influences the health experiences of the marginalized community member.

Social inequalities

Social inequalities refer to the differences between the health rich and the health poor, tapping into the gaps that exist within social systems (both studies conducted under Millen in 2000). The greater the inequality within the social system, the greater the likelihood of healthcare disparity and poorer health in the overall system. In documenting the link between socio-economic inequality and healthcare outcomes, epidemiologists suggest that greater inequities lead to lower levels of social capital within the system, which, in turn, vastly influence the health outcomes of the overall system. In other words, *social capital*, or the level of community cohesiveness and interpersonal trust within the social system, affects the ways in which community members experience health. Lower levels of social capital are marked by greater levels of stress and mistrust, absence of social support networks, and absence of health information resources. These depleted health resources, in turn, produce conditions of poor health outcomes in highly inequitable communities.

Increasingly, a significant body of literature on global health disparities is documenting the widening gaps between the health rich and health poor (Millen, Irwin and Kim 2000; Zoller 2005). For instance, both studies published under Millen in 2000 point out that, whereas in 1960 the poorest 20 percent of the world's people received approximately 2.3 percent of the global income, this share fell to 1.4 percent in 1991, and it further declined to 1.1 percent of the global income in 2000. Similarly, whereas in 1960 the ratio of the income of the wealthiest 20 percent of the people to the poorest 20 percent was 30 to 1, this ratio increased to 82 to 1 by 1995. And whereas the 20 percent of the world's people who live in the highest-income countries have spent 86 percent of the total worldwide private consumption expenditure, the poorest 20 percent account for only 1.3 percent of the worldwide private consumption expenditure. Scholars argue that globalization trends contribute to the increasing gaps between those who have healthcare access and those who do not have access to healthcare, by contributing to healthcare policies that cater to the interests of transnational elites, simultaneously marginalizing the interests of those who have limited access to resources (see also Shakow and Irwin 2000). For instance, although the rhetoric of the free market is utilized by the WTO and IMF to urge relatively poorer countries to open up their economies and adopt free market principles and to open up their economies to unconstrained foreign investment and foreign competition, the reality of the growth of industries in the wealthy countries demonstrates significant uses of protectionist and anti-free-market devices within these countries during the periods in which the fledgling industries were beginning to mature (ibid.). For instance, while promoting the free market rhetoric and the message of unrestrained market freedom globally in the 1980s, President Reagan substantially supported protectionist legislation that safeguarded key American industries and firms from foreign competitors (ibid.). In other words, the rhetoric of free trade is quite a far cry from the reality of the practice of free trade among some of the strongest proponents of the free trade principle in the global economy; the principles of free trade are promoted inequitably by those with access to resources and power, in order to promote their interests globally and to create markets for global corporations located within the wealthiest nations, which have some of the strongest voices (ibid.). The hegemonic power of transnational capitalism is maintained through the creation and implementation of global policies that seek to deliver profits for the centers of power, simultaneously producing conditions of poor health in underserved communities by minimizing government interventions and support in the public health sector. For instance, the World Bank policy document *Investing in Health* emphasizes the privatization of the health sector and recommends "shifting public health expenditures from tertiary to primary care; developing more targeted interventions, such as micro-nutrient programs and early childhood interventions; decentralization; and the use of 'cost recovery' mechanisms, such as user fees" (p. 30). Empirical analysis of the implementation of cost-recovery mechanisms in sub-Saharan Africa demonstrated that the quality of care as reflected in attendance levels at hospitals and clinics had been falling sharply since the 1980s after the cost-recovery mechanisms were introduced (ibid.).

As our discussion of global politics demonstrates, policies are passed by those who have access to power to serve their economic interests; it is this very bias in the formulation of global policies that threatens the health of the global poor. The structural gaps between the higher and lower socio-economic segments are not only reflected in the access to health resources, but also in the access to information and communication about health and in the ways in which we go about practicing health communication. The agendas of health communicators, in other words, are established within these very logics of global capitalism. For instance, a large proportion of the health communication interventions are globally sponsored by USAID; USAID policy documents articulate the ways in which health communication initiatives also serve the economic agendas of the US and US corporations (2002: iv):

> Successful development abroad generates diffuse benefits. It opens new, more dynamic markets for US goods and services. It generates more secure, promising environments for US investment. It creates zones of order and peace where Americans can travel, study, exchange, and do business safely. And it produces allies – countries that share US commitments to economic openness, political freedom, and the rule of law.

To the extent that USAID uses the health communication and the health promotion efforts as tools for creating a free market economy and in order to facilitate the penetration of US corporations in Third World spaces, health communication efforts under the rubric of USAID continue to promote the dominant hegemonic agendas.

Health communication scholars have long demonstrated that health campaigns often maintain health knowledge gaps within communities by contributing to the knowledge and information of the sectors which are rich in resources and by depleting the knowledge and information resources available to the poorer sectors of social systems (Viswanath and Finnegan 1996). In his work, Dutta-Bergman (2004d, 2004e, 2004f) demonstrates how these gaps are created and sustained by health campaigns, with their focus on information-based media which typically remain inaccessible and/or incomprehensible among lower segments of the population with lower socio-economic status (SES). For instance, information-heavy campaign messages placed in newspapers typically miss the underserved segments, as newspapers are minimally consumed by these segments. In other words, this knowledge gap is typically created by an elite bias of the health campaign designers at the center, who develop communication strategies more closely aligned with elite interests rather than addressing the interests and needs of those in the margins.

The dominant discursive framings of health communication continue to perpetrate the inequities of healthcare access by supporting the reasons underlying these access differentials; they justify inequities by framing health problems in the form of individual-level absences. For instance, the emphasis on individual reproductive choices as a solution to poverty backgrounds the problems of resource inaccess and of structural inequities, which underlie poverty. The emphasis on individual-level beliefs and attitudes as sources of health problems shifts focus away from the socio-cultural factors that contribute to the increasing gaps between the health rich and the health poor. This focus on the individual also distracts from basic socio-cultural inequities which contribute to the gaps in the health experiences of those with access and those without access.

Access to structural resources

In the realm of healthcare, structural resources are those basic elements of health systems which make up the capabilities of the system. How these basic capabilities of the system are defined depends upon the ways in which the overall system is approached in the conceptualization of healthcare, and upon the basic elements needed by the individual to survive within the system, being able to maintain health as defined by him/her and by his/her community. Broadly speaking, the basic capabilities of healthcare are defined in terms of food, preventive services, and treatment services. Inaccess to these resources produces conditions of poor health in the community. Typically, inaccess in one area of healthcare is accompanied by inaccess in others.

In Dutta-Bergman's work in rural India (2004a, 2004b), we see narratives of health and pain being articulated in the context of food. Community members in underserved sectors discuss the fact that they have limited supplies of food, and this is fundamentally related to their health. In this context, poverty and health are intertwined through inaccess to food, which is seen as a basic element of an individual's health. Similarly, in his dialogues with Santalis, Dutta-Bergman documents the minimal access to healthcare resources in the form of treatment options and medical supplies available to community members. Patients discussed their inability to get treatment from doctors because doctors at subsidized state hospitals would typically be unavailable. Medical supplies were also typically lacking in these areas, as the medicines got sold at the local clinics and thus made available to those individuals who had the money to buy the medicines. Similar inaccess to medicine is also witnessed in other research contexts where participants discuss the ways in which the social structure limits the options available to them (Farmer 2003). It is within this minimal access that individuals and communities find ways of resisting the structures, of changing them, and of negotiating the impediments posed on them by the structures within which they live their lives.

Structural violence

Structural violence is reflective of the ways in which the socio-cultural structure marginalizes the health experiences of individuals, groups and communities by limiting access to the basic resources considered quintessential to human survival; it is reflected in the lack of the basic physical necessities of life (Abraham 1993; Farmer 1994, 1996; Kleinman 1997).

When structures continue to limit the access to basic health capacities to the members of marginalized communities, violence is enacted through the erasure of the needs of those who are underserved; these needs are erased through talks of development which, rhetorically, are designed to promote the appearance of serving the interests of the marginalized and yet, in reality, serve the dominant interests. Violence is played out through the acts of erasure, through those communicative acts which silence the voices of the marginalized and place them at the peripheries of the socio-cultural system. This condition of being under, of being erased from the mainstream discursive space, is also referred to as subalternity. The marginalized sectors are often spoken *for* by others as targets of interventions; as demonstrated earlier in this chapter, their stories get written up by elite actors to serve their interests. For instance, in earlier sections we have seen the ways in which members of marginalized communities articulated being in the position of feeling silenced. In the realm of the health and development policies that are passed and implemented, violence is reflected in the absence of marginalized groups from those development and policy platforms supposedly designed to help them.

Ultimately, violence is played out in the hypocrisies of global health policies of development and in the disjunctures in these policies (Farmer and Bertrand 2000). This is reflected in the following formulation of Mme Lamandier, a resident of the displaced community of Kay in Haiti. This community was flooded by the building of a dam, which was erected without involving the people it was going to displace and without giving them sufficient warning:

> The rich people, the city people, bribe the bureaucrats so they can have electricity. Water makes electricity, but you need high water. So they flooded us out . . . And it's not the first time they've done such things. Whenever they start talking 'development,' poor people have to be careful. (Mme Lamandier in Farmer and Bertrand 2000: 71)

Mme Lamandier reflects on the violence perpetrated by the status quo while using the discourse of development to push the agendas of the transnational elite. Farmer and Bertrand further point out that the building of dams in the name of development displaced poverty-stricken Haitian people and failed to reimburse them. This deceptiveness of the logic of development is intrinsic to the nature of violence perpetrated in marginalized communities.

> They called an assembly to say that they would be reimbursing everyone for their gardens and land. My friend, that was a lie! They came to measure the lands, and indeed a few people did receive payment – only those who were well educated, those who had secured deeds. (p. 73)

This notion of being lied to and deceived is quintessential to the experience of being violated. For instance, in Dutta-Bergman's conversations with rural Santalis (2004a, 2004b), he points out that Santalis talk about their mistrust for politicians, local doctors, NGOs and the police because they "use" the poverty of the Santalis to fulfill their own interests.

Although promises are made to provide resources, the reality of development as articulated through the voices of rural Santalis demonstrates that these promises are rarely kept.

The erasure from the mainstream discursive spaces is also tied to the absence of education and of the tools needed to participate in these spaces. In the Haitian example of the displaced residents of Kay, the ability or inability to get reimbursed was intrinsically linked to poverty. For instance, according to Mme Dieugrand, "it was the rich peasants who were reimbursed"; powerlessness was deeply entrenched in poverty. Furthermore, the lack of political power was connected to the lack of education, "those who were literate and who had deeds were the only ones to get paid" (Farmer and Bertrand 2000: 74). Marginalized communities are marginalized by civil society platforms by means of those very requirements of literacy and specialized skill sets which condition participation in these policy platforms.

Structural violence in the healthcare context taps into those conditions of health which are marked by the utmost absence of basic resources considered to be the core elements of human survival. Structural violence is also evident in the explicit acts of violence that threaten the health and well-being of individuals and communities (Das, Kleinman, Ramphele and Reynolds 2000; Farmer 2003). At a social level, such violence is evident in wars and riots, which often serve dominant social structures and the needs of those in power. Violence is also evident in the explicit use of force in minimizing the resistance to positions of power, as is evident in the roles of the army and the police, or in the role of the Guantanamo Bay prisons. Violence is evident, again, in the treatment of Iraqi prisoners at the hands of US soldiers and in the pictures of prison abuse that inundated the media. Such forms of violence pose a direct threat to the health of individuals and communities, and are often accompanied by the large-scale destruction of lives. However, violence can also be implicit in the very acts of oppression that limit the possibilities of health for the marginalized. Such implicit violence is contained in the lack of access to food, lack of access to treatment information, lack of access to medical supplies, lack of access to health insurance, and so on.

Whether implicit or explicit, the condition of structural violence is marked by narratives of pain (Das 1997; Dutta-Bergman 2004a, 2004b; Farmer 2003). These narratives emphasize the deeply felt pain that is quintessential to those marginalizing structures within which individuals and communities live their lives. The narratives articulate the lack of resources; they discuss the pain of hunger, the pain of illness, the pain associated with the inability to secure health and medical services for oneself and for one's family, the pain associated with the absence of medical services, and so on. It is through the sharing of these stories that health communication scholars open up discursive spaces for voicing the stories of oppression and violence. It is also through the sharing of these narratives that new possibilities for social change are presented in the discursive space. The narratives foreground the agency of the subaltern participants in emphasizing co-constructed meanings. It is in the discussion of the ways in which meanings are negotiated and the structural impediments are resisted that we see possibilities of social change.

The dominant structures that marginalize are brought to discursive awareness by the very interrogation of the oppression that marginalizes individuals and communities. The silencing essential to the experience of marginalization is put in question through the very presence, in the discursive space, of the voices of the marginalized. In other words, dialogical engagement with subaltern participants who have experienced the violence enacted by dominant structures opens up discursive possibilities of change. The next section presents the role of communication in the realm of marginalization.

Communicative Enactment of Marginalization

Marginalization is intrinsically intertwined with communication, since it is through communication that the positions at the margins are created, enacted, and reinforced. Acts of communication define symbolically the position at the margins, and it is also through these communicative acts that individuals and groups come to be disenfranchised. For instance, the circulation of certain types of messages in the communicative space about the characteristics of the welfare mother continues to reify the marginalized position of mothers on welfare. Similarly, the lack of access to a medical system among the poor is communicatively enacted in the limited amount of time physicians spend with them and in the closed nature of the communication with the physician. Marginalization, therefore, is achieved and reinforced communicatively through the messages that circulate in the discursive space and through the communication processes that are available or unavailable to the members of marginalized communities.

Message-based perspective

The message-based approach to the communicative enactment of marginalization examines how messages directed at marginalized groups minimize the agency of such groups by constructing them as passive actors, in need of interventions designed by those at the center of power. In other words, the communicative construction, through discourse, of marginalized groups legitimizes the flow of power from the centers to the peripheral positions in the margins. For instance, the communicative construction of native Americans as passive and addicted to alcohol provides the basis for alcohol awareness campaigns run by mainstream organizations directed at native Americans. Escobar (1995) exemplifies this form of communicative marginalization in his discussion of Western constructions of the Third World, suggesting that the Third World body is constructed as a homogenized dark mass to be acted upon and to be uplifted by efforts of development led by the developed world. In this context, Escobar questions the very construct of development, suggesting that the ways in which development is communicatively constituted embodies the power of the communicative centers on the marginalized sectors of the world. Such discursive constructions of development provide criteria for the measurement of development, suggesting what it means to be developed and simultaneously offering a prescriptive understanding of what it means to be undeveloped or underdeveloped. In doing so, the actors at the center can then define the meaning of development and offer prescriptive guidelines for interventions targeting underdevelopment. Such marginalizing discourse also sustains the economics of colonial interventions, carried out by the powerful actors through the rendering of the colonized as being in need of the acts of colonization. The interpenetration of discourse and colonialism is most recently evident in the US interventions in Afghanistan and Iraq, which were carried out in the name of promoting democracy; in other words, the discursive constructions of "bringing democracy" and "building a free society" were utilized to support neocolonialism. Images of oppressed people, women and children who needed to be freed circulated widely in the mainstream media to generate support for Operation Iraqi Freedom; US intervention was "necessary" so that these oppressed people could be freed (Dutta-Bergman 2005a).

A similar communicative construction of marginalization in terms of absences and drawbacks is also evident in how policy documents, campaigns, and healthcare services discursively construct the homeless as devoid of agency, lazy, addicted, and mentally ill (Marshall and McKeon 1996). These stereotypical constructions are intrinsically intertwined with the access of the homeless to healthcare services and resources. In inner city neighborhoods, individuals and community members are communicatively constructed as passive, lazy, and prone to violence. Such constructions, once again, drive individually-targeted messages that seek to modify individual-level characteristics, simultaneously ignoring broader socio-cultural elements of the structure that might contribute to the conditions of marginalization.

Gramsci's notion of hegemony provides a conceptual basis for examining how marginalization is carried out through the distribution of messages. Hegemony depicts the hidden forms of control exerted by those who are at the center of power on those other individuals, considered to exist at the peripheries of the social system; control is exerted implicitly, without any need for violence and coercive strategies. Hegemonies are circulated and sustained through messages that support the status quo and the positions of power. Furthermore, hegemonic processes operate within social systems through the co-optation of the resistive possibilities that are likely to be brought about by the evident inequities within the system. For instance, responding to the critique of top-down health campaigns, USAID-funded population control programs in Nepal created participatory platforms in its communities, and yet these platforms were created to support the USAID agendas of discussing ways of controlling the population. Although the community was indeed involved in this case, its community involvement was used to serve the broader agendas of the dominant actors (Dutta and Basnyat, in press). Health communication messages sent by dominant actors at the center often maintain the dominant configuration through the hegemonic portrayal of the marginalized communities as devoid of agency and therefore in need of the uplifting messages sent from the center. The framing of health matters and risks as problems of individual-level behavior, as opposed to problems of structural inequities, further continues to sustain the status quo. For instance, much of the emphasis of the National Cancer Institute on health disparities discusses campaign messages directed at the behaviors of underserved communities, and not at the structural inequities underlying these disparities. In addition, the portrayal of absences in the marginalized communities continues to maintain the power of the dominant groups (Kreps 2006).

Process-based perspective

The process-based approach to marginalization asks how communication processes contribute to the experiences of being marginalized. Communicative processes typically refer to the ways in which communication is deployed and negotiated in the areas of policy, implementation and evaluation (Wallack 1990). Marginalization in the realm of communicative processes, therefore, typically refers to the array of communication outlets and structures which are typically made unavailable to the members of marginalized communities by virtue of their existence at the peripheries of the dominant communicative structures. Therefore individuals and communities who are typically marginalized do not have avenues for engaging in the communicative processes which are essential to dialogue in the sphere of policy and its implementation.

Process-based marginalization is, once again, deeply connected to structures of power and to the ways in which the dominant structures of power maintain their control over the discursive and material spaces. The discursive and material spaces are deeply intertwined, and the relationship between them is both simultaneous and interactive. In other words, the very nature of the material space affects the discursive space, and, conversely, the very nature of the discursive space affects the material space. Not having access to economic resources and structures affects the ways in which individuals and communities can participate in communication platforms, and, in turn, the condition of not having access to communication platforms impacts on the ways in which economic and healthcare resources are distributed in the community.

Existing research in health communication demonstrates that process-based marginalization typically happens in the form of minimal access to the communication outlets which present the policy; inaccess to the language used in these policy platforms; inaccess to communication tools such as forms, protocols, and steps that need to be taken in order to influence the policy; and inaccess to those political processes that shape the outcomes for the marginalized sectors (Dutta-Bergman 2004a, 2004b, 2004c, 2004d, 2005a, 2005b; Dutta and Basu 2007; Dutta and Basnyat, in press). Furthermore, communicative inaccess is also manifest in the day-to-day experiences of marginalized community members: in the context of the language used in physician–patient interactions, in the forms that need to be filled out during the visits, in the level of literacy required for processing the health information presented, in the ways in which the availability of resources is communicated to community members, in the availability of health communication technologies in communities, and so on.

Communication processes often participate in the hegemonic co-optation of the participatory potential of marginalized communities by appropriating those communication platforms and avenues that would otherwise serve as conduits of resistance. One such example of hegemonic co-optation in the realm of health communication is the deployment of participator entertainment education (E-E) programs which use the rhetoric of participation and engage participatory platforms in the diffusion of the agendas of dominant actors such as the United States Agency for International Development (USAID) (Dutta-Bergman 2004e; Dutta 2007; Dutta and Basnyat, in press). In their example, Dutta and Basnyat (in press) demonstrate how community meetings and folk theater are utilized to serve the USAID agenda of population control; in this instance, participation is used as a mechanism of control, as a tool that further lends the subaltern space to the exertion of control by the dominant actors. Similarly, civil society efforts that are targeted toward building participatory fora for subaltern voices have been critiqued for co-opting the participation of the subaltern classes to serve the dominant agendas (Dutta-Bergman 2005a). In this instance, non-governmental organizations (NGOs) were supported and funded by USAID to promote pro-US sentiments and pro-free market public opinion and to sustain the rule of the local elite, thus co-opting the opportunities for transformative politics and structural change. The participatory nature of resistance is framed within the goals and objectives of transnational elites.

Conclusion

In conclusion, this chapter presents the various facets of marginalization, documenting the plethora of ways in which individuals and communities are marginalized in healthcare contexts. The review presented here suggests that marginalization is constructed both communicatively and materially. One of the ways in which individuals and communities get located at the margins of social systems is through silencing. Silencing is communicatively enacted in the context of access to power; those with access to power have the opportunity to define the agendas and priorities of the healthcare sector, whereas those without access are left in positions of exclusion. Power, in turn, is connected with access to resources, placing

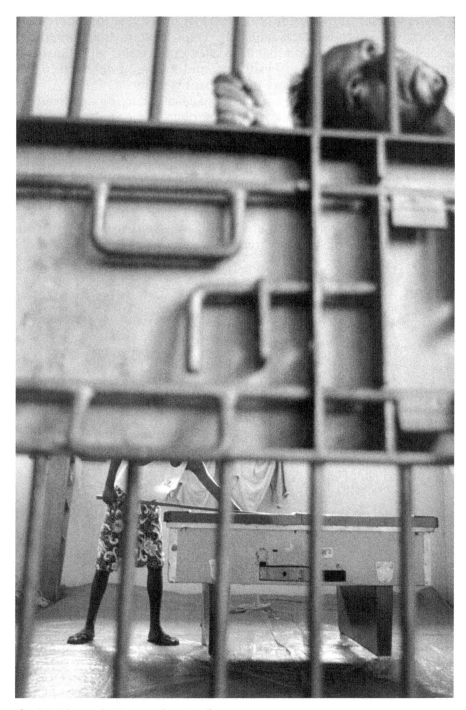

Fig. 6.2 Prisoners in Manaus prison, Brazil
© Alvaro Leiva @ Panos Pictures

marginalization in the realm of a variety of underlying indicators such as social class, gender, race, nationality, etc. Those in the margins are excluded and this exclusion manifests itself in increasing global inequalities, increasing inaccess to healthcare, and increasing injustice in the realm of the structural violence of dominant systems.

Communication plays a major role in marginalization through the recirculation of messages and processes that contribute to the fundamental inaccess to resources experienced in marginalized communities. Furthermore, communicative messages and processes co-opt the resistive opportunities in marginalized communities by incorporating the participatory processes into the dominant agendas of the transnational hegemony. Ultimately, the very marginalization of subaltern sectors of the globe exists in a dialectical tension with the possibilities of change and resistance. Chapter 11 will discuss the ways in which communicative agency is enacted in its resistance to the dominant socio-cultural structures.

7 Health Experiences in Marginalized Sectors

Chapter objectives

In this chapter, we will:

- further examine what it means to be marginalized in specific contexts
- study marginalization in the realm of race, age, income, and gender
- examine marginalization in postcolonial contexts

The discussion of marginalization in chapter 6 provides the theoretical foundation for exploring the health experiences of certain segments of the population on the basis of their existence at the peripheries of the healthcare system. Four critical markers that have typically dictated much of the experiences of marginalization are gender, race, age, and socio-economic status. These four markers will be compared and contrasted, in order to identify the similarities and differences between these different populations in terms of how structure enacts violence by limiting the availability of basic resources to marginalized communities, and the ways in which structure creates conditions of healthcare disparities. Although it is important to articulate the fluidity of shifting cultural contexts within which identities and experiences are embodied, the socio-demographic categories discussed in this chapter provide a foundation for understanding the material bases for healthcare disparities. The discussion of women's health will examine patriarchy in the realm of women's experiences of the healthcare system. The ways in which race acts as a marker and conduit of marginalization will be discussed in the next section, followed by a discussion of the interplay between power and marginalization in the context of age. The chapter will conclude with a look at the socio-economic disparities in healthcare.

Experiences at the Margins

What does it mean to be marginalized? What are the ways in which marginalization plays out in the lived experiences of the people who are marginalized? How do the dominant socio-cultural systems justify and propagate the limited access to healthcare experienced in marginalized communities?

Box 7.1 The story of Sarah

As a single mother of four children, Sarah finds it very difficult to juggle her job and her family. She lives in constant fear that the folks from the child protective services are going to come and take her children away, finding her to neglect their needs. She survives on her welfare checks and the food stamps, but these are not enough for Sarah to support a family of five. It is difficult for her to keep a job, especially with the responsibilities she has with her children. She does not have health insurance and mostly works part time, switching from one job to another.

  Sarah worries about what she might do if her children were to fall sick. She does not have the money to pay hospital fees and fees for the doctor. She just goes from day to day, hoping and praying that things will be alright, and that God will take care of her and her children. She also does not trust the doctors at the local hospital. She feels as though they look at her with mistrust, as if perhaps she does not belong there. Her interactions with the nurses are not pleasant either, and each time she comes away feeling upset at how they talk down to her.

Sarah's experience as an African American woman in her late twenties living in the inner city of Chicago taps into the healthcare disparities that continue to manifest themselves across the United States. These health disparities reflect the broader socio-cultural disparities within the country. Demographic markers such as gender, race, age, and socio-economic status determine the access an individual will have to the healthcare system, health information and communication infrastructures, and the extent to which he/she will have a participatory voice in the shaping of discursive and material realities. In this section, we will examine the different elements of the experience of marginalization in the areas of basic health capacities, prevention programs, health services usage, and access to communicative infrastructures.

Discussion point 7.1

- What do you understand by marginalization?
- Please select a community that you think has been marginalized in terms of healthcare.
- Why do you think this community has been marginalized? How has it been marginalized? How has the marginalization of the community played out in the realm of health?

Basic health capacities

Basic health capacities refer to the basic resources that make up what it means to be healthy. One of these basic resources is food (Dutta-Bergman 2004a, 2004b, 2004c, 2005a, 2005b). Therefore, communities that exist at the margins of the healthcare system typically experience minimal access to food. For instance, African Americans in the US discuss the limited access they face in securing healthy food. Similarly, rural communities in the US experience lack of access to fruits and vegetables. In fact, one of the critical barriers to the consumption of fruits and vegetables is the limited access, in marginalized communities, to fruits and vegetables – which are typically expensive. In marginalized communities in the South, the minimal access to food is a critical health problem. Existing research documents the widespread malnutrition and starvation in marginalized sectors. In his conversation with Santalis, Dutta-Bergman (2004a) points out that their ability to secure food for themselves and their children depends upon their ability to find work on a day-to-day basis. In this context, then, access to basic health capacity is limited by the inability to find work and participate in the production system of the economy. The increasing demands on local jobs further complicates the situation, with minimal number of jobs available to the local workers. Shelter is yet another basic health capacity that protects individuals, groups, and communities from natural disasters, diseases, infections, and various forms of violence. The importance of shelter to healthcare is evident in the experiences of the homeless in the US. The lack of a stable shelter exposes individuals to a variety of direct health threats, including threats of violence posed to them and to their whole communities. Finally, yet another basic health resource is adequate availability of health services and medical supplies.

Discussion point 7.2

- Do you agree with the position articulated in this section, that it is important for health communication scholars to theorize and develop applications around basic capabilities? Why? Why not?
- How would you go about using health communication principles and concepts to build basic capabilities of healthcare in marginalized communities?

Prevention programs

Prevention programs offer health information and health resources that are directed toward the prevention of disease and illness. Such programs are typically run in the form of health information campaigns targeted toward communities and their members. Research on knowledge gap theory (Viswanath and Finnegan 2002) suggests that prevention interventions typically increase the gaps between the health rich and the health poor rather than mitigating these gaps. In other words, individuals from higher socio-economic status groups learn more health information and gain greater preventive knowledge from health information campaigns as compared to individuals from the lower socio-economic segments of society.

Box 7.2 The story of Jim

The Centers for Disease Control and Prevention ran a health promotion campaign in North Dakota (ND) that sought to promote the consumption of at least five servings of fruits and vegetables in the state. This campaign was based on the fruit and vegetable consumption trends in North Dakota, accompanied by the cancer prevalence rates in the state. The campaign was run on news programming in local television channels in Fargo and Bismarck, ND, which are two of the largest cities in the state. After the campaign evaluations were conducted, the results suggested that the mean rate of fruit and vegetable consumption in the state had indeed increased.

Jim, a 62-year-old patient who was recently detected with cancer, however, does not recall having heard anything about five servings of fruits and vegetables. Jim lives in rural North Dakota and primarily watches the sports channel on television. He does not read the newspaper and does not visit the doctor's office unless he absolutely has to. With his retirement payments of about $850 a month, Jim says that he wouldn't be able to afford the five servings of fruits and vegetables even if he had the information that eating at least five servings of fruits and vegetables prevents cancer.

Knowledge gaps are created because of the minimal access to communication infrastructures in marginalized communities (Dutta-Bergman 2004a, 2004b; Kreps 2005a, 2005b). Also, prevention campaigns often suffer from elite biases in their choice of information-heavy communication channels that have fairly limited use among lower socio-economic segments, among ethnic minorities, in immigrant communities, and so on (Dutta-Bergman 2004a, 2004b, 2004c, 2004d, 2004e). The experience of Jim presented here is reflective of the broader inaccess to the prevention campaigns among members of marginalized communities (Dutta-Bergman 2004a, 2004b, 2005a; Kreps 2002, 2005a, 2005b). Information-heavy health campaigns typically remain inaccessible to these communities, as members of underserved communities typically are not equipped with the communication infrastructures and communication capacities to access the preventive messages (Dutta-Bergman 2004a, 2004b, 2005a, 2005b).

In addition to facing limited access to prevention information, members of marginalized communities also report experiencing minimal access to the resources that are prescribed in the preventive programs. For instance, although the five-a-day program launched by the National Cancer Institute recommends that individuals eat five or more servings of fruits and vegetables a day in order to minimize their chances of cancer, access to fruits and vegetables is particularly limited among marginalized community members, who do not have the financial resources to purchase fruits and vegetables.

Similarly, programs that recommend exercising are often limited in their reach to marginalized communities because it is expensive for community members to access exercise facilities. Programs recommending walking are not particularly suitable for inner-city neighborhoods that

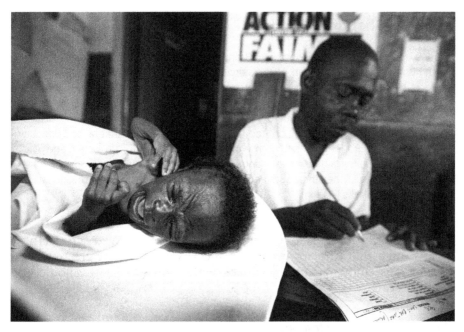

Fig. 7.1 Malnourished child in a feeding center in Uganda
© Sven Torfinn @ Panos Pictures

do not have easily accessible and safe walkways and parks. Programs that recommend screening for cancer need to take into account structural barriers such as the costs of the screening program, the amount of time taken by screening options, and the availability of such time for the community member, who might be juggling multiple jobs to make ends meet.

Health services usage

Yet another domain of resources in which marginalized communities experience poorer access is healthcare services (Agency for Healthcare Research and Quality 2004; Perloff 2006). Healthcare services comprise the array of services for detecting and treating illnesses and the variety of treatment options which are typically available to patients and communities. Individuals belonging to poorer social classes also experience greater access problems in the area of health services. Individuals without health insurance have fairly limited healthcare choices as compared to individuals who have health insurance (Perloff 2006). Furthermore, barriers to healthcare are not only experienced at individual level but also at community level.

Existing research suggests that communities with lower levels of education and income at an aggregate level are also communities with minimal access to a plethora of healthcare services (Agency for Healthcare Research and Quality 2004; Perloff 2006). For instance, Perloff points out that a White child growing up in Appalachia will live a shorter and less healthy life as compared to her/his White counterpart growing up in Orange

Box 7.3　The story of Rodney

Rodney is 22 and Black. Growing up in Bronx, New York has brought him face to face with his identity as a Black man. He was first pulled over by the cops when he was sixteen; he was beaten up and incarcerated. His experiences with health have also borne witness to similar stories of pain. Time and again, he has been turned away from the local hospital because he did not carry insurance. At other times, the local health clinic asked for him to fill out too much paperwork, which that he had difficulty wading through. Rodney has felt a sense of despair at the healthcare system and wonders when things are going to change. He talks about the racism which is deeply entrenched in the US healthcare system today and denies access to basic healthcare to him and other Blacks like him.

County, California. This access differential is also observed across ethnic groups, such that African Americans and Hispanics report greater access problems as compared to Caucasians within the US (Dutta, Bodie and Basu, in press).

Communicative infrastructures

Communication infrastructures refer to a range of communication channels and outlets that serve as platforms for exchange of information, including health information, social support, and healthcare services. Communication infrastructures are critical in healthcare delivery, as these structures serve as the conduits through which health information is exchanged among community members and services are offered to patients. Health information here refers to information about prevention, health maintenance, treatment, health services, and a variety of health resources. Social support refers to the types of emotional and physical support that community members offer to one another. In addition to learning about illnesses and ways to prevent them, communication infrastructures serve as resources that direct community members to the appropriate sources of health services, as well as to the appropriate policy and judiciary platforms that determine accessibility to healthcare services. Not only do underserved communities experience the effects of marginalization in their access to healthcare services and preventive resources, but they are also typically impoverished in the communication infrastructures present within the communities (Dutta-Bergman 2004a, 2004b, 2004c, 2004d, 2005a, 2005b; Kreps 2005a). As a result, members of such communities continue to exist in information vacuums with limited access to health communication resources.

Discussion point 7.3

• Think of HIV/AIDS in the US. What role does communication play in creating marginalizing discourses? How so?

- Please identify one communication infrastructure that you believe is inaccessible to certain communities in the US. How does the inaccessibility to this infrastructure influence the lives of these communities?

Structures of Violence

As articulated earlier in the book, structure refers to the social, cultural and political elements of social systems that determine what is and what is not accessible in communities (Das 1995). Structures serve as conduits of violence by limiting human agency and by constraining the possibilities of health available to community members. Violence here refers to explicit forms of aggression, tied to health as well as to those conditions of daily oppression which are marked by the absence of the basic resources that constitute what it means to live a healthy life, with human dignity and respect (Bourdieu 1993; Farmer 2003; Kleinman 2000; Scheper-Hughes 1992). The conditions of violence might be linked with the direct use of force in wars and civil strife, or might be more implicit in the day-to-day experiences of individuals, as they continue to struggle with the minimal resources available to them.

Violence becomes structural when it is enabled by the socio-cultural differences in the distribution of power and is constituted by this power differential. This distribution of power is sometimes so largely uneven that the ways in which power and control become exerted constitute oppression.

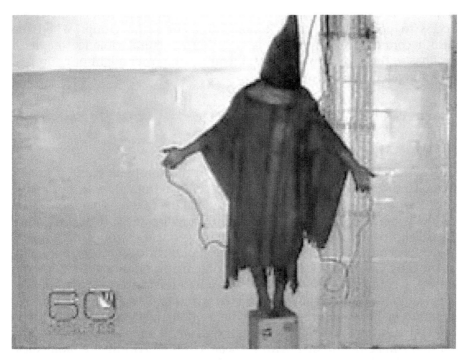

Fig. 7.2 Photograph from mobile camera of prisoner abuse in Abu Ghraib

Structural violence manifests itself in the forms of high rates of disease and death, hunger, thirst, bodily pain, lack of education, homelessness, unemployment, stigmatization and loss of identity, and the lack of access to communicative spaces (Kleinman 2000). Violence is multilayered and affects people in many ways, crosscutting a variety of socio-demographic indicators such as social class, race, gender, and age.

The structures which are central to the enactment of violence vary in their scope and in the levels at which they operate. On the one hand, individuals and groups that are marginalized often face experiences of marginalization at the local level in the form of inaccess to local structures such as local hospitals and treatment options. On the other hand, the experiences of individuals with the local structures are connected with national level structures such as national policy bodies, legislative assemblies, and judiciary organizations; and global-level structures, for instance global policy organizations like the World Bank, the International Monetary Fund, and the World Health Organization – organizations that implement health policies and provide funding for local level implementations, and global platforms for social justice such as human rights organizations. In addition, explicit structures of violence are often connected with vastly unequal distributions of power at the local, national, and state levels. For instance, the genocide in Rwanda was a structural violence connected with the unequal distribution of power between the Hutus and Tutsis in Rwanda. Similarly, the structural violence in Iraq is connected with the unequal distribution of power between nation-states in global politics. Ultimately, structures of violence exist because of differential access to positions of power among different social groups. Therefore health communication programs targeting structural violence ought to emphasize the ways in which such inequities in power might be addressed and mitigated.

Markers of Marginalization

Gendered experiences

The ways in which health is constructed in the dominant cultural system demonstrates its privileging of a set of gendered practices as normative (Agency for Healthcare Research and Quality 2004). The biomedical model is based on the notion of identifying diseases and health conditions, and treating them rationally, playing out a discourse of warfare, which is gendered in its very construction of techno-scientific rationality as the only viable solution to health problems. The notions of health and illness, accompanied by the ways in which illness is addressed in the biomedical model, are socially constructed within a patriarchal framework.

Patriarchy here refers to a social system of organizing and communicating which is built around masculine norms, and operates to support and reinforce male dominance within social systems. Within the biomedical system, the dominance of patriarchy is witnessed at the very roots of the model and its early practitioners. Within the biomedical model, the emphasis on masculine ideals has imposed a view of illness as a condition to be removed and conquered by this model, creating a healthcare system which is typically aggressive in its manner of approaching health, illness, and disease.

Rudy (1997) points out that one of the central concerns of feminists today is the mechanization of the reproductive process. The "natural" process of childbirth has been taken over by a variety of new technologies designed to enhance and ensure fetal health. Pregnancy, as a result, has been transformed into a mechanized affair, further serving as a conduit for exerting the control of men over women – because most of these technologies are controlled by men. Furthermore, the mechanization of the reproductive process has served the interests of capital, as reproductive health has been commoditized. In other words, reproductive technologies are foregrounded as the solutions, thus creating an entire market around the reproductive needs of women. More and more couples are testing out new interventions such as in vitro fertilization, artificial transfers, amniocentesis, chronic villus sampling, fetal ultrasonography, percutaneous umbilical blood sampling, and fetal biopsy. The discursive and material practices around childbirth have therefore been shifted from the domain of women to the realm of precise technological control; the fetus has been privileged as the site of reproductive care, whereas the needs, desires, and powers of women have been ignored.

Yet another realm in which feminist scholars have interrogated the role of patriarchy is plastic surgery and its male-dominated industries, where the commercial producers of medical devices and the plastic surgeons are privileged as actors who exert control and benefit economically from the patriarchal constructions of women's body images (Musick 1997). One specific area of recent examination has been that of the dominant constructions of breast implants, both in medical and media discourse. In the 1980s, the American Society of Plastic and Reconstructive Surgeons (ASPRS), a lobbying group of over 4,500 surgeons, submitted a group memo to the FDA, declaring that having small breasts is a deformity, which may be classified as a disease because it affects the well-being of women (Regush 1992). The categorization of having small breasts as a disease not only legitimized patriarchy in the socio-cultural system by using male-dominated views of the ideal female body image; it also legitimized the male-dominated nexus of physicians, product manufacturers, pharmaceuticals, lobbies and policy-makers (Bird 1979; Schaef 1981; Soffa 1994).

Of particular concern here is the limited information available to female patients about the unreasonable risks and limited efficacy of breast implants. As the political economy of the breast implant industry continues to be supported by the broader regulatory and political system, the benefits of breast implants are foregrounded, while the limitations, side effects, and costs of such implants are simultaneously obscured. For instance, Musick (1997) points out that the American Cancer Society (ACS) continues to support the manufacturers and surgeons working with breast implants by recommending the uninterrupted use of saline-filled silicone implants and by suggesting that such implants respond to a strong public health need among women. Furthermore, the ACS continues to commend the FDA for its role in ensuring the well-being of cancer patients in spite of a three-decade regulatory negligence of FDA of the 91,000 reported breast implant-related injuries and 71 of the deaths between November 1994 and 1996 (Musick 1997). A feminist criticism of breast implants becomes especially relevant when one considers the implants that cancer patients go through after having gone through mastectomy – which is itself critiqued for its violent roots in patriarchy, its limited efficacy, its side effects, and the fact that it ignores the bio-psychosocial causes of breast cancer (Pavalko 1988; Soffa 1994). Originating from a male-dominated standpoint, the disease is localized and approached through invasive technologies built to deal with it, simultaneously ignoring the whole person and her needs.

In discussing how women have resisted the traditional patriarchical construction of health, Hayden (1997) cites the example of the Boston's Women Health Collective, which started with a small group of women coming together to discuss "women and their bodies" at a women's liberation conference. In discussing some of the key issues facing women at the time, the group discovered that, although they had first-hand knowledge and direct experience of many of the topics of women's health and sexuality, they had very little health information on these issues and topics. The information void sparked off the decision to do research on critical issues related to women's health, which resulted in group papers, discussions at weekly meetings, and subsequent offering of a course based on the women's experiences. The participants in the group found that the health information became more relevant when weaved in with the women's experiences, and the group membership solidified as the course was re-offered, which resulted in the Boston Women's Health Course Collective (BWHCC). The increasing popularity of the papers written by the collective led to their publication as a book, *Our Bodies, Ourselves*, which covered a variety of issues tied to women's health and sold more than three million copies.

In analyzing the discursive style of this volume, Hayden (1997) points out that the book not only challenged patriarchy in the healthcare system by discussing its modes of objectifying women and of privileging masculine principles, but it also did so communicatively, by adopting a feminine rhetorical style that placed human experience and human voice at the core of knowing rather than adopting a distanced stance of objectivity through the presentation of grand theories. One of the key resistive strategies of the book was to emphasize knowledge articulated through the personal experiences of women (ibid.). This is spelled out in the following excerpt from the chapter on sexuality:

> We are experts on our sexuality in the sense that we are women sharing our experiences and insights. This process has been more helpful and informative to us than all the how-to-do-it and what-is-it-all-about books we have ever read. (Boston Women's Health Book Collective 1973: 23)

The above excerpt demonstrates how the collective privileged the personal experiences of women as conduits to knowledge rather than simply relying on medical explanations and facts. Hayden (1997) further points out that the book communicates in the feminine style by establishing peer relationships between its authors and between its authors and readers; by using a personal and tentative tone; by inviting the audience to participate; and by adopting inductive arguments. The book ends with a call for collective mobilization, suggesting that there are many ways for women to get together to raise critical questions about major health issues that impact them.

The presence of the voices of women in the discursive space offers an opening for social change. As pointed out in our early discussions of the culture-centered approach, these voices provide pathways to knowledge through the expression of individual experiences. It is in the articulation of these individual experiences that we witness the day-to-day interactions between structure and agency, played out in the realm of culture. The presence of the voice which has traditionally been silenced in the discursive space draws our attention to those acts of marginalization which contribute to the health experiences of women.

Structures of inaccess.   In their day-to-day experiences of health, women regularly experience limited access to a healthcare system that is dominated by men, funded and supported by a healthcare industry that is run by men, and regulated by policy-makers who are mostly men (Tong 2002). Such structures include: material inaccess due to lack of financial resources; inaccess due to lack of time because of household commitments; inaccess due to the epistemological construction of a medical system that is unresponsive to women's personal experiences; inaccess due to fundamental differences in communication expectations and goals of patients and their providers. Limited access also becomes a key issue in the realm of women's access to adequate and healthy food, spaces for exercising, participating in screening programs, and the like. Worth noting are the ways in which race and class interact with gender to marginalize the health experiences of women even further.

Health communication scholarship engaging with issues of gender ought to interrogate in greater depth the ways in which policy discourse is created so as to support conditions of gendered inaccess. Furthermore, we need to engage with questions regarding the role of communication in addressing gendered inequities in healthcare: How can policy-makers be approached with meaningful communication strategies, which draw their attention to the gendered inaccess in healthcare? How can healthcare providers be trained in communication processes that are responsive to the gendered characteristics of healthcare? What communication processes and strategies might be applicable in mobilizing communities around issues of gendered inaccess to healthcare resources?

Gendered violence.   The discussion of plastic surgery and mastectomy presented in the earlier section documents avenues through which the modern medical system continues to enact violence on the woman's body. Violence is gendered, and is constituted by a social system which regards the female body as the locus of enacting violence. This violence of the social system is embodied in society's modes of constructing the feminine ideal and in the values attached to the ideal of the feminine body. The objectification of the feminine ideal and the necessity to modify and alter the female body so as to make it fit into the dominant normative ideals of patriarchy enact violence on women: the woman is set as a subject to be worked on, operated on, and treated. She never is the ideal, but aspires instead to reach the ideal through tools created by the modern biomedical system. The biomedical enterprise of plastic surgery industry survives economically through the process of the creation and constitution of the feminine ideal.

Racial experiences

Race serves as yet another site where violence gets enacted in the healthcare context, marked by experiences of inaccess and struggle among members of minority groups (Perloff 2006). Illness and life expectancy are differentially distributed across racial and ethnic groups (Kreps 2006; Perloff 2006). Members of minority groups, especially African Americans, experience significantly greater mortality and morbidity rates than the members of the racial majority. For instance, comparing the different health experiences of Blacks and Whites, Marmot (2004) observes that, whereas two out of three Black 15-year-olds on the streets of New York will not see their sixty-fifth birthday, three out of four Whites in Michigan will.

Threats to health are more likely to be concentrated in minority contexts, and are likely to be structurally reinforced by community characteristics (Kreps 2006). For instance, published scholarship documents the higher levels of exposure to various types of crimes experienced by members of minority groups such as African Americans and Hispanics in certain geographical contexts, where racial communities tend to be clustered. These higher levels of violence in certain ethnic communities are correlated with lack of infrastructure, absence of adequate opportunities for growth, and lack of employment. The lower levels of trust and social support in these underprivileged communities further contribute to the climate of violence. Also, African Americans and Hispanics are more likely to be incarcerated and subject to harassment by law enforcement officials than Caucasians within the US. This opens up spaces for the enactment of violence in obvious ways, as communities become sites of violence and prisons serve as spaces of violence, marginalizing the health experiences of racial minority groups, and continuing the system of racial violence both inside and outside prisons.

Race also operates as a site of differential access in terms of the preventive resources and health services that are offered to patients. For instance, African Americans have lower levels of access to preventive services as compared to Caucasians. The health disparities between ethnic groups continue to exist even after controlling for differences between ethnic groups in income and health insurance status (Kreps 2006; Woolf et al. 2004). The quality of care received by patients varies significantly by race even after controlling for access-related factors. In addition to facing the direct problems of limited resources, patients from underprivileged races typically experience stigma in terms of attitudes of healthcare professionals toward them, of the manner in which healthcare professionals communicate with them, and of their sources of information on prevention and on the service options available to them.

In discussing cancer-related risks and health outcomes among minority groups, Kreps (2006) points out that African Americans carry the highest cancer burden among any of the US racial and ethnic groups. Not only are the incidence rates of cancer higher among African Americans, but they are also 33 per cent more likely to die from cancer than Whites (Shavers and Brown 2002; Underwood 2003). Kreps (2006) further points out that the cancer disparities are often likely to co-exist along with other conditions that constitute areas of health inequities such as heart disease, diabetes and stroke. In discussing the factors that contribute to the cancer-related health disparities among African Americans, Kreps (2006) draws our attention to poor socio-economic status, low levels of educational attainment, and racial prejudices toward African Americans.

Proposed health communication solutions to problems such as cancer-related disparities typically focus on developing messages and campaigns that would promote preventive and screening behaviors in the underserved population. Public health communication campaigns are developed and targeted that are tailored to the cultural factors of the group, for instance culturally tailored message strategies effective in influencing cancer prevention and screening behavior among low-income African Americans. In terms of channel strategies, Kreps suggests that the use of familiar, trustworthy, and engaging communication channels such as radio and television programs accompanied by the use of interpersonal networks is particularly effective for reaching at-risk groups. Kreps suggests that persuasive health communication campaigns need to be "strategic and persuasive to overcome audience resistance to promotion and screening goals, encourage personal acceptance of health messages, and reinforce the adoption of health promotion and screening behaviors" (2006: 766). It is worth noting that culture in this framework falls under the culture-as-barrier or cultural sensitivity approach, discussed earlier in this book. Relevant characteristics of the culture are identified and subsequently communication strategies are developed to respond to these characteristics. Interrogating this approach from a culture-centered perspective suggests that, although the addressing of preventive and screening behaviors is commendable, such a persuasive design strategy does not touch on the underlying factors of disparity.

In addition to developing communication strategies that promote preventive health behaviors and screening, communication scholars have also started exploring questions of *digital divide* in the realm of inaccess to communication technologies among racial minorities (Kreps 2002, 2005a, 2005b). Those consumers who typically suffer from the greatest health risks are also the ones who have minimal access to key communication channels that provide health information. It is also this same segment that has minimal access to healthcare resources. Thus health disparities are structurally reinforced, both in terms of direct access to healthcare and in terms of access to the communicative resources of health. In order to address such information disparities, the National Cancer Institute funded the Digital Divide Projects, to test new strategies for developing communication and information infrastructures in underserved communities (Dervin 2005; Kreps 2002, 2003, 2005a, 2005b).

Yet another communicative avenue for healthcare disparities focuses on developing appropriate interpersonal and group communication strategies which are responsive to the needs of racial and ethnic minorities. Kreps (2006) eloquently points out that healthcare providers typically contribute to racial disparities by bringing in cultural biases to their interactions with patients and by communicating in ways that are culturally unresponsive and prejudicial (Burgess, Fu and van Ryn 2004; Kagawa-Singer 2001). He suggests greater need for developing culturally sensitive health communication that minimizes the communication of biases, is built upon respect for others, and develops a collaborative healthcare relationship. Such communication uses language, examples, and descriptions that healthcare consumers can understand, and feedback for evaluating current levels of understanding in order to guide future interactions (Parker and Kreps 2005; Kreps 2006). The ultimate goal is the development of effective intercultural communications in the delivery of healthcare through the use of a variety of culturally sensitive materials that support health promotion, health education, and treatment decision-making. Worth noting, once again, is the emphasis of the cultural sensitivity model on developing communication strategies that are responsive to the culture. This attempt is different from that of the culture-centered approach, which would call for examining the underlying epistemologies that drive systems of curing and healing, with the goal of ultimately developing dialogical spaces that are open to multiple meanings and interpretations.

From a culture-centered approach, it would be critical not only to develop communication strategies that adapt to the cultural characteristics of diverse cultures, but also to question the underlying communicative processes through which health inequities are created, recreated and sustained. For instance: in the case of health problems related to disparities, what role does their discursive construction, under the cultural sensitivity framework, as behavioral problems play in shifting the focus away from the question of deeper underlying structural inequities? Communication scholars ought to go a step beyond the development and deployment of culturally adaptive messages targeted at underserved communities, to developing communication processes and strategies targeted at policy-makers and implementers of policies that address the root causes of the healthcare inequities. For instance, how do policy-makers and health agencies justify the differential access to the basic capacities of healthcare within communities? How do policy-makers use discourse to justify the absence of healthcare infrastructures in underserved communities? The implications of such questions became amply clear in the case of Hurricane Katrina and its consequences on lower income African American communities.

Healthcare in this respect is perhaps reflective of deeper structural disparities within social systems, and, for health communication scholars to address these health disparities in a fundamental way, the structural disparities among racial and ethnic groups would need to be resolved. Communication strategies may be developed that focus on addressing unhealthy policies, which breed structural violence, with the goal of bringing about changes to these unhealthy policies. There is also a greater need for understanding health communication in the realm of activism that seeks to transform the unhealthy structures that breed disparity and inequality.

Additionally, much of the existing health communication work targeted at racial and ethnic minorities embodies a top-down framework: it focuses on developing and diffusing messages that serve the dominant agendas, therefore suggesting that more work is needed to develop communicative spaces and create openings for a dialogue with those voices that have typically been left out. From a culture-centered perspective, one of the critical tasks ahead of communication scholars is in the articulation of the structural violence in the healthcare system through co-constructive participation with marginalized groups. The sharing of stories of structural violence becomes a way of resisting the dominant structures of oppression and of creating openings for social change within systems.

Age

Yet another socio-demographic context within which marginalization gets enacted is age. A significant body of literature has developed which interrogates the ways in which age is socially constructed and how this phenomenon continues to create positions at the peripheries of the healthcare system, marginalizing certain communities through the creation of dominant discourses of "normalcy" and "deviance." Of particular relevance are the communicative strategies through which age is stigmatized in certain contexts, and the embeddings of the social construction of aging within the social structures. Estes (1999) suggests that a multilevel framework would be relevant to understanding the discursive and material constructions of aging if it were to examine the roles played by the financial and industrial capital, the state, the "aging enterprise," the medical-industrial complex, and the public. In this framework, aging is seen as a process which is structurally situated within a social system and is constituted through cultural symbols and meanings rather than simply being an individual biological and psychological process. From a culture-centered approach, aging is situated within the social structures that constitute it, is communicatively constructed through the participation of various stakeholder groups who give it a meaning framework, and is enacted through the day-to-day experiences of the aging population.

Aging is experienced as a heterogeneous process, with the status, resources and health of the elderly being determined by the location of the individual within the social structure and the economic mode of production within this structure. The elderly are constructed as dependent, and this dependency is tied in to the logic of the market and of the social relations produced by it (Estes 1999). The experience of aging varies as this variable intersects those of gender, class, and ethnicity; thus aging is part of a multilayered socio-cultural system. The structures surrounding aging determine the policies that are constituted, passed and implemented, and they do so through the diffusion of certain ideologies that privilege the dominant structure. For instance, aging is constructed around the key question of independence versus dependence; hence the worth of individuals is seen in terms of their capacity to contribute to the economy as productive participants in the labor force, as purchasers in the marketplace, and as independent caretakers who would not absorb the resources of the state. To the extent that individuals need forms of support, they are constructed as abnormal and deviant.

The critical structures which dictate how policies are passed and executed exist at the intersections of state and capital. The state in a capitalist economy exists to serve the interests of the capital as its very existence depends upon the growth of private wealth; growth in private wealth and private economy finance the state in such situations. In the realm of aging, the state serves the capital through its continued construction of aging as an individual and medical problem, thus legitimating the existence of managed care where medical services are sold for a profit, and focusing on the aging individual as a problem without addressing the structural and cultural issues around aging. Furthermore, the elderly are seen as non-contributing, non-productive vestiges within the socio-cultural; they are constructed in terms of dependence. The stigma of dependence continues to support the framework of property-bearing individuals and productive participants in the capitalist mode of production.

As suggested earlier, the discursive construction of aging is multilayered. For instance, Nelson (1982) suggests that the process of devaluation varies with class and gender. Working-class elders and minority elders, for instance, are devalued more rapidly in the labor market than members of other classes. Similarly, Estes and Binney (1997) suggest that aging women are less valued, because they are socially constructed as unproductive. Essential to the marginalization of the elderly is the socio-cultural construction of aging as an individual problem, drawing upon the individualistic roots of the culture. The discursive construction of the elderly as "dependent" is framed within the taken-for-granted notions of the value of the independent and productive individual who contributed to the economy by actively participating in it. The conceptualizations of old age as an illness and as an economic crisis are socially created by dominant groups of experts, policy-makers, the media and the biomedical enterprise, which exist in positions of power within the social system and continue to benefit from this construction. For instance, the entire "aging industry" of nursing homes, medical services for the elderly, and biomedical technologies targeted toward the elderly depends upon the construction of old age as an illness. It is the crisis of illness that after all feeds the commercial growth of new biomedical products and services designed to serve the elderly.

Many of the efforts of application targeted toward the elderly are oriented toward seeking to modify individual psychological and/or behavioral processes, without attending to the social, cultural, and economic structures within which aging is constituted. In being oriented this way, the dominant discourse shifts attention away from those structures which sustain the conditions of marginalizing the elderly. In contrast to this individual-level approach to aging, the culture-centered approach suggests that aging should be located at the intersection between culture, structure, and agency; that those structures should be examined that underlie the marginalization of the aging population. Therefore, instead of suggesting individual-level solutions for the elderly such as counseling and individual services, policy implications that derive from a culture-centered approach pay attention to the fact that structures create unhealthy policies for the aging population in order to serve the interests of the capital. The goal therefore is to alter these structures of production through the interrogation of discourse, such that openings might be created for policy change.

Socio-economic status (SES)

Finally, as discussed earlier in this chapter, socio-economic status (SES) is one of the critical indicators of structural violence, and plays out its role in the realm of healthcare by limiting access to a variety of healthcare resources that are considered basic for human survival (Agency for Healthcare Research and Quality 2004). Individuals living in poorer communities are directly exposed to violence through the absence of basic infrastructures and opportunities and through the presence of a variety of threats to the health of the individual. Social class is a critical indicator of health capacity in underserved communities, poorer communities having lower health capacity as compared to communities with higher levels of income. The basic health infrastructure in such communities is either absent or minimal, with limited number of providers, limited medical supplies, limited healthcare technologies, limited transportation, and limited access to preventive resources. In addition to affecting the distribution of resources at a community level, SES fundamentally impacts individual health by determining the amount and types of healthcare services that are available to individuals. Class contributes to a culture of poverty that is built around narratives of pain, struggle, and resistance. It is through these narratives of suffering and survival that we gain insights into the agency of marginalized communities, and the ways in which communities make sense of their limited structural resources.

The SES of an individual directly determines the types of preventive services, healthcare services and communication infrastructures he/she would have access to (Agency for Healthcare Research and Quality 2004). Higher SES groups are more likely to have better access to a variety of health-related services than lower SES groups. For instance, individuals from higher SES have greater access to providers as compared to individuals from lower SES groups. Similarly, higher SES individuals have greater access to cancer-screening resources as compared to individuals who belong to lower SES groups. Furthermore, disparities exist between higher and lower SES groups in the realms of access to policy platforms, access to civil society forums, access to health delivery organizations, and access to organizations that evaluate the ways in which policy gets implemented by healthcare organizations. Also, the quality of communication experienced by individuals varies with their SES such that low SES individuals are more likely to experience unpleasant interactions with their providers.

Whereas higher SES groups typically can afford a plethora of preventive services, lower SES groups are limited in their access to preventive services – limited in terms of costs of these resources, effort needed to access them, and time consumed in individual-level attempts to take such steps. In addition, higher SES groups typically live in resource rich communities, who also have greater levels of access to preventive resources of various types – including parks and walkways for physical exercise, easily accessible screening facilities, easily accessible food resources, and so on – than low SES groups. In addition, higher SES groups also have greater access to hospitals and medical centers, physicians, nurses, and a variety of treatment options (medicines and surgical options). Of particular concern in the realm of SES is the health of those who are not covered by health insurance, the health of the working classes, the health of homeless populations and the health of individuals who live in rural communities. Each of these segments of the population is marked by its inaccess to basic healthcare resources.

Discussion point 7.4

- What are the ways in which education and income influence health?
- What role does communication play in reinforcing structures of violence in the context of education and income?
- How would you propose we change these unequal structures that marginalize lower SES groups?

The uninsured. According to published scholarship on health services usage, an increasing number of Americans do not have health insurance coverage (Hellander et al. 1995). Between 1989 and 1996, the number of uninsured persons in the United States increased by 8.3 million, such that by 1996, 41.7 million Americans lacked any health insurance coverage (ibid). The absence of health insurance coverage has been shown to be correlated with a decreased likelihood of obtaining preventive services and having a usual source of care (Mainous et al. 1999). The uninsured are more likely to face major barriers to healthcare utilization and to report poorer physical and mental health (Hahn and Flood 1994; Short and Lair 1994; Wu et al. 2003). Existing research suggests that the uninsured are also less likely to have access to communication infrastructures that are typically taken for granted in health communication work. For instance, the uninsured are less likely to have access to, and use, the Internet for health-related purposes as compared to individuals who are insured.

Homelessness.   Homelessness is a key problem facing the United States, with the late 1970s and the 1980s seeing a surge in the number of homeless people across the country. Because they lack permanent housing and are often among the poorest members of a community, with restricted access to resources and services, the homeless have unique health needs and problems that merit the attention of health campaign and public health researchers (Markos and Allen 2001). The lack of structural resources and social networks marks this segment of the population as marginalized. Also, lack of access to primary health services works hand in hand with lack of access to communication resources (Markos and Allen 2001). While efforts to improve the health of the homeless have more or less centered around service delivery – providing emergency shelters, soup kitchens, detoxification clinics, and even permanent housing (ibid.) – the role of communication in helping the homeless scale barriers to health is largely undermined in literature on the subject. The marginalization of the homeless is reinforced through the stigma which circulates in dominant media messages and through their limited access to communicative infrastructures. The nature of marginalization in the US runs parallel to experiences of marginalization enacted globally.

Marginalization in a Global Context

By the end of the nineteenth century, most of the globe was under European control, which had important consequences for the spread of disease, its effects on the colonies, and the way diseases were approached. Imperialism, on one hand, created a climate for the diffusion of certain diseases, and, on the other hand, pushed Western solutions to control these diseases. In other words, the dialectics of diffusion of disease and its control was integral to the colonial enterprise, creating a condition of dominance within which Western solutions became the critical solutions for the development of the colonized spaces. This Western dominance in the postcolonial world continued to recreate positions of power on the basis of the universal logic of biomedicine.

Culture is central to the logic of colonialism, since it is the portrayed inferiority of the native culture and its "need" for colonial expansion that justifies the imperialist expansion. Theorists working with the culture-centered framework of health communication are specifically interested in how voices of marginalized communities are silenced through the attempts at universalizing the mainstream biomedical model, which brands alternative cultural systems and forms of knowledge as inferior, "underdeveloped," and "Third World" systems (Dutta-Bergman 2004a, 2004b, 2005a: Dutta and Basnyat, in press). Culture in postcolonial contexts serves to maintain the status quo, so that concepts like development and modernization might be used to retain the discursive and material conditions of privilege and underprivilege. What is evident here is the use of the term culture to locate the "other," who exists outside the realm of normalcy, and therefore ought to be targeted through interventions. It is this act of othering that maintains the positions of colonizer and colonized, by discursively creating points at the margins that ought to be acted upon and transformed. To the extent that the actors in these locales at the margins continue to participate in the discursively constituted position of inferiority ascribed to them, the colonial logic maintains itself.

The beliefs and behaviors of these others are categorized as culture, and hence are targeted as objects of health communication interventions. The goal in such instances is to address the inherent cultural beliefs as barriers and to change them, such that the population could be shifted toward the acceptance of desirable health behaviors that are promoted through interventions. In such instances, the cultural beliefs are categorized as traditional and in need of interventions, and the values of science and rationality are presented as universally desirable markers of modernity. Central to this impetus for categorizing other ways of knowing is the political economy of the global enterprise, where the legitimacy of the biomedical model and its widespread diffusion is legitimized by the depiction of these other forms of knowing as inferior. In other words, colonialism in the global arena is maintained through the construction of the Third World as an inferior space that needs to be saved through the scientific technology of modernity.

Communication plays a critical role in maintaining colonial relations. After all, it is through discourse that the positions of marginality are created, sustained, and recreated. Scholars such as Airhihenbuwa (1995) and Dutta-Bergman (2004a, 2004b) argue that the discursive marginalization of Third World cultures is essential to the colonial logic of hegemonic systems, and health plays a key role in this discursive marginalization. The Third World is constructed as a space that is elsewhere, exotic and imbued with negative traits, which need to be transformed through the proselytizing actions of the Western savior. The culture-centered approach interrogates this very construction of the Third World as another space in need of interventions; it questions the very logic of interventions. Of specific interest to cultural scholars are the material manifestations of this discourse and the interrogation of material conditions of inaccess that are linked with the so-called projects of modernization.

Imperialism and Disease

Imperialism refers to the condition of control held by a nation-state over another nation-state, with the goal of drawing economic benefits from the nation-states that are controlled and occupied. Essential to imperialism, therefore, is the economic logic according to which there are economic benefits to be obtained from imperialist interventions (Comaroff and Comaroff 1992). In the context of the development of imperialism, medicine and medical technology emerged as tools for control that allowed the imperialists to exert it and to derive economic benefits from the colonies. Therefore the logic of benefits is central to the relationship between modern medicine and imperialism, and this relationship continues to be echoed in current health communication programs in the areas of population control, HIV/AIDS and so on (Comaroff and Comaroff 1992; King 2002).

Of particular interest to the health communication scholar is the construction of culture in the realm of health: How do health communicators construct culture, and what role does this phenomenon play in the broader discursive space? How does culture get formulated in the design and development of communication solutions directed at marginalized spaces? The dominant rhetoric of health communication framed in the context of development ultimately serves the bases for imperialism by creating a sense of need of interventions developed by the colonial powers. Imperialism becomes a much-needed solution to tradition and underdevelopment.

Box 7.4   The story of Kini

As a member of the Okigbo community in Sub-Saharan Africa, Kini remembers the campaigns and messages that have been targeted at her community over the last several decades. She remembers the times when United Nations workers would come to her community, and they would round up people to hold meetings and to get them to participate in immunization camps. She also remembers the times when volunteers came from door to door, gathering people to participate in these camps. A few years would pass, and the enthusiasm of the UN personnel would decrease, and then, all of a sudden, they would have left the community. A few years later, another set of volunteers and doctors would come, with a new agenda and with the goal of diffusing a new health intervention. Kini remembers how she learned very quickly not to trust really the sustainability of any of these programs. They only lasted for as long as there was enthusiasm among the UN staff. These interventions never really solved the problems of food and basic health supplies, problems that were more fundamental to Kini and her neighbors in the community.

The above excerpt captures the frustration felt by subaltern groups at their exclusion from mainstream health communication programs that typically decide the key health agendas; in these instances, the imperial logic of decision-making is based on the notion that the intervened spaces and people need outside experts to make the decisions for them. They need the mantras of enlightenment showered upon them by these experts. Kini and her community members learned not to trust the UN and USAID-led programs because these programs were more clearly dedicated to pursuing a top-down agenda of the funding agencies and were not really concerned with the real problems of the community as articulated by community members.

Historically, imperialism was driven by European interests in expanding colonies to other parts of the globe, with the goals of controlling the resources within these colonies and of utilizing the resources, so as to feed into the industrialist economies of the European nation-states. Essential to imperialism was its close ties to the industrial revolution. The colonies occupied by Europe served as resources for raw materials and as markets for the industrial revolution. In other words, the transformation of the globe during the period of modernity is marked by the existence of colonies and colonizers; the economic logic of modernity was built on this very relationship in some fundamental ways.

In spite of the overt economic interest of Europe in exploiting colonies for economic gains, much of the discourse of imperialism was hidden under the chador of "civilizing the native." In this broader discourse which circulated around imperialism, it was argued that the colonized people needed the intervention of the imperialists in order to be civilized and brought under the umbrella of modernity. Inherent in this logic was the portrayal of the colonized people as barbarians who needed the proselytizing acts of the invaders. This discourse, of the barbarianism of the native people, was particularly relevant in the realm of health: health in the colonies was portrayed as primitive, unhygienic, and in need of the interventions deployed by the colonizers. In other words, imperialism was necessary for the purposes of ensuring development in the occupied colonies. The imperialist function served by this rhetoric of "need to be civilized" is well illustrated in the following excerpt:

> Development help inherited the missionary idea, with its accursed crusade to win converts and mania for redemption. The message of salvation has been secularized compared to the missionary idea, but that is precisely the reason why the condition of "not yet partaking" appears in the shaming form of a deficit. However emphatically cultural particularity and historically evolved multiplicity may be discussed, the modern missionary idea still declares that a shortfall of civilization must be remedied, an incorrect historical development corrected, an excessively slow pace accelerated. (Gronemeyer 1993: 66)

The deficit of the native culture portrayed in the discourse of health campaigns served as the basis for penetrating the native culture (King 2002). Development and modernization came to be taken for granted as necessary goals that served the civilizing efforts of the West. This logic of Western medicine, which justified imperialism as an altruistic exercise, is evident in the following excerpt from King's analysis of postcolonial discourses of health (2002: 765):

> Europeans contrasted their own medicine and public health, symbolizing rationality and modernity, with putatively superstitious and primitive indigenous medical beliefs, which they denigrated and sought to eliminate as part of the larger "civilizing mission" of colonialism. The medical modernization of native populations, via export of Western medical theories and practices, was part of the "ideology of colonial healing," that justified colonialism as an ultimately humanitarian endeavor.

Discussion point 7.5

- Identify a current health issue that lends itself particularly well to the postcolonial context. Demonstrate how this issue is impacted by the politics of postcolonialism.
- More specifically, demonstrate the role of communication in constituting and reinforcing the postcolonial politics of health with respect to the issue that you picked.

Imperialism, disease and control

The colonies in the imperial projects were exotic spaces with immense economic benefits and profits; however, they were also dangerous spaces rife with life-threatening diseases and illnesses. Therefore, if the imperial project were to work and the economic benefits were to be reaped, these exotic spaces needed to be monitored, the disease threats needed to be identified, and solutions needed to be developed. Colonial medicine developed as a disciplinary body of work targeted at controlling diseases in colonies. The expansion of the colonialists into the native spaces was dependent upon the control exerted by medicine. Furthermore, the diffusion of disease and the introduction of new diseases in erstwhile colonies are deeply related to the ways in which imperialism operated (Marcovich 1988). The growth in imperialism meant that goods and people were continually circulated between geographical areas. This continuous flow of people also opened up the geographical spaces to the diffusion of disease. The entry of bureaucrats, merchants, and soldiers into the colonies and the disruption of the existing ecological relationships were accompanied by the introduction of new diseases, foreign to the native spaces.

The colonial encounter with "new" tropical diseases in the colonies and the rapid spread of certain disease types that accompanied imperialism came along with the development of public health infrastructures, primarily for the purposes of servicing and protecting the bureaucrats, merchants, and soldiers who were posted in these colonies; furthermore, colonial medicine was needed to ensure the supply of laborers from the colonies, who were integral to the expansionist project. In other words, the development and diffusion of healthcare services in the colonies occupied by Europe was marked by the reciprocal relationship between colonialism and disease. Essential to the imperial machinery was the need to control the disease and to contain its diffusion in the colonies.

The biomedical project therefore became a tool for European expansionism across the globe, as it gave the imperialists the power to stop sickness (Marcovich 1988: 109). The work of Louis Pasteur, the bacteriological studies of Koch, Yerson, Kitasato and Ehlrich, and the use of vaccines and serums put important tools in the hands of colonialists. Marcovich further writes:

> A basic idea began to develop: that once nature had been mastered at a global level, western scientific culture could inevitably be adopted everywhere and by all. The struggle to dominate nature was therefore transformed into an instrument of colonization, of economic growth and of new possibilities for settlement. The power able to stop a sickness from spreading or which could resolve a sanitary problem would be able to impose its domination all the more easily and would therefore be able to exploit the wealth of occupied territories. (Ibid.)

Hence medicine became a tool that allowed the colonialists to operate in their territories and to reap the economic benefits in these territories. By controlling the spread of disease, the exotic and dangerous spaces in the colonies could once more be tamed, so that the economic benefits of these spaces might be harvested. Marcovich notes:

> The conquest of sickness was a basic condition for colonial expansion and development. Conquering the Indochinese forests, for example, raised the problem of coping with malaria. The construction of new railway lines, roads, and canals, not to speak of the development of agriculture in regions that had never been exploited, could only be carried out by using 'native' laborers who were exposed to the risks of malaria. (Ibid.)

In order to expand the territories, the colonialists needed the medical enterprise to control the threat of disease. Medicine offered a solution to the problem of underdevelopment in the colonies, and it allowed the colonies to expand their control further. The role of medicine in serving the state's economic and political interests continues to be echoed in modern discourses of global health (King 2002). Connecting the link between modern public health and the economy, King argues that modern public health has had a history that directly links it to interests of national security and international commerce.

Discussion point 7.6

- What are the ways in which imperialism plays out in current discourses of HIV/AIDS?
- How do health messages constructed in the realm of global health interventions constitute economic interests of dominant power structures? Please illustrate your argument with an example.

Western knowledge as a solution

Western knowledge was seen as the basic and exclusive solution to disease, and the way to control the diffusion of disease was to spread Western knowledge of modern medicine rapidly into the communities. The scientific rationalistic mode of thinking was proposed as the universal and logical solution to disease, and it was juxtaposed in the backdrop of the traditional systems of the colonized communities. Knowledge systems within the traditional communities were typically considered to be primitive and culturally determined. The notion of culture was closely tied with these practices of healing and curing, and the lens applied to the understanding of such practices developed on the basis of an outsider's understanding of culture in terms of an exotic other, who lay outside the realm of the mundane.

The cultural location of the native practices has historically been co-present with the depiction of the rationalistic practices of modern medicine, presented as distinctly different from traditional forms of healing and curing. Modern medicine, strictly located in the compass of science, was depicted as a system which rises above and beyond the narrow limits of culture, and is applicable universally because of its appeal to scientific reasoning and empirical observation. For the modern medical model to succeed in the colonies, the traditionally rooted cultural practices needed to be examined and eradicated. In this context, culture was equated with tradition, and was depicted as a marker of the primitiveness of the savage, who needed to be tamed.

This dichotomization of tradition versus modernity continues to drive current discourses in health communication, particularly in the realm of current constructions of health communication projects in former colonies. These colonies today are largely identified as the Third World or as the underdeveloped world, continuing the colonial legacies of colonialism into the current global climate. The characteristics of this Third World are marked by the lack of development and modernization and by the apathy of the populations within these spaces to the projects of modernization.

The dichotomization of tradition versus modernity is critical, as it serves to support the logic of colonialism, where messages and interventions from the positions of power are directed toward the so-called inferior positions at the periphery. For instance, the analysis, conducted by Dutta-Bergman and Basnyat (in press) of the Radio Communication Project in Nepal demonstrates how the categories of tradition and modernity are evoked in the radio dramas, with Nepal being depicted as a traditional space in need of the modernist interventions led by Johns Hopkins University (JHU) and funded by the United States Agency for International Development (USAID). The argument for the necessity of modernity is based on the description of tradition as primitive and savage; culture here is seen as a category that needs to be transformed in order to make way for the rational, scientific role of modern medicine, which has supposedly risen above culture and therefore offers universal solutions for human health problems. Further analysis, however, demonstrates that the model of modern medicine, i.e. the biomedical model, is itself situated within the realm of culture, and is deeply tied to the Enlightenment project and the industrial revolution in Europe.

Postcolonial Experiences

The ways in which health continues to be negotiated in the fragmented and yet seamless web of cultural dialectics in former colonies tap into the postcolonial nature of health communication in a globalized world. The negotiation of health meanings in these postcolonial spaces reflects the ways in which power and control continue to be exerted and are dispersed through the communicative outlets of a global healthcare system.

Ideology of dominance

Fundamentally, the health communication discourse of the biomedical model is embedded in an ideology of dominance. Inherent in this ideology is the idea that health can be controlled, monitored and manipulated, and that the desired targets of health interventions need to be persuaded to engage in the proposed health behaviors, which hold the key to better health. The emphasis here is on treating health as a commodity that can be harnessed through the uses of modern medical technology. Modern medical technology provides universal solutions to healthcare problems on the basis of its ability to conceptualize problems and to develop solutions derived from empirical observations and rational thinking. The claims to objective truth made by the biomedical model underlie the privilege accorded to the model, accompanied by the simultaneous downplaying of alternative models as inferior and primitive.

The ideology of dominance is also tied to an economic logic where health is treated as a commodity in the marketplace. The commodification of health is achieved through presenting health solutions that ought to be purchased at competitive prices. The large-scale global growth of the pharmaceutical industry attests to the rapid diffusion of the market ideology; health products and health technologies offer the solutions to health problems in this marketplace. The emphasis is on the individual, and health is his/her individual resource. Therefore the ideology of dominance is played out at individual level, simultaneously ignoring other critical questions about healthcare resources and about their distribution within collectives.

Taming the savage: Development campaign

Much of the health communication discourse of the dominant paradigm is embodied in the development campaigns directed at the Third World.

Such campaigns are typically based on the assumption that Third World populations are in need of interventions offered by the developed world. Inherent in the campaigns is a power differential that puts the First and Third World in the corresponding relationship of sender and receiver. Inherent in the logic of such campaigns is a notion of development based on the differences in power between the involved actors. This difference in the distribution of power determines who gets to develop and evaluate messages targeted at whom. The taken-for-granted assumptions driving the flow of such campaigns revolve around the inherent superiority of the sender of the message, who could proselytize the receivers through the messages of development targeted at them.

Health in the postcolony

In spite of the continuing discourse of assistance and development embodied in the health communication campaigns targeted at postcolonial spaces, the material gains of the modernization projects seem to go beyond the scope of the individuals, groups, and communities of these sectors. In other words, the material conditions of inaccess to basic healthcare continue to plague the communities, in spite of the so-called efforts of development that are directed toward them. The very paradox of the so-called modernization projects is that they are unable to serve those segments of the global population that they continue to stigmatize through their individual-level campaigns.

For instance, individuals in the rural communities of West Bengal are constructed as primitive and traditional because they visit the *ojhas*, and yet these very same individuals have limited access to modern medical facilities (Dutta-Bergman 2004a, 2004b). Most of such facilities are located in towns that are hard to access because of the absence of adequate transportation; they do not have adequately trained doctors who would treat the patients; and they do not have adequate medical supplies that should be available to the patients. Therefore the material conditions of health in the postcolony are marked by the absence of the very resources of modernization that are touted as the solutions to the problem of primitiveness within these spaces.

The projects of modernization which continue to construct the postcolonial spaces as traditional and underdeveloped simultaneously limit the access of such spaces to modern healthcare facilities and to resources by locating the problem at the level of the individual and by backgrounding questions of resource reallocation and of redistributive justice in the context of the health problems faced by the community. The silencing of the voices of community members is achieved through the circulation of discourse that continues to construct the community as passive and voiceless, and advances policies without the participation of the community. The absence of the community from policy fora is justified by the modernist discourse which constructs the community as passive and incapable of participation.

Positions of Subalternity

As discussed in the Introduction, the condition of subalternity refers to the silencing of certain groups within social systems (Dutta 2006). This form of disenfranchisement happens at multiple levels within social systems, being marked by inaccess to a variety of basic resources and disparities between the "haves" and the "have-nots" of society. Subaltern positions are communicatively created and reinforced through the articulation of discourse which continues to position subaltern subjects in places of inferiority. In other words, the material lack of access is reinforced by lack of access in the realm of communication.

At national level, conditions of subalternity are reified by the interests of the national elite, which wants to maintain its positions of control in writing the history of the nation-state, and by the international stakeholders, who want to write the narrative of colonization drawing upon the construction of the subaltern as the passive subject, in need of the interventions carried on by the actors in positions of power. In both of these instances, the politics of knowledge production is driven by parties interested in projecting a dominant narrative that strips the subaltern of his/her agency and celebrates the emancipatory role played by the actors writing the history. What, then, is absent from this broader discourse is the voice of the subaltern and the writing of the subaltern narrative.

In the realm of health, subalternity is maintained by the interests of national and global elites, who continue to present the modernist project of development as the only viable path to healthcare, and simultaneously construct the subaltern subject in positions of inferiority. The complicitous relationship between the national elite and the international stakeholders is particularly critical here, because it is this very relationship that continually locates the subaltern in the position of periphery. The conglomeration of elite actors at the national and international levels is referred to as transnational hegemony, and this hegemonic configuration consists of global and national funding agencies, national and global monitoring organizations, multinational corporations, and national and international leadership at various organizations such as public health agencies, medical organizations, universities, etc.

The interests of the transnational hegemony are driven by the need to create continuous flows of capital, goods, and markets that would sustain transnational capitalism. In order to maintain the flow of capital and markets, the emphasis of the transnational hegemonic configuration is on creating communication strategies which invite the opening up of economies to the free market and highlight the individualization of property, which drives the free market economy. Therefore, in this configuration, health is portrayed as a commodity that must be purchased, and the responsibility of health is shifted to the level of the individual. Health interventions pushed by transnational hegemony focus on individual-level solutions to health resource problems in marginalized contexts, thereby ignoring questions of inequity and inaccess which are primordial in the current global configuration.

The individual-level interventions proposed by those in positions of power at the center continue to look at health as a commodity, emphasize the need for individual-level behavior change in order to ensure greater health in marginalized contexts, and simultaneously remove any type of discussion about redistributive justice and structural access to resources from the discursive space. In doing so, the dominant health interventions targeted at the marginalized sectors continue to reproduce the stigmatization of subaltern groups, and simultaneously limit possibilities of structural change for greater health among subaltern groups. What is missing from health communication about the marginalized sectors is the very presence of the subaltern voices in the articulation of health problems and of relevant health solutions.

Subaltern rewriting of health communication

Rewriting health communication theory, research, and practice from a subaltern perspective suggests that discursive openings be explored that open entryways for listening to subaltern voices. As a starting point, a subaltern rewriting of health communication calls for health communication students, researchers and practitioners to interrogate the positions of privilege they bring to the table and to engage with subaltern participants in order to listen to their voices about critical healthcare policies and about their implementation. Engaging with the position of subalternity, therefore, begins with reflexivity on behalf of the researcher, who interrogates the taken-for-granted positions of power and privilege embedded in the ways in which health problems are defined and health solutions are targeted toward the subaltern sectors of the globe. In writing histories from below, the health communication scholar needs to start by engaging with the very suppositions and taken-for-granted assumptions that drive his/her work.

Subaltern rewriting of health communication suggests the importance of questioning normal definitions of problems and proposed solutions within communities. For instance, for campaign promoters working on population control programs in the subaltern sectors of the world, engaging with the subaltern position involves questioning the very normalcy of population control as the obvious solution to problems of (under)development. Rewriting the subaltern narrative brings forth underlying power relations and hegemonic interests that drive health solutions such as population control. When attention is paid to what is not spoken and to what remains unsaid within the discursive space, openings for reflexivity emerge from within. It is through these openings of reflexivity that alternative health communication problems and solutions have opportunities to emerge. It is only through this reflexivity that the health communication researcher and practitioner can start opening up to the possibilities of alternative epistemologies, understandings, and interpretations of health problems.

Therefore the very starting point of the subaltern rewriting is the interrogation of healthcare policies for the presence and/or absence of subaltern voices. A recent example of such interrogation is the controversy surrounding the human genome diversity project. The question regarding the commoditization of the indigenous gene has led to debates about the presence of subaltern voices in the way the policies were decided and would be implemented. These voices draw our attention to the questions of power, structure, agency, and voice in ways that are typically omitted in the mainstream discourses of health communication. For instance, the very act of listening to subaltern voices draws our attention to the active participation of groups in day-to-day healthcare decision-making, even in spite of the minimal resources that are available to them. Furthermore, engaging with the subaltern voices draws our attention to the configurations of problems that are typically not envisioned within the broader health policy discourse.

Conclusion

In conclusion, this chapter demonstrates that the health experiences of the marginalized sectors are marked by inaccess to health services, poor quality of healthcare even in situations where access is less of an issue, inaccess to preventive and screening services, and inaccess to communication infrastructures that serve as conduits of health information. Furthermore, the chapter underscores the critical role played by communication in maintaining disenfranchised positions within social systems. Positions at the margins are maintained through messages which continue to ignore questions of inequity and injustice and focus instead on individual behavior change, further stigmatizing individuals from underserved sectors. The analysis presented in this chapter documents the fact that the dichotomous categories of tradition versus modernity continue to inform the mainstream discourse of health communication targeted at the underserved segments of the world. As an entry point to an alternative approach to health communication, this chapter suggests that one needs to question the dominant discourse with respect to its deliberate ignoring of matters of structure and its stigmatization of underserved populations through the circulation of discourse. This questioning will simultaneously open up the discursive space to articulating the voices of marginalized groups, through which the narratives of structural violence might be heard. This very hearing of the narratives creates a space for social change.

8 Culture, Social Capital, and Health

Chapter objectives

In this chapter, we will:

- understand the role of social capital in the realm of health
- connect social capital to income inequalities
- understand the role of community processes in health communication
- address processes for engaging the community in culture-centered applications

Health is not only a resource that is possessed by the individual, but it is also a resource of the community. The culture-centered approach draws our attention to the intersection between structure, culture, and agency where health is constituted, suggesting that communities are constitutive spaces where the relationships between structure, culture, and agency are played out (Dutta-Bergman 2004a, 2004b, 2004c, 2004d, 2004e, 2004f, 2005a, 2005b; Dutta and Basu 2007). The community, also referred to as the neighborhood, is defined here as the geographical space within which the individual and his/her family resides. In this sense, the community is spatially located and is tied to certain markers and material resources such as streets, schools, educational institutions, transportation services, telecommunications facilities and hospitals, which define the boundaries and assets of the community (Dutta-Bergman 2004d, 2004e, 2004f, 2005b; Kawachi et al. 1999). It is the spatial setting where the health experiences of the members are constituted; also, it is in the realm of the community that cultural meanings create constitutive spaces for interpreting, working with, and challenging the structures and structural disparities (Dutta-Bergman 2004a). The basic material resources constitute community capacity and are reflective of the structural features of the community; they become meaningful to community members as these participate in meaning-making through the use of cultural symbols, languages, and processes. The physical constitution of the community is also tied to its communicative construction as a cohesive and interconnected space where members live and come to define their relational ties. This chapter focuses on discussing these relational ties within communities and the role of communities in the realm of health.

The nature of the community fundamentally influences the health of community members (Dutta-Bergman 2004d, 2004e; Kawachi and Kennedy

1999). Communities that have greater access to a variety of health-related resources are better able to sustain the health of their members (Dutta-Bergman 2004d, 2004e). Furthermore, communities that enjoy higher levels of reciprocal trust among their members and have greater social ties are also more likely to have better health results, as they are better able to mobilize the resources for optimal health (Dutta and Basu 2007; Kawachi and Kennedy 1999). In such communities, members find greater access to health resources, face lower number of health-related barriers, and are also more likely to experience minimal stress and increased social support. Sociologists studying community characteristics in terms of their health enhancing or health depleting effects have typically employed the concept of *social capital* to tap into the characteristics of the community. Social capital refers to the ability of a community to mobilize its collective resources and secure maximum gains through its network of relationships and social structures (Putnam 1993). It is built upon the foundations of community participation, interpersonal trust, and the collection of all social, collective, economic, and cultural resources to which a community has access. The idea of social capital taps into the extent to which community organizations involve the members of the community and help the formation of bonds of reciprocity within the community that facilitate cooperation for mutual benefit (Coleman 1990; Putnam 1993).

That social capital is integral to the health of a community has been substantiated in a growing number of studies on the sociology and epidemiology of health (Kawachi et al. 1999). Health communication scholarship has built upon this line of work, to argue that health communication efforts ought to focus on building community social capital, because forms of social capital ultimately lead to greater health in the community (Dutta-Bergman 2004d, 2004e). This chapter interjects culture in the discussion of social capital, positing that culture is intrinsically intertwined with participatory processes in communities, providing the symbols, stories, and languages for interpreting the structures and for challenging them through participatory action. Through examples of cultural mobilization at local levels, folk theaters, and community participatory processes, it elucidates the ways in which culture works with community processes in garnering social change; it is through their interactions with cultural processes that communities participate in challenging unhealthy structures. On the basis of the articulation of community participatory processes, it concludes by discussing the culture-centered approach to community organizing.

The Community as an Organizing Framework

Communities are sites within which health is played out through the availability of material and communicative health resources that are used by individuals and their families (Dutta-Bergman 2004e, 2004f). They offer the social bonds that foster the health of individual members through the sharing of information and resources, social support, and communication. In other words, communities provide the contexts for

Box 8.1   The story of Sarah

Sarah is a 34-year-old woman living in downtown Chicago, in what is considered the inner city. After her husband lost his job at one of the local grocery stores, Sarah has had a difficult time finding even enough money to buy food for the family. The entire family lives without health insurance, and so do most of Sarah's neighbors on Oxford Street, who are struggling for daily resources and to find a job to make ends meet. The neighborhood does not have a stable source of income and has recently experienced a surge in its already high crime rate. The youth in the neighborhood have been incarcerated for violent crimes and occasional shootings are fairly common. In fact, recently a 6-year-old girl was killed in a street fight that involved drugs and erupted from disagreements between two factions of youth in the neighborhood. Sarah is very concerned about the safety of her children and is not sure about their health.

What do we learn from Sarah's story about marginalization and the way it plays out in the lives of individuals who are structurally deprived? What is the relationship between individual-level marginalization and structural marginalization in the spheres of neighborhood and community?

the enactment of health through the provision of a wide variety of health-related resources and through the exchange of communication among members of the communities.

Sarah's narrative presented in the above excerpt demonstrates the community linkages of health. The neighborhood on Oxford Street presented above comprised Sarah's community. Both the material resources within communities and the communicative ties among community members are critical to the constitution of the community. Health promotion efforts often are directed toward fostering these social ties among community members and toward harnessing the benefits of these social ties within communities in order to promote health-enhancing behaviors. In other words, the goal of these health promotion efforts is, typically, to use the community ties to diffuse health behavior within the community.

Discussion point 8.1

- What are the ways in which the community offers health benefits?
- How does communication within the community help secure material resources for the community?

Community organizing

Community organizing efforts focus on building community ties in order to foster positive health outcomes within the community, and using pre-existing community networks to diffuse health interventions within communities. In these situations, community networks are mobilized to diffuse preventive behaviors such as healthy eating and exercising. In other instances, community organizing efforts are often also directed toward achieving social change in the context of the distribution and availability of health resources, the implementation of health-related policies, and/or the formulation of such policies. Community organizing efforts ultimately focus on strengthening the community ties and on involving community members in participatory processes that are directed toward a particular goal. The ultimate goal is to harness the participatory platforms of community organizations to bring about opportunities for communicating about health.

For instance, in Dutta-Bergman's study of communities in rural Bengal (Dutta-Bergman 2004a, 2004b; Dutta and Basu 2007), it was observed that community members often participated in rallies and marches in order to protest the lack of health resources such as medical supplies and doctors. In such instances, mobilizing the participation of community members serves the purpose of providing a platform where issues may be raised in the context of healthcare policy and its implementation. Similarly, in their study of HIV/AIDS prevention efforts among migrant farm workers, Ford and Yep (2003) discuss the ways in which the participation of the community is mobilized in order to foster the use of condoms.

Fundamentally, participatory processes in the community are harnessed with the objective of achieving specific community-based objectives for health interventionists. In mobilizing community participation, health communicators identify an issue or a set of issues which would need to be addressed; they identify community points of contact who serve as opinion leaders; they select communication avenues where participation might be generated; and they identify a series of steps that might be put into place in order to achieve the community outcomes. Communities typically present a variety of participatory platforms that are available to the members, ranging from meetings, street theater, folk dance, and protest marches to mass-mediated community platforms such as newspapers, newsletters, radio programming and television programming. With the advent of the Internet, communities are also using this medium toward the goal of addressing specific health outcomes. In the following sections, we will specifically discuss community-based health interventions and community-based social change efforts. Whereas community-based health interventions address individual health behaviors within the community, community-based social change efforts seek to alter the structures within the community that limit the community's access to fundamental healthcare resources.

Community-based interventions.   Community-based interventions are directed at using communities for the purposes of promoting health-related behaviors. The community, defined as a group of individuals who share a common space, social, cultural and economic milieu (Airhihenbuwa 1995), plays a critical role in health promotion efforts. Health behaviors are often embedded within this social milieu. As a result, health communication scholars have become increasingly interested in the role of the community as an avenue for promoting positive health behaviors (Dutta-Bergman

2004c, 2004d). They have consistently noted that community participation generates systematic changes in the population through citizen involvement and active participation in identifying the health needs of the community and in implementing initiatives for the improvement of health of the community and its members (Fawcett et al. 1993). The importance and usefulness of community participation is underlined in its use in a variety of health campaigns, like heart disease prevention, smoking, HIV prevention, healthy eating and road safety (Dutta-Bergman 2004d; Person and Cotton 1996; Kennedy 2001). Stephens, Rimal and Flora (2004) point out that, since participation and membership in community organizations are voluntary, health messages that come out of the organizations are likely to be considered with greater trust. Scholars like Rappaport (1987) and Repucci, Woolard, and Fried (1999) note that individual-level preventive efforts should be complemented with community-based approaches.

According to Merzel and D'Afflitti (2003), the rationale for the community-based approach to health promotion stems from the notion that individuals cannot be considered separate from their social milieu, and that context is interdependent with the health and lives of individuals in the community and hence with the community as a whole. Campbell and Jovchelovitch (2000) state that participation allows community members to formulate strategies that are based on the barriers they face and their perceived health needs. As a result, health program messages and program implementation procedures are created from within the community, enhancing their chances of eliciting the desired results. Related to this articulation is the notion of empowering the community. Communities with actively participating members are likely to perceive that they are more in charge of their lives. Hence they are also more likely to take control of their health, engage in health enhancing behaviors, and actively seek out health resources (Campbell and Jovchelovitch 2000). A conglomeration of individuals with such high loci of control will result in a community that ranks high on a scale of being healthy and of engaging in health promotion practices. In other words, situating a health communication model within a participatory community-based framework empowers members of the community to articulate their needs, map the resources available, mobilize them in the production of positive health outcomes and engage in health sustenance behaviors (Dutta-Bergman 2004d).

The theory of reasoned action (Ajzen and Fishbein 1974) and Bandura's social cognitive theory (1986) also substantiate the link between community participation and health outcomes. Extrapolating from these theories, it can be stated that individuals are more likely to engage in healthy behavior if the behavior or norm seeps through the web of the community, and if the behaviors, similar or dissimilar (Rimal et al. 2005), are being enacted by trusted peers and community leaders.

Inherent in these conceptualizations of community participation is an underlying sense of social commitment (Dutta-Bergman 2004d; Tocqueville 1999; Scheufele and Shah 2000; Veenstra 2000). This sense of commitment leads members of the community, and hence the community as a whole, to partake in health promoting behaviors. In a way, then, a community characterized by a high sense of social commitment among its members (reflected in high participation) is likely to be better off in terms of practicing healthy behaviors. In articulating this link between community participation and health, researchers and practitioners in the field consistently evoke the concept of social capital. It is also not uncommon to find the terms community participation and social capital being used interchangeably.

Community-based social change efforts.   Community-based social change efforts are directed toward addressing the structural constraints within the community that minimize the access to health resources. Examples of such barriers might include inadequate transportation to community clinics, lack of adequately trained physicians at the clinics, lack of preventive and treatment-related resources such as immunizations, medical supplies and so on. Community mobilizing efforts in these contexts focus on ways of addressing such structural barriers. Community members typically engage in a variety of communicative platforms such as street theater, folks performances, protest rallies, letters to the editor or programming in the local radio in order to draw the attention of others and to present their voices in the relevant outlets.

The locus of change for the initiative might cover local, national, and /or international contexts. Increasingly, health communication scholars are demonstrating the link between local level politics and politics at the global level. In this realm, community-based social change efforts develop with the goal of impacting local, state, national, and global policies. Communication scholars have started investigating the ways in which multilevel stakeholders might be addressed through efforts of social change.

Public Sphere and Health

The previous section discussed health communication efforts at the community level that are directed toward altering those social structures that constrain the health capacity of communities. Health here is seen as a resource that is limited in its accessibility to community members, and therefore, community-based efforts are directed toward altering the fundamental structures that limit healthcare access among community members. Public sphere refers to the publicly available community spaces where issues can be raised, debated over and communicated about. In this sense, public spheres are the grounds where debates are played out and where various stakeholder groups engage in communication. They typically serve as the sites where broader policy issues and their specific implementations get discussed.

Although public spheres are intended to provide accessible platforms for communities, extant scholarship suggests that communities and members within communities differ in the extent to which they have access to the public sphere. Marx (1975) argues that the subaltern classes of society have minimal access to the public spheres where the critical policy issues are discussed. In a healthcare context, members of underserved communities such as the homeless are typically absent from the communicative spaces of the public spheres where the issues regarding homelessness and the health of the homeless are discussed. In such an instance, decisions are made with respect to the public sphere without engaging the members of the groups who are directly impacted by the policy.

Social Capital and Health

The extant literature on the social capital linkages of health directs our attention to the role of community ties and cohesive linkages in fostering health within communities. Whereas Bourdieu (1993) described social capital as investment in social connections through valuable social relationships, the concept was highlighted in the scholarship of political scientist Robert Putnam (1993, 1995). Putnam (1995: 66) defines social capital as "features of social organization such as networks, norms, and trust that facilitate coordination and cooperation for mutual benefit". According to Pilkington (2002), Putnam's analysis of social capital had four characteristics: the existence of community networks, civic engagement, local identity, and a sense of solidarity and equity with other community members, and trust and reciprocal help and support. Coleman (1990: 302) states that "social capital inheres in the structure of relations between persons and among persons." McMichael and Manderson (2004: 89) refer to social capital as those factors that contribute to well-being and those that capture "how people use and gain from voluntary associations, interactions with others in their neighborhoods, and the contacts that friends and relatives provide." Operationalizing social capital in an effort to measure it has been varied. While Weitzman and Kawachi (2000) operationalized social capital in terms of an individual's average time committed to volunteering over a period, the Health Development Agency (HDA) in the UK developed a 54-question matrix within five topic areas (view of local area, civic engagement, reciprocity, and local trust, social networks, social support) to measure social capital. Despite this diversity in defining/operationalizing social capital, there is little evidence to deny the relationship between social capital and health (Pilkington 2002).

With its emphasis on participation, social capital assumes a lead role in instituting positive health behavior change through the mobilization efforts of community members. Social capital has often been considered an antecedent to health indicators in a community, in a way that relates health outcomes to social capital. While a community rich in social capital enjoys good health, one that is low in social capital suffers from disease and mortality. This link is played out consistently in several studies (Baum 1999; Campbell and Jovchelovitch 2000; Dube and Wilson 1996; Dutta-Bergman 2004d; Kennedy 2001; Person and Cotton 1996; Rappaport 1987). The February 16, 2004 issue of *Health and Medicine Week* quoted a series of studies in Sweden stating that there is a relation between social activity – social, cultural and religious participation, political empowerment – and coronary heart disease. Participation in community activities and friendships has been shown to improve conditions related to mental illness (Marcovic and Manderson 2002). While these studies leave no doubt about the link between social capital and health promotion, several explanations are offered to lay out the mediating processes involved in the link.

Theoretical approaches

The theoretical foundation of the social capital literature links it to income disparities, and to the socio-economic gaps that exist within communities (Kawachi and Kennedy 1999). Social capital serves as a mediator between the disparities within communities and the health outcomes experienced by these communities (Kawachi et al. 1999; Kennedy, Kawachi and Prothrow-Stith 1996; Wilkinson 1994). Several cross-national studies have pointed out that the degree of income inequality in a given society is strongly related to the society's level of mortality (Wilkinson 1996). Within the United States, the degree of income inequality within each state has been reported to be positively correlated with total mortality rates as well as deaths from specific diseases such as coronary heart disease, cancer, and infant mortality (Kennedy, Kawachi, and Prothrow-Stith 1996). Communities with greater disparities typically experience poorer health, and the link with in-community inequality and health outcomes in the realm of these disparities is offered by the research on social capital (Atkinson and Micklewright 1992; Kawachi et al. 1999; Kawachi et al. 1994; Kennedy, Kawachi and Prothrow-Stith 1996; Wilkinson 1994). Social capital, as described earlier, taps into the interconnected ties that link community members and the bonds of cohesiveness within communities. Therefore communities with higher levels of disparities typically experience lower levels of social capital, because of the mistrust generated by the inequitable distribution of resources within these communities; the growing gap between the rich and the poor in these communities has led to disinvestment in community organizations and in the norms of reciprocity. This link between poverty, income inequality and falling social capital is expressed in the following excerpt from an interview with a participant in Moldova (Narayan et al. 2000: 223):

> Poverty has created rifts in communities . . . between former friends and neighbors. People are cynical, suspicious, and jealous of other's success, which they most often attribute to dishonest and corrupt behavior. In their own communities, the poor feel ashamed and constantly humiliated in their encounters with former neighbors and friends who have prospered . . . Although poor people extensively rely on each other, at the same time frequent mutual suspicions and animosity, as well as fear of those in authority, often prevent people from cooperating on a community scale to help each other more effectively and improve community conditions.

According to this body of literature on the health effects of social capital, communities that experience greater levels of socio-economic disparity are also communities with lower levels of social capital (Kawachi et al. 1994, 1999). In this sense, social capital mediates the link between income inequities and health outcomes. Social capital influences a variety of health outcomes and is, in turn, a manifestation of the inequalities existing within communities. In their analysis of state-level social capital, Kawachi et al. (1999) demonstrated that the size of the gap between the rich and the poor led to lower levels of investment in social capital; this disinvestment in social capital, in turn, led to increased levels of mortality.

Discussion point 8.2

* What is the role of social capital in the realm of community health? How does social capital connect health inequities with population-level mortality?
* Think of a community where the healthcare disparities are evident to you. Comment on the specific ways in which healthcare disparities in this community play out in the realm of community social capital.
* How would you develop a community health effort that would address the inequities in the community?

Health outcomes of social capital

Health outcomes of social capital cover a wide range starting from heart–health related outcomes to outcomes related to diseases such as cancer and diabetes (Kawachi et al. 1999). Ultimately, the extent to which the community is cohesively connected influences the types of health outcomes its members are likely to experience. In developing the theoretical link between social capital and health outcomes, health communication scholars suggest that the degree of the ties within a community directly influences the levels of psychological stress and social support experienced by its members. To the extent that community members have higher levels of social support, they also report higher levels of perceived health. Furthermore, community ties serve as communicative links which provide health information to community members and reinforce health-enhancing behaviors through community networks. In this context, the community serves as a repository of health-enhancing behaviors, which get further reinforced by the participation of individual members in health-enhancing lifestyles.

Discussion point 8.3

* How specifically does social capital influence health outcomes?
* Imagine you are a healthcare researcher who is interested in studying health inequalities and the connections of health inequalities with income inequalities. You want to convince policy-makers that income

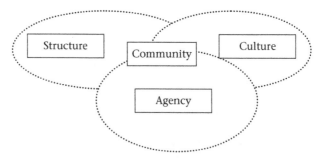

Fig. 8.1 The relationship between structure, culture, agency, and community

inequalities ultimately influence not only health inequalities but also the population level mortality of the community. How would you go about developing your argument?

Culture and Social Capital

Social capital is embedded in the local context as it taps into the communicative bonds and ties within the community. These bonds and social ties are embedded within the social context and therefore are intrinsically intertwined with the culture of the community (Dutta-Bergman 2004a, 2004b, 2004c, 2004d). In this sense, culture provides a lens through which the community comes to constitute itself and define the parameters of its actions.

Cultural mobilization

Efforts of cultural mobilization draw upon the distinct characteristics of the community in order to foster the social cohesiveness that exists in the community and to provide communicative platforms where members might engage in dialogue. Cultural mobilization builds upon the inherent strengths of the community to articulate spaces and opportunities for change. Mobilization therefore is fundamentally based on identifying the community capacities that are intrinsic to the community and define its strengths. For instance, a planning grant project described by Baker and Motton (2005) used community coalitions to address structural features of the physical environment, such as parks and safe walkways, as well as to develop capacity for planning and implementing community change projects. In this case, the community was mobilized through the creation of participatory processes and mechanisms that allowed the community to voice its concerns about issues and to develop community-based solutions to these issues.

Discussion point 8.4

• What specific strategies would you use if you were asked to build community capacity in your own community?

- What barriers do you anticipate in your community capacity-building efforts? How would you go about addressing these barriers?

Folk theater.   Folk theater provides a platform for participation through culturally meaningful participatory processes and through the enactment of culturally situated narratives that foreground the contextual elements of the culture. As a platform for community participation, folk theater is particularly powerful because it engages with the narratives of the community and resonates with the stories which circulate within it. Furthermore, folk theater engages with the problems that are typically closer to the needs of the community, as community members get involved in co-creating meaningful narratives they consider to be important. As a form of participation which directly engages the voices of cultural members, folk theater offers the opportunity for articulating culturally situated problems within the discursive space.

Community participatory processes.   Community participatory processes refer to a variety of platforms within the community which are available to community members for articulating their needs and concerns (Freudenberg, Rogers, Ritas and Nerney 2005; Israel, Eng, Schulz and Parker 2005; Lopez, Eng, Robinson and Wang 2005; Minkler and Wallerstein 2003; Wallerstein, Duran, Minkler and Foley 2005). The types of participatory processes available within communities vary from community to community and depend upon the contextual factors within the community. Some communities with strong interpersonal community ties might offer the strongest avenues of participation in the form of informal gatherings that take place at the homes of community members. In such instances, the pre-existing strong networks within the community are informally tapped into for the purposes of generating greater health. In other communities, more formal networks such as churches might offer entry points for communicating with community members about critical health issues. The participatory processes that emerge within communities depend upon the cultures of the communities and on the meanings attached to various community organizations. Some community cultures might be drawn toward pre-planned organizing that is done in a systematic way, yet other community cultures might engage in participatory avenues in more of a spontaneous fashion and without much planning.

Power and resistance in communities.   The dispersion of power across and within communities is typically fragmented (Dutta-Bergman 2004a, 2004b). Communities at the margins of social systems typically experience disenfranchisement, because of their locations at the peripheries of dominant social systems. In such circumstances, cultural symbols and meanings are circulated within the discursive spaces that support the dominant positions of power, simultaneously silencing those communities that exist at the peripheries of the dominant systems. Similarly, within communities, power is differentially distributed in terms of who has it and who does not, who gets to speak and who does not, who gets to constitute community agendas and who does not. It is within this inequitable distribution of power that resistance gets enacted.

The possibilities of resistance, in other words, are intrinsic to the very inequities perpetuated by the unequal distributions of power within and across communities (Dutta-Bergman 2004a). Inequities and differential distributions of resources create the openings for resistance. Within communities, the structural disparities bring about the possibilities of challenging these very inequities. The resistance of community members to inequitable practices is observed in a wide variety of community-based platforms. The community becomes a site through which resistance is enacted and the voices of members are heard. It is also in the realm of the community that problems continue to be articulated as members collaboratively engage in the discursive articulation of key problems and accompanying solutions.

Ultimately, culture and social capital are intrinsically intertwined, because it is at the cultural level that communities come to define shared identities, platforms, rules, and roles in order to achieve desired outcomes. It is in the realm of culture that communities come to be formed through the articulation of shared meanings, interpretations and values among community members. Community members are drawn together through the contextual elements of the culture. It is also in the realm of culture that meanings are articulated in participatory processes.

Box 8.2   The story of Bob

Bob has lived without a home for the past five years or so. Bob moves from one street corner to the other in downtown Minneapolis and goes into the Food Kitchen at the corner of Hennepin and First Avenues to get food and shower. For Bob, it is difficult to access any form of healthcare resources, and he feels completely disconnected from any community. Being homeless has meant that Bob is not connected to any particular neighborhood and therefore he does not really have a sense of a cohesive community that stands behind him and is supportive of his health. He does not also have a network of friends and family members on whom he can fall back. Bob's life is lonely and he lives isolated from others.

   Why do you think Bob feels isolated from any sense of community? What aspects of his structural situation contribute to his sense of isolation? What, according to you, are the possibilities for engaging Bob in a community? How do you think such forms of engagement offer possibilities for individuals such as Bob, who have been disenfranchised from the mainstream system? What are the ways in which Bob can resist the social structure that marginalizes him? What community platforms are available to Bob for engaging in these acts of resistance?

A Culture-Centered Approach to Community Organizing

The culture-centered approach emphasizes the context within which communication is enacted through the participation of the members of the culture in processes of structural and social change that are meaningful to the members of the culture. In this context, the culture-centered approach to community organizing emphasizes cultural meanings that are driven by the participation of cultural members in the process of meaning-making. It is through the active engagement in interpreting culturally situated problems and the solutions to these problems that community members come to engage in participatory processes within the community. The community becomes a site for engaging in solving those problems that are considered to be critical from within the community.

Therefore dialogue is a critical component of the culture-centered approach such that opportunities are created for the participation of members in opportunities for change through processes that allow them to articulate their needs, concerns, and perceived solutions to the felt needs. Central to the engagement in dialogue is a commitment to a two-way communication process, through which community needs are presented to key stakeholders and solutions are collaboratively developed. In this sense, culture-centered community organizing originates in response to a certain set of felt needs within the community. In other words, community members play a central role in need identification and in the development of pathways for solving these felt needs within the community.

Theoretically, culture-centered community organizing is built upon the two concepts of agency and context. Agency refers to the capacity of individuals within the community to engage in socio-cultural processes which challenge those conditions and problems that limit the lives of cultural participants. Therefore agency is fundamentally reflected in the culturally situated avenues of participation through which community members go about securing access to structurally constrained resources. In this realm, the culture-centered approach begins with the notion that members of communities are active participants by making sense of their lives and by attempting to live in the context of the structural impediments that they face on a daily basis. Agency is not something injected in the community from outside by an external source, but is already present within the community and visible in the various forms of community processes that members engage in.

Context refers to the collection of socio-cultural elements of the community which constitute the lived experiences of its members. Therefore context is embodied in the lives of community members. In this realm, health issues are best understood when located in the realm of the lived experiences of community members. Efforts of community organizing that build on the culture-centered approach focus on the lived experiences of cultural members. These lived experiences are articulated through a dialogical stance, through community-based participatory processes that create openings for the sharing of culturally situated stories and narratives. It is also through these stories that cultural members articulate possibilities of change.

In other words, culture-centered community organizing privileges the local context in the realm of community-based efforts. An example of community organizing built on the local context is the SHIP project in Sonagachi, India (Jana et al. 2004). The project focused on meeting the health needs of sex workers in Sonagachi, and was built to address the structural factors surrounding sex work such as the need for money, the availability of economic opportunities, and the role of clients in the realm of negotiating the use of condoms. The participation of the sex workers in the project created an opening for the articulation of problems from within the community, and for the development of solutions that sought to address these community-based problems.

Also important in culture-centered community organizing is the role of the external agent and/or the researcher. The external agent typically acts as a facilitator and catalyst who engages in dialogue with the community to identify key problems, develop collaborative solutions, and find resources for addressing these problems. The position of the agent shifts from one of an expert who provides the inputs into the problem and solution configurations to one of a co-participant who shares the narrative space with the participants, and, in the process of sharing these narratives, co-creates opportunities for the community. This stance of the researcher as co-participant also suggests that the power inherent in the role of the researcher needs to be reframed into a stance of solidarity and friendship built upon the foundations of mutual respect.

Conclusion

The culture-centered approach to the community context of health communication highlights the linkages between community organizing and culture. Culture provides an intertwined web of meanings within which the community comes to exist. The structure of the community is constituted through the participation of cultural members in the rituals, practices, and meaning-making acts that are drawn from the culture. In other words, the culture supplies the template for community cohesiveness. Community members come together on the basis of shared identities, shared meanings and shared values, and these identities, meanings, and values are created in the realm of culture. Culture, therefore, is central to the social capital of the community. The community participatory processes become meaningful when understood in terms of the cultural context within which they are created and of the cultural symbols and meanings that provide the interpretive framework for these participatory processes. For instance, the participatory processes of the sex workers in Sonagachi become meaningful only through their interactions with cultural processes and the cultural contexts within which they are embedded.

Drawing upon the culture-centered approach, this chapter highlights the importance of context and agency in community organizing. Community organizing begins with the active participation of community members in community platforms, and the impetus for such organizing has to be generated from within the culture. The interpretations of these participatory processes are also dependent upon the meanings that circulate within the culture. Therefore this approach is critical of an empowerment-based model that seeks to empower communities from the outside, on the basis of the agendas of external actors. Arguing that cultures have the capacity to organize and to identify critical resource needs within the community, it suggests the relevance of looking at discursive openings and of listening to the voices of cultural participants in the community-organizing processes which are being enacted in many communities across the globe.

9 Culture and Resistance

Chapter objectives

In this chapter, we will:

- understand the ways in which individuals, groups, and communities resist dominant structures
- examine the role of communication in resisting dominant structures
- study the micro and macro practices of resistance
- study the relationship between culture, communication and resistance

---

Earlier in this book we have examined the ways in which structures marginalize the health experiences of subaltern groups by fundamentally limiting healthcare resources, communicative resources and other critical resources that are available to the privileged actors in social systems. The conditions at the margins are sustained through communication through the unavailability of communication channels, and through the circulation of discourse that continues to stigmatize underserved communities, thus justifying their locations at the peripheries of healthcare systems. This chapter builds on the earlier discussions of the marginalizing role of structures that constrain the health capacities of communities, and explores the role of resistance in the context of experiences of marginalization, locating resistance within the broader context of power and control. Resistance here is defined as a process of enacting agency in opposition to the structures that constrain the access to basic resources of life, including the fundamental resources of healthcare (Dutta-Bergman 2004a, 2004b).

Resistance is intrinsically tied to communication. It might further be argued that it is ultimately communication as it is through communication processes such as rallies and demonstrations, messages and silences that existing structures are challenged, pointing toward the ways in which the structure contributes to the creation of marginalized positions and underserved communities and creating spaces for bringing about shifts in these structures (see Chuengsatiansup 2001; Das and Kleinman 2000; Kleinman, Das and Lock 1997: ix-xxvii; Dutta-Bergman 2004a, 2004b; Dutta and Basu 2007). Resistance offers an avenue for social change through the enunciation of those modalities that contribute to marginalization; it creates discursive openings for social change by bringing forth alternatives to the mainstream discourse that marginalizes (Guha 1982). Resistance is a key communicative act through which members of marginalized communities participate in health communication processes, with the goal of transforming those structures that limit their lives (see Dutta-Bergman 2004a).

How do individuals, groups, and communities participate in communication in order to critique the dominant social system that contributes to their marginalization? What discursive openings do marginalized communities create for articulating opportunities of social change such that greater structural access might be secured for these communities? What are the ways in which communities offer cultural meanings that resist the stigmatizing messages that continue to be circulated in the culture to justify the conditions of subalternity? This chapter engages with these critical issues with the goal of understanding how marginalized communities enact their agency and, hence, offer opportunities for structurally altering a system that sustains their positions at the margins.

This chapter articulates the various ways in which cultural members enact resistance and participate in social change processes around health-related issues. In doing so, it seeks to draw our attention to the enactment of agency, the participatory capacity of marginalized individuals and groups to exercise their choices in response to the constraining structures. Building on the interplay between structure and agency, the chapter draws upon the dialectical tensions that operate in marginalized settings in order to discuss ways in which community members mobilize cultural symbols and artifacts to resist the dominant structures. We will begin by examining the role of communication in the realm of resistance. This will be followed by a discussion of the micro and macro practices of resistance and of the ways in which resistance brings about possibilities for social change. We will conclude by examining how culture serves as a basis for resistance, and how culture is resisted.

Communicating Resistance

Resistance is intrinsically communicative as it communicates certain meanings about the social structure. It serves its objectives through the communication of certain meanings to the intended audience. Every act of resistance is ultimately a communicative act, as it seeks to constitute a meaning (Dutta-Bergman 2004a, 2004b; Farmer 2003). Resistive acts open up spaces of social change by creating new meanings and by offering alternatives to the dominant discourses which marginalize certain sectors of society.

Box 9.1   The story of Radheshyam

Radheshyam lives in the village of Gobindopur, which is about 60 miles from the railway station of Panskura in the eastern Indian state of West Bengal. Radheshyam does not really have a stable source of income and has to travel to Panskura each day to find a source of income. In the month of June in 2005, it was a hot summer day when Radheshyam's son Jonglu started throwing up and complaining of intense stomach pains. Radheshyam took his son to the local homeopathic doctor, who prescribed some medicine for Rs. 5 or so, but Jonglu's condition kept getting worse. On the third day, he decided to take his son to the state hospital in Panskura. However, his son could not be admitted into the hospital because of the long queue, and was not attended by a doctor. After two days of waiting, Jonglu passed away. Incensed at this incident, the men and women in the village of Gobindopur decided to march to the hospital and find an answer to why Jonglu could not receive proper treatment in adequate time. The approximately 70 or so men and women surrounded the house of the chief medical officer of the hospital, and demanded answers.

What do we learn from Radheshyam's story about the possibilities of resistance in marginalized settings? How does resistance go about changing social structures? How do individuals and groups come together in resisting unequal social structures that underlie marginalization?

As Radheshyam's narrative presented above demonstrates, members of marginalized communities participate in communicative processes which challenge the marginalizing practices that limit their life possibilities. Resistance here is defined as the collection of communicative processes that covertly and/or overtly challenge the dominant structures and seek to transform these. Resistance is an act of communication as it embodies meanings and interpretations, and it seeks to achieve a desired set of objectives through messages. Therefore inherent in resistance is the notion of alternative constructions of discursive spaces, which leave openings for transforming the structures that impose limits on the health experiences of individuals, groups, and communities. Resistance offers an opportunity for reorganizing the spaces of marginalization, and in these reorganized spaces, it brings forth a new set of meanings, through the participation of subaltern voices. Ultimately, resistance co-exists with the structural disparities that create and sustain the conditions of marginalization. In the realm of health, the fundamental deprivation from the basic necessities of a physical life brings forth the necessity for resistance. This relationship of resistance to structures of inequity is well articulated by Farmer (2003):

Some ask why we decided to begin now, if we were prepared before. The answer is that before this we tried other peaceful and legal roads to change, but without success. During these last ten years more than 150,000 of our indigenous brothers and sisters have died from curable diseases. The federal, state, and municipal governments' economic and social plans do not even consider any real solution to our problems, and consist of giving us handouts at election times. But these crumbs of charity solve our problems for no more than a moment, and then, death returns to our houses. That is why we think no, no more, enough of this dying useless deaths, it would be better to fight for change. If we die now, we will not die with shame, but with the dignity of our ancestors. Another 150,000 of us are ready to die if that is what is needed to waken our people from their deceit-induced stupor.

Resistance here is a structural response. It is a response to the basic deprivation of health that has continued to plague the community over years. As articulated by the excerpt, mainstream civil society platforms turn deaf ears to the plight of the marginalized, and hence there's a realization for the need to identify and utilize alternative forms of communication beyond these mainstream civil society tools.

Resistance is communicated in a variety of ways. As a communicative act, resistance serves as an entry point for challenging the status quo, for questioning the taken-for-granted assumptions that drive the hegemonic practices of social systems. In this sense, resistance challenges those communicative practices that are typically assumed to be essential to the operation of the status quo. For instance, the questioning of their unfair treatment by medical professionals is a resistive act in subaltern groups. The very formulation that "I am mistreated because I am poor" is an act of resistance as it draws attention to the taken-for-granted notions of the dominant system that typically go unnoticed.

This act offers a point of reference for questioning the dominant ideologies that drive the daily practices of social systems. In the medical context, resistance to the dominant biomedical discourse offers a space for interrogating its power and, ultimately, for shifting this enactment of power. Therefore, fundamental to resistance is the transformative potential of communication that would shift the ways in which power is distributed in the dominant system. Resistance is embodied in the choices of a Hmong immigrant not to take the medicine prescribed by the physician. In this form, resistance offers other possibilities. In the case of the Hmong immigrant, it offers possibilities for engaging with systems of knowledge that exist outside the biomedical system.

Resistance to dominant systems is offered via a wide variety of communicative actions and strategies (Dutta-Bergman 2004a, 2004b; Farmer 2003). These communicative actions take on different forms depending upon their goals, the time frames and contexts within which they operate, and the level of involvement of community members in such actions. Examples of communicative actions include participation in street protests, participation in *gheraos* (*gheraos* are fairly common in India, where a health official or an administrator is surrounded by the public and answers are demanded), hunger strikes, rallies and protest marches, folk performances, and so on. Each of these actions is a communication channel and all are rife with meanings, bringing forth opportunities for interpretation and reinterpretation. Irrespective of their differences, what is central to these actions and strategies is their existence in opposition to the dominant structures of power within social systems, and their desire to transform the ways in which things are practiced within the dominant system. The communicative nature of resistance is well articulated in the following excerpt from the narrative of Yolanda Jean, an HIV-positive Haitian refugee detained on Guantanamo who led a hunger strike on January 20, 1992 (Farmer 2003: 64–5):

Before the strike, I'd been in prison, a tiny little cell, but crammed in with many others, men, women and children . . . Snakes would come in; we were lying on the ground, and lizards were climbing over us. One of us was bitten by a scorpion . . . there were spiders. Bees were stinging the children, and there were flies everywhere; whenever you tried to eat something, flies would fly into your mouth. Because of all this, I just got to the point, sometime in January, I said to myself, come what may, I might well die, but we can't continue in this fashion. We called together the committee and decided to have a hunger strike. Children, pregnant women, everyone was lying outside, rain or shine, day and night. After fifteen days without food, people began to faint. The colonel called us together and warned us, and me particularly, to call off the strike. We said no.

Hunger strike here is both a material act (in the choice to "give up" food) and a communicative act, as it sends out a message that challenges the marginalizing structure encompassing the community and its experiences of being marginalized.

Resistance in the realm of the culture-centered approach is continuously transformative (Farmer 2003). In other words, resistance continues to emerge and evolve as it engages with the structures that limit the life experiences of subaltern groups. On one hand, it exists in relationship with the structure it seeks to change; on the other hand, it exists within the contextual climate of the culture within which it is constituted. Resistance is meaningful in the realm of the structure that it responds to. In other words, it is on the basis of their material inaccess that the members form a set of shared meanings they communicate.

Cultural members participate in co-constructive processes in order to constitute resistive acts, and they impart meanings to these acts; what is going to be resisted, what messages are going to be picked for the acts of resistance, what acts of resistance are going to be enacted are all open to negotiation through communication among members of the culture. Therefore, resistance takes up from within the culture the symbols and communicative markers that serve as indicators of resistance. In other words, resistance is contextually embodied and is meaningful in the context that surrounds it. For instance, labor movements resisting the unhealthy structures in factories pick up communicative markers such as slogans, banners, and songs that mark the identity of the movement, and communicate their resistance to these dominant structures. These songs, slogans, banners, and speeches continually evolve as the movement shifts focus in responding to the structural processes.

Resistance in the context of healthcare is played out at both micro- and macro-levels. Micro-level resistance refers to the daily practices of individuals as they continue to live their day-to-day lives (Dutta-Bergman 2004a; Prakash 1992). Micro resistance focuses on everyday acts of resistance, on day-to-day acts that individuals engage in. At the micro-level, resistance is played out in the individual choices that community members make in response to their marginalization. Such choices might involve non-compliance with the recommendations of the dominant biomedical system. The decision of a Hmong community member to not undergo a surgery is a micro practice of resistance, as it fundamentally questions the biomedical system within the framework of the patient's choices. Cultural members might choose a different course of action for treating an illness because they have a different epistemological under-standing of its cause and of the way it ought to be treated; these choices are embodied in modes of knowing which, in turn, are situated within the culture and its mores. In doing so, they resist the dominant interpretation of the mainstream biomedical system, which seeks to impose its domi-nant epistemological understandings on the community.

Similarly, micro practices of resistance may be enacted in reframing the discourse around health and illness. For instance, Santali community members in Dutta-Bergman's work (2004a) resist the dominant construc-tion of illness by suggesting that illnesses are caused by the disruption of nature and natural processes. In articulating alternative epistemologies that provide different sets of interpretations and explanations, cultural members offer alternative sets of vantage points. In the realm of health communication discourses that seek to identify problems and correspon-ding sets of solutions to these problems, resistance is offered in marginal-ized communities by offering alternative formulations to problems that challenge the mainstream epistemic problem configuration. For instance, members of marginalized communities typically discuss unhealthy poli-cies, corruption, and elite interests, which underlie their inaccess to poor health services, in opposition to the dominant framings, which suggest issues such as contraception and population control underlying this lack of access to healthcare resources (Dutta-Bergman 2004a, 2004b; Farmer 2003; Narayan et al. 2000). Similarly, in the realm of solutions to health problems, the dominant framings are interrogated and challenged. For instance the discourse on population control, which dominates much of the health communication scholarship targeted at the southern nations of the world, is challenged by subaltern participants, who discuss the rel-evance of having more children in resource-deprived conditions in order to ensure higher chances of survival for the children, gain greater support in the family, and ensure greater safety for the future (Dutta 2006). Here's a resistive articulation by a participant from Armenia in Narayan's *Voices of the Poor* project (Narayan et al. 2000: 111):

> I had a prescription for free medicines. I went to a pharmacy and they told me that they had none. I found the medicines in a pharmacy near the Ministry of Health. I didn't want to pass as a hooligan, so I dropped in to the Ministry and clarified whether I could get the medicine free with this prescription. They said yes. So I asked, "If they don't give it to me, can I take it by force?" They said, "If you can, take it." So I went to the pharmacy and asked to see the box of medicines to verify the expiration date. I took the medicines and said that I was leaving with it. They wanted to stop me. I told them, "I am not a hooligan, if you want, let's go together to the Ministry of Health and we can ask there. If I am not correct, they can take me to the police." No one came after me.

In addition to the micro practices of resistance, community members in marginalized settings also participate in political and social processes at the macro-level, which seek to transform the structures within the communities, nation-states, and global configurations that limit their access to healthcare resources (Dutta-Bergman 2004b; Farmer 2003). Such macro practices of resistance are visible in the form of political processes that individuals, groups, and communities participate in. Through their involvement in political platforms, members of resource-deprived communities seek avenues for changing those structures that limit their access to healthcare resources. Community members also seek to mobilize their communities in order to raise critical healthcare issues such that policies and their implementations might be impacted.

In addition to participating in mainstream avenues of civil society organizations, members of marginalized communities also seek out alternative communicative channels. Such channels become particularly relevant when the mainstream civil society platforms are inaccessible to the community. One example of an alternative channel of enacting resistance is local mobilization and the barricading of the office of the chief medical officer at the local hospital. In some instances, such forms of resistance include violence directed at the hospital administration and staff. The demonstration of violence is indicative of the lack of communicative access to other possible platforms for participation, which community members think would be worthwhile. In yet other instances, members of marginalized communities engage in resistance by participating in protest marches, street theaters, folk theaters, and so on. Resistance ultimately seeks to transform the communicative structures that lie at the root of the oppression of subaltern groups. The next section draws the link between resistance and social change.

Discussion point 9.1

- Think of a marginalized community that you have familiarity with. What are the ways in which you see resistance being enacted in this community?
- What are the differences between micro and macro practices of resistance?
- How meaningful are micro practices of resistance?

Resistance and Social Change

It is through resistance that transformative openings are made visible within social systems and alternative possibilities are opened up for cultural participants to transform the very structures that constrain their health experiences (Dutta-Bergman 2004a, 2004b; Farmer 2003). First and foremost, communicative acts of resistance foreground the taken-for-granted assumptions that underlie the mainstream discourse, and by foregrounding these taken-for-granted assumptions they suggest alternative discursive and material possibilities. The ideological premise underlying the dominant discourse, which is widely circulated, is brought to the attention of policy-makers and implementers of health communication programs. By doing this, such acts of resistance challenge some of the fundamental tenets of existing healthcare systems.

Resistance is enacted at a wide range of levels and with a variety of goals, from the day-to-day acts of resistance enacted in the ways of living of the marginalized, which are referred to as micro practices of resistance, to more overt forms of resistance, which openly challenge the structures and seek to change them at the macro-level. For instance, in describing her total replacement surgery and her relationship with her surgeon, Sharf (2005) eloquently discusses how she fired the surgeon. She writes: "Dr Rigor and I were at ideological odds about our relationship; he declined any attempts I initiated to negotiate with him. To remain as his patient would have meant conceding all control of decision making to him, the scenario that ostensibly provoked my dilemma" (pp. 340–1). In this instance, Sharf challenged the traditional assumptions of what marks a doctor–patient relationship, and, in doing so, she discursively and materially shifted the relational distribution of power with her surgeon. The choice to fire her surgeon embodied the "sense that one can influence the course of one's own experience of illness and health seeking" (p. 341).

This form of resistance to the biomedical model at the micro-level, by not complying with the recommendations of the physician, fundamentally challenges the dominant assumption about the unquestionable authority of the biomedical system over the life of the patient. By introducing alternative epistemologies, such acts of resistance create discursive openings for considering alternatives to the dominant ways of knowing and practicing healthcare. The dominance of the biomedical model is thus challenged and inroads are made, leading to transformations in the social system. Social change therefore is made possible through the continual introductions of alternative and multiple discourses into the public sphere.

Macro practices of resistance refer to forms of communicative resistance that overtly challenge the dominant structures and seek to transform them (Dutta-Bergman 2004a, 2004b; Farmer 2003). In the realm of structural inaccess to resources, such practices challenge the communicative processes already in place within the dominant structures and encourage individuals, groups, and communities to think beyond these structures and the constraints imposed by them. Communicatively, such forms of resistance open new discursive spaces by bringing to attention possibilities that have typically been omitted. Materially, these forms of resistance are directed toward securing structural access and toward shifting those barriers that limit the life experiences of marginalized individuals and communities. Hence resistance to structural barriers creates openings for an equitable and accessible healthcare, which would be available to members of marginalized communities.

Examples of such forms of resistance are evident in Dutta-Bergman's work with Santali communities (2004a, 2004b), where community members participate in a range of political platforms with the goal of shifting them. In several instances, community members discuss participating in political rallies, protest marches and community-wide discussions, in order to articulate their voices with respect to those issues that are critical to them. Community members also discuss practices such as questioning local politicians and policemen about the gaps in policy, or pointing out that none of the declared health schemes really reaches them. Possibilities of resistance are articulated in the following excerpt:

> Can't we do it? They did it ... You can't listen to the babus. Sidhu and Kanhu (referring to Santali leaders who led a revolution) led all Santals, in the plains, in the forests, in the mountains to come out and fight. We can do it. But where is the leader? Something needs to happen. (Dutta-Bergman 2004b: 1117)

Worth noting here is a sense of urgency, and it is around this urgency that the community discusses the necessity to organize as a collective. Community mobilization occurs in the backdrop of awareness of the structural inequities and acknowledgement of the necessity to shift these inequities and transform the structures.

In their work with sex workers running the Sonagachi Health Information Program (SHIP) campaign in Sonagachi, Basu and Dutta (2007) report narratives of resisting the dominant structures, which marginalize sex workers through organizing. Sex workers discuss the ways in which they have created a socio-cultural climate in Sonagachi such that clients are resisted if they try to create pressure around not using condoms; pimps and money lenders are confronted when they seek to use sex workers for financial gains; and local politicians and police are confronted for their corrupt practices.

Resistance also occurs in the form of challenging local, national, and global politics, as is evidenced in participation to resistive strategies among indigenous communities on the banks of the river Narmada, in the form of the Narmada Bachao Andolan (NBA), which resists the building of dams that would displace these communities. In all these forms of resistance, the dominant structure is challenged through active participation of community members, and ultimately social change is achieved through the reconfigurations of policies and the manners of implementing them.

Box 9.2   The story of Illeana

Illeana works as a maid servant in the town of Cardes. In Cardes, the only form of employment for youths is part-time work at the coal mines. Illeana was married to her husband Hernando when she was sixteen, and they had their first child when she was seventeen. Hernando died in an accident at the mines about four years back and Illeana has since had to struggle in order to feed her four children. Last year, Illeana's daughter Rosanna was suddenly taken ill. She decided to wait it out a few days as she could not take time off from her work to take Rosanna to the clinic, which is located about three bus trips away and would require almost half a day to get to. When Illeana brought Rosanna to the clinic, the doctor suggested some medicines and asked Illeana to come back if things got worse. Things did get worse by the time Illeana brought Rosanna to the clinic; the doctor ordered a chest X-ray and detected pulmonary tuberculosis. However, the doctor could not offer medication as the clinic was out of its supplies. He suggested that Illeana feed Rosanna and bring her back to the clinic. Rosanna passed away within a couple of days. Frustrated and angered by the scenario, Illeana lodged a complaint with the local clinic's lack of medicines. She also filed a complaint with the block development officer. Months went by and nothing happened with the complaints she had launched. Unable to read and write, she also didn't know how to navigate the legal system and get around it. Frustrated with her situation, Illeana started talking to other mothers who had lost a child to TB, and put together a women's activist group "Mothers of dead children." The group would put together plays and organize protest marches, with the goal of drawing the attention of policy-makers and key politicians.

What do we learn from Illeana's experience about the nature of resistance and the ways in which resistance is constituted?

Illeana's story presented here documents the limits imposed upon resistance by the mainstream civil society platforms, with their requirements for literacy and knowledge of the normative tools of civil society organizations. In such instances, marginalized communities develop alternative spaces of resistance which challenge the very foundations of the organizations that exclude them from participation. In the next section, we will examine the ways in which culture intersects with communication in the realm of resistance.

Discussion point 9.2

- What are the ways in which subaltern groups resist dominant structures beyond the normative tools of dominant civil society organizations?
- What is the role of communication in the realm of bringing about social change?
- What functions do you think can health communicators play in resisting dominant social structures and in transforming them?

Culture in Resistance

In the last few sections we have learned about the ways in which resistance is enacted in response to the structural constraints within which marginalized individuals live their lives, but this enactment of resistance is played out in the realm of culture (Dutta-Bergman 2004a, 2004b; Dutta 2006). In other words, it is through the exchange of cultural values, symbols, and meanings that communities participate in resistive acts. Resistance becomes meaningful when enacted within the contextual framework of the culture. Therefore, in this section, we will explore the interplay between culture and resistance: How does culture offer a vantage point, or a lens, for participating in resistance? What are the ways in which the structural inequities enforced by cultural conditions are resisted?

The notion of culture as a source of resistance and as an object of resistance exists dialectically. Whereas, on one hand, the marginalization of cultures provides the recipe for mobilizing cultural symbols in resisting the dominant structures, on the other hand, the marginalizing role of culture and its complicitous relationship with structures of inaccess and inequity suggests possibilities for social change and cultural transformation. This dialectical tension between the concepts of "culture as resistance" and "resisting culture" is a key theoretical concept in the culture-centered approach, highlighting the notion of culture as dynamic and transformative, with both the retentive and the trans-generative elements playing valuable roles in shaping our theorizing and understanding of culture in health communication.

Culture as resistance

Culture provides a substratum for resisting dominant structures that marginalize them and create conditions of oppression and deprivation in the underserved segments of social systems (Dutta-Bergman 2004a, 2004b). In this sense, culture is used as a metaphor to construct the "other," who can be discursively and materially managed and controlled through health interventions sent out by the dominant actors at the center and serving the interests of these dominant actors. As put in chapter 6, culture is marginalized through the discursive symbols and meanings that circulate in the dominant spaces of social systems, and it is through the circulation of these dominant framings of culture that individuals and communities are placed at the margins, justifying the inequities that underlie such marginalization. It is in the dominant constructions of culture that marginalized spaces are imbued with markers of passivity and lack of agency, thus justifying the power and control exerted by the center (Dutta-Bergman 2004a, 2004b; Escobar 1995; Farmer 2003).

Such constructions render marginalized communities as agency-less homogeneous masses that need to be constructed as targets of health interventions, without any heed paid to the values, goals, and sensibilities of the community. Therefore it is in the realm of culture that resistance is played out when the dominant meaning configurations are challenged by members of marginalized communities. Cultural meanings are mobilized to present alternative understandings of culture that challenge the dominant constructions. For instance, in their discussion of their profession, sex workers in the Sonagachi red light district in Kolkata suggest the relevance of alternative cultural articulations of the very profession of sex work (Dutta and Basu 2007). They suggest that it is through the foregrounding of these alternative meanings that the oppressive forces surrounding the sex worker community can be meaningfully dealt with. Cultural meaning and symbols are thus mobilized with the goal of changing the fundamental structures which mark sex work as a stigmatized profession.

Similarly, in their discursive constructions of cultural norms, the sex workers of Sonagachi suggest the relevance of shifting those norms that contribute to the stigmatization of subaltern populations. Subaltern resistance is witnessed in the very return of the subaltern gaze toward the observer, who is supposed to be objective and therefore outside the realm of discourse. The subaltern gaze situates the objective–rationalistic viewpoint of the observer within the very space of discourse, suggesting that this approach of science is also culturally situated and embedded within the political, social, and economic institutions that make up social systems. It is this act of locating Europe and its centers of knowledge production within a cultural space that challenges the very notion of culture being elsewhere and hence being the subject of rationalistic–universalistic approaches to healthcare (see chapter 7). The location of the discourse of science within the realm of culture opens up the discursive space to dialogue, where scientific innovations and biomedical technologies become contested sites. It is at these contested sites that cultural meanings are continuously recreated and circulated.

The narratives of immigrant communities within the US that resist the biomedical model and demonstrate their preference for culturally meaningful forms of healing is yet another example of the ways in which culture operates as a resistive site. Similarly, when Native American individuals and families resist certain treatment options that are typically taken for granted by the proponents of the biomedical model, their resistance embodies the mobilization of culture, its values, meanings, and epistemologies. What such resistance documents is the fragmented nature of health communication. It brings forth the cultural location of the biomedical model and draws our attention to the disjunctures where the model fails to offer meaningful solutions.

It is also in the realm of culture that dominant meanings imposed by external stakeholders are challenged. For instance, Dutta (2006) demonstrates that population control campaigns imposed on marginalized spaces were resisted through the circulation of alternative meanings. Similarly, cultural meanings are drawn upon in order to craft messages that resist the dominant structures. For instance, when rural community members organize protest marches and hunger strikes against a healthcare system that limits their access, they do so by drawing upon cultural meanings associated with protest marches and hunger strikes. The messages they use and the languages they construct are also tied to these cultural meanings as they draw upon them (Escobar 1995).

Resisting culture

In other instances, practices within the culture are resisted as they embody conditions of power inequity and structural inequity which continue to privilege certain actors and marginalize others within the discursive and material frames (Das 1995). For instance, patriarchy is often embedded within socio-cultural spaces such that the marginalization of women is carried out through the gendered norms and practices within the culture. In this realm, those structural elements of cultures are resisted that continue to serve as sites of oppression and reinforce oppressive messages, values and practices. In other words, culture values, meanings, and practices in this context serve to reinforce the inequities that exist within the structures.

Forms of resistance, as noted in the culture-centered approach, are introduced by stakeholders from within the culture with the goal of altering the cultural practices. The impetus for change comes from within, through the articulation of alternative possibilities by unsatisfied members of the communities. In these instances, resistance is embodied in the questioning of the taken-for-granted assumptions within the culture that constitute the cultural traditions. Existing traditions are challenged through their interrogation by cultural members. Through engagement with the long-held assumptions about acceptable practices within the culture, marginalized groups members draw attention to the need for change and open up possibilities for it.

The practices of resisting culturally valued norms are enacted at a variety of levels that range from micro to macro, and often include some combination of both. For example, in their work with female dairy farmers in India, Papa, Singhal and Papa (2006) document how these women came together to articulate the need for women's clubs in villages, despite opposition from men and village elders. Here's an excerpt from one of the women participants in the project: "I will question why the men oppose the women's club. I will explain to them that if women unite it will be beneficial for the village. So why should men oppose? With their cooperation, we will establish the women's club" (p. 138). In this instance, the community platform offers an opportunity for questioning the gendered practices within the community, and for interrogating the values that underlie these very practices. In other words, the creation of a participatory platform also served as a space for bringing forth questions that typically were not asked; further, it created a space for enacting agency that was typically minimized by the dominant structure. The presence of the participatory platform gave the women the courage to interrogate the opposition put up by men to the listeners clubs started by women. Furthermore, it also provided a space which called for the participation and cooperation of men.

Yet another instance of resisting cultural norms is evident in the participation of Indian women in movements against the exchange of dowry, the practice of paying money to the groom's family. In a recent incident in 2003, Nisha Sharma, a postgraduate in the satellite city of Noida, gained national attention for calling the dowry cell and getting her groom-to-be arrested for demanding dowry. In this instance, a culturally circulated norm was questioned by an individual member. The voicing of this question created a space for further discourse and dialogue around the question of dowry, drawing the attention of the media and generating further public discussion. In this instance, resisting a culturally constructed norm at an individual level created the space for wider public and media discourse around that norm.

These forms of resistance presented here attest to the various ways in which cultural members enact their agency in seeking to transform the structures that limit their lives and impose constraints on them. In doing so, they point out that cultures are transformative and open to multiple possibilities of change from within. Instead of being visualized as a stable box that contains a set of characteristics, culture is constituted in meanings. As new meanings and interpretations emerge, cultures go through changes, thus bringing forth new opportunities for communicating about health. It is this transformative potential of culture that is crucial for health communicators to understand as they communicate health. The narratives of resistance presented here also tap into the possibilities of cultural change from within, and suggest the relevance of cultural activism in resisting the dominant structures that continue to marginalize subaltern groups within social systems.

Discussion point 9.3

- What are the differences between the "culture as resistance" and "cultural resistance" approaches? What are the similarities between them?
- What is the relationship between the "culture as resistance" and "cultural resistance" approaches? Think of a health policy within the United States which in your view fundamentally marginalizes some groups. In this context, please suggest ways in which the "culture as resistance" and "cultural resistance" approaches interplay with each other.

Conclusion

In conclusion, this chapter documents the various ways in which culture serves as a site of resistance in health communication. Culture provides the template for the constitution of meanings. It is after all through the circulation of cultural artifacts and symbols that meanings are constituted and reconstituted. These cultural meanings exist at the intersection between structure and the agency of individuals, families, groups, and communities. It is after all in making sense of the structure and in attempting to change the structural constraints that are imposed on them that individuals engage with culturally circulated meanings. These meanings, therefore, provide the template for individual action.

We have learned in this chapter that resistance is practiced both at the micro-level, through the day-to-day practices of the cultural participants as they engage with various avenues of healthcare delivery, and at the macro-level, through the questioning of the broader structures that limit the basic access to resources. Whereas micro practices focus on creating new meanings through alternative interpretations offered by the individual, macro practices are enacted at the broader level of the social structure, with the goal of altering that very structure and thus of removing the barriers to healthcare experienced by individuals and communities.

Furthermore, this chapter also documented the notions that culture can serve both as a site of resistance and as a target of resistive strategies. Cultural symbols may be mobilized to alter the very structures that impede access. In other instances, however, individuals and groups resist these cultural structures with the goal of bringing about social change. Here, culture is resisted and the communicative act of resistance focuses on providing new meanings and on articulating new entry points for the culture. These two dimensions, of culture as an ally and culture as a site of resistance, tap into the traditional and transformative characters of culture. Whereas on the one hand culture becomes the blueprint for the enactment of communication, it also becomes the site of change and introduces new openings for the community. Ultimately, the culture-centered approach suggests that resistance exists at this very discursive opening, where culture continually interacts with structure and agency and takes on new meanings while at the same time constituting itself on the basis of the existing meanings that are part of its history and tradition.

10 Health, Culture, and Globalization

Chapter objectives

In this chapter, we will:

- understand globalization processes and the ways in which globalization has influenced health
- examine the link between transnational corporations and global health
- study the linkages between global and local health
- understand the ways in which global and local activism are interconnected

In the previous chapters we have studied the ways in which structure and culture interact to create conditions at the margins. This chapter further builds on that discussion, to understand how globalization processes have shaped the health experiences of individuals, groups, and communities, both locally and globally. *Globalization* here refers to the period of economic liberalization brought about by the view that economic growth, in and of itself, is good for everyone and is optimized when governments refrain from interfering in market principles and operations (Millen, Irwin and Kim 2000). Globalization has been accompanied by neoliberalism, a broader pattern of economic theory which asserts that the market, if allowed to operate unhindered, will bring optimal outcomes for the society as a whole (Shakow and Irwin 2000). Neoliberal theory draws on the ideas that the privatization of economies and resources, strict limits on government spending, and minimal interference from government policies create conditions of optimal economic growth, optimal employment levels, and optimal allocation of resources (Millen, Irwin and Kim 2000; Shakow and Irwin 2000).

Globalization in this sense is connected to the global operations of large corporations, also referred to as transnational corporations (TNCs), which operate across national boundaries, in multiple countries, and facilitate the flow of raw materials, labor, manufactured products, and communications across national boundaries (Korten 1995; Millen and Holtz 2000). Furthermore, in the realm of globalization, three key institutions have emerged as key players in the international economy: the International Monetary Fund (IMF) strives to eliminate trade restrictions and to smooth the way for international commerce; the World Bank offers loans for economic reconstruction and development and lays out conditions for economic restructuring underlying the deployment of loans; and the World Trade Organization (WTO) seeks to reduce tariffs and other barriers to trade (Gershman and Irwin 2000). The economic policies accompanying globalization, the operations of TNCs, and the global flows of raw materials, labor, manufactured goods, services, technologies, and communications have had significant effects on health, particularly that of marginalized populations. The goal of this chapter is to examine the linkages between globalization and health, drawing upon the culture-centered approach.

The argument put forth in this chapter is that health is deeply connected with economic questions at the global level, bringing forth the role of structures in influencing health (Gershman and Irwin 2000; Millen and Holtz 2000). The basic capacities of healthcare, which are fundamental to the lives of poverty-stricken communities, are tied to the policies made by global actors, and the life experiences of individuals and communities are determined by policy-makers in far-removed global spaces. This chapter explores the ways in which globalization processes interact with health and global economic policies have health consequences. In doing so, the culture-centered approach locates health within the realm of the global economic structures, which are fundamental to the ways in which health is experienced within local community contexts.

One of the key arguments for the study of culture focuses on the role of globalization in the realm of health, making it imperative for scholars to theorize about the variety of ways in which global processes interpenetrate health communication processes and practices. The interaction between global structure and individual agency enacted at the local level is played out through the lens of culture. Culture offers the entry points for meaning-making through which communication is possible. It also offers a framework for enacting agency among community members and for offering resistance to the structures of power at the global level. Culture offers the communicative space through which the marginalized experiences of individuals are rendered meaningful and are placed within the broader global politics of health.

This chapter will draw the reader's attention to those globalization processes which have redefined health practices, and to meanings that are of interest to health communication. The discussion of marginalizing global policies will be located in the context of communicative practices of resistance, which connect multiple stakeholders across national boundaries in resisting those global structures that create conditions of marginalization. In discussing globalization, the present chapter will elucidate the experiences of indigenous communities in the realm of traditional knowledge systems and the ownership of such knowledge systems, the role played by the technical–medical–capitalist complex of transnational hegemony, the growth of transnational corporations, and the increasing number of global policies that continue to breed inequities. In the backdrop of this discussion, the chapter will focus its arguments on the ways in which cultural members enact their agency and offer resistance to global structures. Ultimately, the chapter will offer theoretical and practical insights into the ways in which the dominant structures may be challenged in the context of health experiences of cultural members.

Introduction: Defining Globalization

Globalization is manifest in the flow of goods and people across national boundaries (Millen, Irwin and Kim 2000). Health in the global arena is fluid, marked by the multidirectional interpretations of health meanings at multiple levels. In the global realm, the health of nation-states and national cultures is embedded within the broader, macro-level policies of global actors. The local in the present context exists in a continual relationship with the global. Identities, relationships, and actions at the local level exist in relationship with global level policies and actions of global actors. The lives and lived experiences of local community members are influenced by the ways in which global policies are constituted and implemented.

As suggested earlier, globalization is embedded in the neoliberal logic that drives much of the current international economic impetus; this phenomenon started with the economic restructuring during the Reagan and Thatcher years. The rest of this chapter will interrogate this interplay between the global and the local in the construction of meanings of health.

Sumirah's story appeared in the Jakarta Post in the aftermath of the Indonesian economic crisis, and brings forth the interactions of the local and the global. The crisis was a result of the economic response of Indonesia to the global free market economy (Gershman and Irwin 2000). When, in the midst of the Asian shake-up of 1997, foreign investors

---

Box 10.1 The story of Sumirah

Sumirah is daydreaming. The 36-year-old mother is wishing that the days when she could properly feed her two under-five children were back. "Every day I ask myself what I can give my children to eat," she said numbly, while watching the children, aged 2 and 4, play in front of their house in Rembang . . . [Sumirah's] husband is a pedicab driver who earns a mere Rp 3,000 (30 US cents) a day. The income is far from enough to support the family of four with the price of rice having soared as high as Rp 4,000 per kilo. "Often my husband and I have to eat cassava so that we can get money to buy rice and tempeh for the children," she said. "We will do everything to ensure they don't get skinny." (As appeared in the *Jakarta Post*, October 11, 1998, as quoted in Gershman and Irwin 2000, p. 41)

What do we learn from Sumirah's story about the relationship between health and the economy? How is this relationship played out in the realm of globalization processes? How do you think globalization has impacted the health of marginalized communities? More specifically, think of a local community the health of which is impacted by globalization.

started withdrawing their hot foreign capital investments in Indonesia, the economy went through a rapid downturn, which resulted in widespread job losses, increase in poverty, and the re-emerging public health threat of massive child malnutrition. The Indonesia case demonstrates the interlinkages of the global economy and the way in which globalization processes are intertwined with the health of populations within the local contexts. The policy decisions that are made at the local level by national actors are embedded within the global political economy, and with the goals of global politics. The next section further discusses the linkages between globalization and health.

Discussion point 10.1

- What is globalization?
- What are the characteristics of globalization?
- How has globalization influenced you?

Globalization and Health

The global location of health is exemplified in the ways in which global policies impact local actions. The local context of healthcare exists within the realm of these global policies which determine the availability of resources in communities, the distribution of resources to communities, the regulations around healthcare that are set up, and the attitudes, values and behaviors that are promoted within communities. The health of local actors within local cultures is intrinsically tied to the framing of health at the global level and to the ways in which health is constituted globally.

For instance, the framing of severe acute respiratory syndrome (SARS) globally was intrinsically tied to the Chinese government and media response to the disease, and it further had an impact on the global reputation of China. The case demonstrated that how a local actor responds to a crisis such as SARS is intrinsically linked with the ways in which the actor is constituted in the global discourse, which in turn influences global policies of healthcare. The issues and agendas that receive attention globally play out the interests of key actors in the global arena and, in turn, influence the varieties of policies at local levels, further influencing the flow and distribution of health-related goods, resources, and services within and across nation-states.

Furthermore, scholars of globalization argue that the globalization process plays out to reflect the interests of the dominant actors within the system. In the realm of globalization, these dominant actors frame issues of health as problems of security and economy. The interests of global health are tied to the interests of the nation-state and of the powerful global actors, particularly transnational corporations supported by the nation-state. Especially important is the role of the nation-states at the center, which continue to exist in harmony with the transnational corporations and constitute the center of power. This configuration of elite nation-states at the center, accompanied by the transnational corporations, is also referred to as transnational hegemony. Inherent in the transnational hegemonic configuration are the mutual interests of the elite national actors and of the profit-driven organizations that seek to generate a stable economy to support organizational performance.

This link between the elite interests in the issues of security and economy in the global arena is visible in the global framing of HIV/AIDS. In 2000, the Clinton administration presented HIV/AIDS as an emergent threat to national security, suggesting that it threatened the basic security of US actors both globally and locally (King 2002). Clinton's articulation of HIV/AIDS as a national security threat was further reiterated by the National Intelligence Council (NIC) when it stated that HIV/AIDS is likely to "endanger US citizens at home and abroad, threaten US armed forces deployed overseas, and exacerbate social and political instability in key countries and regions in which the United States has significant interests" (Noah and Fidas 2000). The NIC document reiterated the connection between the public health interests of global actor that are typically constructed, in discourse, as humanitarian interests, and the fundamental interests of national security and international commerce.

The explicit association between US public health interests and issues of American security and economy resulted in federal support not only through traditional health organizations, but also through the Defense Department, and in the housing of the most sophisticated laboratories and public health surveillance systems within the Defense Department (King 2002). This also made explicit the economic–military–sanitary complex that constitutes the global health agenda in the twenty-first century. In this global health agenda, issues of security and economy are continually linked with questions of health. The uncertainty around health relates to the deep-seated anxiety regarding the contamination of positions at the center with pollutants from the underdeveloped periphery. The threat of the Third World is no longer that of a distant entity in another space, encountered through colonial invasions, but it is everywhere as geographic boundaries become fragmented and interpenetrate in the global context.

Therefore health is continually framed in terms of a global discourse which continues the colonial threads of the nineteenth-century discourse of health where the colonies in the Third World were identified as the sites of contamination. Fear and anxiety abounded in the colonial discourse as new lands were brought under colonial rule. What emerged from these fears of contamination with the reservoirs of infection was the necessity to develop systems of surveillance such that the places or populations could be adequately identified. Furthermore, strategies of avoidance, segregation, and development of sanitary cordons were put in place, so that the contamination could be avoided. The globalization discourse of the twenty-first century functions similarly, to identify Third World spaces that are sources of disease and biomedically to insulate the United

States and its allies from the economic periphery of developing nations that are the potential and actual sources of global pandemics such as HIV/AIDS, tuberculosis, West Nile Virus, Ebola, and dengue (King 2002; Noah and Fidas 2000).

King (2002) argues that the solution proposed to this territorialization of the globe was a form of de-territorialization, linking vast networks of information and risk management that would identify and manage risks before they became epidemics. In this worldview, because the flow of people and goods is inevitable in the global landscape, it is critical to develop global response systems that effectively manage risks across borders. King quotes a 2001 report generated by the Centers for Disease Control and Prevention (CDC), stating that "increased international engagement has stimulated CDC to rethink its infectious disease priorities, keeping in mind that it is far more effective to help other countries control or prevent dangerous diseases at their source than to try to prevent their importation" (CDC 2001: 5).

The development of such global information and risk-management infrastructures connects in turn with the political economy of funding global corporations, think tanks, and academic enterprises that would support the creation of a large-scale network. In other words, the very anxiety of contamination inherent in globalization feeds fuel to large-scale corporations and to the transnational hegemony supported by globalization. For instance, the National Academy of Science's Institute of Medicine (IOM) published a report in 1997, *America's Vital Interest in Global Health: Protecting our People, Enhancing our Economy, and Advancing our International Interests*, that documented the need for the efficient production, distribution, and consumption of biomedical products such as vaccines and other pharmaceuticals, thus opening up new markets for the transnational pharmaceutical industry and feeding into American economic growth. Here's an excerpt from the IOM (1997) document that captures the notion of expanding markets under this framework:

> The global market for pharmaceuticals, vaccines, and medical devices is a large one. Expenditure on pharmaceuticals was $220 billion, or $40 per capita, in 1992, while expenditures on vaccines were about $2 billion and those for medical devices and equipment were about $71 billion. In this global market, the share of the developing countries is surprisingly significant. In 1992, for all developing countries combined, the public and private sectors together spent $44 billion. This amount represented 10–30 percent of public-sector recurrent costs in developing countries, second only to expenditures on health personnel. In industrial countries, by comparison, drugs and vaccines represent 5–20 percent of health care spending . . . Thus, for the foreseeable future, the introduction of new drugs and vaccines in developing countries will be dependent on the pharmaceutical and vaccine industries in the United States and other industrial countries . . . The question is how to make it economically feasible for the best of American science, technology, and industry to address major global health problems and to enable US industry to profit, rather than suffer losses, by that engagement.

What is evident in this excerpt is the framing of this global health crisis as an opportunity for US science and technology, coupled with commercial organizations, primarily the pharmaceutical industry. Health becomes a commodity that enters into the exchange system of the global economic order and is bought and sold in the marketplace, generating substantive profits for international pharmaceutical organizations.

The goal, as outlined in the IOM document, is to make it economically feasible for international pharmaceutical organizations to operate successfully in these developing markets, without suffering losses. The document proposes a few strategies in order to accomplish this goal, including the "acceleration of international synchronization of regulatory standards regarding safety, quality control, intellectual property and piracy" (King 2002: 776). The goal here is to create global markets that are segmented on the basis of demand and ability to pay for the pharmaceutical products. Health and human suffering is conceptualized as a commodity that may be exchanged between international actors. Health is negotiated and traded in the international markets, where the buyers and sellers enter into negotiation of pricing strategies, invest in resources, and develop effective marketing plans. With its commitment to generating maximum profit for the international pharmaceutical organizations operating globally, this framework privileges innovative production, efficient distribution and global consumption of pharmaceuticals (King 2002).

Discussion point 10.2

- How do you think globalization has influenced the landscape of healthcare?
- What are the ways in which globalization has influenced cultures? How has the interaction between globalization and cultures influenced human health?

Global policies and health

Global policies therefore continue to serve the global economic interests, simultaneously ignoring the needs of the underserved segments of the globe. This is particularly evident in those global policies that are supported by the key actors at the center. The material marginalization of subaltern populations is witnessed as a global phenomenon, as the gap between the health rich and the health poor continues to increase globally. Millen, Irwin, and Kim (2000) argue that the aggregate statistics demonstrating health improvements mask the fact that these improvements are largely unevenly distributed across the globe, with 90 percent of the disease burden of the world being carried by the developing sector and with poorer countries having access to approximately 10 percent of the global resources allocated to health. Therefore, although economic growth in terms of indicators such as GDP promotes a vision of development, the distribution of the economic growth has been vastly uneven, and the benefits of economic growth have not materially trickled down to the poorer sectors of society, as suggested by the proponents of neoliberal principles.

Neoliberal ideology asserts that economic growth, in and of itself, is good for everyone and the benefits of economic growth spread widely within social systems; furthermore, economic growth is optimized when governments refrain from interfering in markets. Manifest in the "Washington Consensus" or the "new policy agenda," neoliberal ideology was first promoted by the leading political ideologues Reagan and Thatcher, and was reflected in a set of economic reforms or policies that sought to promote minimal government interventions in global market operations. Such reforms included cutting tariffs and other trade barriers, reducing government intervention in the economy, cuts in social spending, reducing or eliminating subsidies that provided benefits for the poor, privatizing public enterprises and services, and emphasizing exports as the engine of growth (Korten 1995, 1999; DeSouza et al., in press).

Neoliberal ideology is most evident in global trade policies and agreements. Scholars (Labonte 2001; Labonte and Torgerson 2002) argue that what distinguishes this globalizing era from previous ones is the scale of movement of financial capital and the establishment of binding rules through global institutions, such as the World Trade Organization or the World Bank and their trade policies.

The documentation of economic growth patterns in the context of neoliberal trade policies demonstrates that the growth's benefits have not gone to those living in dire poverty, who constitute almost 25 percent of the globe (Millen, Irwin and Kim 2000). The rates of growth have been concentrated in the hands of those who are already well off. For instance, Millen and his collaborators point out that the economic benefits in developing countries have flown to the most affluent 20 percent of the population and to foreign investors, corporations, and banks, whereas the health of the poor has continued to decline (ibid.). Access to basic healthcare continues to be a core problem in marginalized sectors, with a United Nations Development Program (UNDP) report suggesting that less than 4 percent of the combined wealth of the 225 richest individuals in the world would provide and maintain access to basic education, basic healthcare, reproductive healthcare, adequate food, safe water, and adequate sanitation for all people living on the planet.

Neoliberal trade agreements have been associated with negative health and dependency patterns in developing regions of the world. Clarkson (1999) concurs that nation-states today often find themselves locked into neoliberal principles by structural adjustment programs in the South and by international agreements and international institutions in the North. Scholars (Harris and Seid 2004; McMichael and Beaglehole 2000) argue that the principal promoters of the contemporary market-based economic system advocate development strategies that often impair population health in countries affected by the strategies and reforms. According to Labonte (2001), globalizing influences such as enforceable trade agreements and various forms of international development affect the national context of health through effects on labor rights, food security, the provision of public goods and services, and environmental protection.

Poverty has grown substantively with neoliberal reforms, underscoring the illness, suffering, and premature death of those in its grasp (Gershman and Irwin 2000). As a direct cause of lack of food, clean water, sanitation, curative drugs and other treatments, poverty is the major contributor to reduced life expectancy, starvation, handicap and disability, mental illness, suicide, stress, family disintegration, and substance abuse. The per capita income in almost 100 countries is lower than what it used to be over three decades ago, with the average household in some instances consuming 20 percent less today than it did 25 years ago (ibid.). The poorest 20 percent of the world's people received only 1.1 percent of the global income in 2000 compared to 2.3 percent of the global income in 1990; the poorest 20 percent account for only 1.3 percent of the world-wide private consumption expenditures whereas 20 percent of the world's people who live in the highest income countries account for 86 percent of the worldwide private consumption expenditures. These data document the increasing inequality and poverty in the global landscape in the face of the neoliberal trade policies which directly influence the economic strategies both at local and at global levels.

This discussion demonstrates that health is squarely located in the realm of economics, and how economic decisions are made depends upon access to power. The economic decisions are embedded in political processes, thus revealing the intrinsic links between health, economics, and politics. The differential between those who have the power and those who don't becomes the determining factor in shaping how resources will be allocated and policies will be formulated. As the scholars Gershman and Irwin (2000) argue, decisions are made by elite actors in poor countries to allocate limited resources to purchasing new military weapons or to making payments on staggering foreign debts instead of allocating them to construct local health clinics that would increase healthcare access among underserved populations. The political nature of economic and healthcare policies is particularly critical for health communicators to explore, as they deal with questions of how principles of communication might be engaged in addressing advocacy and activism (Zoller 2005, 2006).

Also evident from the discussion presented here is the absence of the sub-altern voice with respect to questions of equity and access. As global policies get framed under the umbrella of aggregate economic growth, questions of access and quality are omitted from the discussion. As global economic policies continue to be formulated, greater attention needs to be paid to questions of structure and structural access in the realm of health-care. Drawing upon the culture-centered approach, it may further be argued that creating dialogical spaces for entering into conversations with the underserved sectors of social systems is critical to health communication processes of the twenty-first century. It is through this commitment to dialogue and conversation that global policies would respond to the needs of cultures and communities at the local level.

Transnational corporations

As suggested in the previous section, transnational corporations (TNCs) play a major role in the realm of public health in the twenty-first century. TNCs are global corporations that operate across national boundaries and trade in goods and services at a global level, participating in the global economy through the exchange of commodities across national boundaries and simultaneously operating in multiple nation-states (Gershman and Irwin 2000). These transnational corporations are the key beneficiaries in the realm of globalization, as national governments are pushed more toward favoring privatization and toward reducing the regulations of foreign trade and investment, and play a pivotal role in promoting free trade agreements (Gershman and Irwin 2000; Millen, Lyon and Irwin 2000). TNCs have been actively involved in the electoral, legislative and judicial processes both nationally and internationally by hiring professional lobbyists and lobbying firms (Millen, Lyon and Irwin 2000; Miller and Kehler 1996). TNCs sponsor entertainment events and fund raisers, as well as fund national ad campaigns targeted toward influencing voters and policy-makers (Miller and Kehler 1996). For instance, in 1994, when the Clintons sought to reform the healthcare system, corporations paid through special interest groups to combat the reform launched advertisements designed to inform the average American about the dangers inherent in the proposed reform (Miller and Kehler 1996). The insurance industry played a key role in blocking the healthcare reform bill (Miller and Kehler 1996).

According to Millen, Lyon and Irwin (2000), the mostly corporate-backed lobbying industry grew by 37 percent between 1997 and 1999, spending approximately $1.42 billion in 1998 to influence legislators. Similarly, the Archer Daniels Midland Company (ADM), the world's largest agricultural commodities firm, invested approximately $3 million in the campaign funds for both Republicans and Democrats in the US Congress, in return receiving more than $3 billion in corporate welfare in the form of ethanol tax breaks and other government subsidies (ibid.). Furthermore, Millen and his collaborators note that TNCs and their lobbyists (ibid., p. 227):

> Keep abreast of, and try to influence, any legislation that might impede corporate efforts to minimize costs. Labor laws such as the minimum wage, workers' entitlements and benefits, worker health and safety rules, environmental protection, and food and drug safety regulations all fall under this rubric. Even when the public strongly support proposed legislation, as in efforts to improve air and water quality, corporations can foil a bill's passage by simply outspending those who support it. Between 1990 and 1994, some 267 political action committees for many of the largest and most environmentally destructive

American TNCs, such as Chevron Corporation, Dow Chemical, Exxon, and Freeport-McMorRan, contributed over $57 million to political candidates. Their investment paid off; the TNCs were able to limit the authority of the Environmental Protection Agency (EPA) and erode many US environmental laws including the Clean Water Act.

Unhealthy environmental policies are passed because those that have access to economic resources and therefore have access to power are able to dictate the agendas of policy-makers and the ways in which they vote. Therefore national policies are ultimately shaped by the powerful lobbies, which, in turn, are sponsored by the powerful TNCs. Similarly, lobbies supported by major pharmaceuticals dictate policies regarding intellectual property rights and access to drugs.

Hence the voices that influence national and global policies are the voices of the TNCs, of those with economic power and access, not those of the ordinary citizens. This elucidates one of the key arguments outlined in the culture-centered approach (Dutta-Bergman 2004a, 2004b) – that the voices of those with access to power are central to the ways in which policies are mapped out and implemented, simultaneously erasing the voices of marginalized communities.

With the impetus on privatization, more and more of the health needs of marginalized communities in global spaces are being rearticulated within the realm of the corporate logic, and are being driven by the profit motives of major TNCs (Millen and Holtz 2000). For instance, globalization policies ensure that transnational corporations have access to the local markets of HIV/AIDS patients, simultaneously ensuring that the prices remain competitive, and thus reducing the growth of local manufacturers of HIV/AIDS drugs and curtailing the opportunities of receiving treatment among the social classes in developing countries, who cannot afford the highly priced drugs manufactured by the TNCs. In the realm of health, the effects of the TNCs are experienced primarily through the policies, objectives, and control of the pharmaceutical industry over global health conditions (Millen and Holtz 2000; Millen, Irwin and Kim 2000; Millen, Lyon and Irwin 2000). Additionally, global corporations such as Monsanto control the global agribusiness through the supply and exchange of seeds, fertilizers, and agricultural products on a global scale (DeSouza et al., in press). This has contributed to the driving up of prices of food products, accompanied by the loss of jobs among local farmers who relied on the local economy to support themselves. Thus the growth of TNCs has further contributed to inaccess to food, which is one of the basic resources of life.

TNCs have also contributed to the loss of jobs among local workers as new technologies have been brought in, making human labor irrelevant to the production process within local economies. The job losses, in turn, have significantly contributed to the poverty of the marginalized sectors of the globe, leading further to poor health in these sectors. Voices of participants in these marginalized settings narrate the suffering and violence brought in by the new boom of technology. They express the view that, in the name of development, new projects have only created fewer opportunities for the poor.

Discussion point 10.3

- Please take a health issue of your choice. How do you think this particular issue is impacted by global politics?

Local rights

Yet another realm where health is questioned is the area of indigenous health and the rights of indigenous communities, in the realm of knowledge production in the context of globalization. In the global landscape, knowledge and its ownership are widely contested, as questions of ownership over nature arise. Neoliberal policies such as TRIPS, which seek to patent plants and herbal products that have been part of indigenous healing systems for centuries, bring forth important questions regarding the ownership of nature (DeSouza et al., in press). Whereas the supporters of global patenting rights suggest that the patenting is really concerned with the process of production of the manufactured product from the raw materials, the experience of marginalized communities speaks otherwise. The patenting of food products such as Basmati and turmeric has driven up the prices of the seeds, fostered market monopolies for global seed producers, and made subaltern communities dependent upon TNCs for agriculture and for cultivating crops that were part of the cultural history for centuries. Similarly, recent years have seen debates around the notion of patenting the knowledge of gene pools, particularly those of indigenous communities. Indigenous communities have protested at the notion that the indigenous identity is reducible to a set of genetic codes, and further patentable by expert geneticists who are dominant social actors. Worth noting are the ways in which knowledge is constructed within the realm of ownership, tying the production of knowledge to capitalist interests and to the interests of the market economy.

Global and local processes

As our discussion earlier in this chapter suggests, health is both a local entity embedded in the very context within which it is articulated and a global commodity as it is exchanged in the international network of markets on the basis of market demands and of the capability of buyers to pay for health. Health today is a commodity in the global marketplace; it is constituted by the marketing strategies of TNCs, which play critical roles in determining the global health agendas and the policies that support these agendas. The local meanings of health that are situated in the local culture and are contextually embedded gain relevance in their interactions with the global policies within which they are constrained.

The narratives of health of a Mequilodora worker in Mexico who has lost his job and is struggling with poverty are embedded within the transnational politics of global corporations, global agencies, and national governments which are, in turn, embedded within this global politics. The experiences of an individual living in Haiti is deeply connected with the global policies that are passed and implemented. Politics at the local, state, and national levels today are intertwined with global policies, and this is the reality within which health communication strategies and solutions ought to be delivered.

Communicating Globally about Health

Global health communication today is embedded in the intersections of power and structure in the global arena. As the analysis in the previous section demonstrates, the health communication problems in the global arena exist at the intersections of structure and culture. Structure is manifest in the mode of articulation and enforcement of economic policies in the global arena. The political process that underlies the deployment of economic policies is enacted through the discursive construction of the policies and through the framing of the policies in favorable ways.

Culture here is the local context within which these political processes are played out and the policies are approved, implemented and reinforced. Therefore one of the key tasks in front of health communication scholars is to interrogate the communicative practices through which the policies are politically supported and reinforced. What strategies are used by political actors in the global landscape to discuss the global economic policies of neoliberal trade and to generate support for such policies? What communication strategies are used by key political actors to background, discursively, the problems of poverty and healthcare inequality?

Furthermore, applying the culture-centered approach to the question of globalization opens up the discursive space to alternative voices that have been traditionally absent from globalization discourse. Much of the globalization talk focuses on the economic question, demonstrating with numbers the success or failure of global economies. However, the falling stock prices and the shrinking corporate profits in the global realm also have human aspects, aspects that connect with the life experiences of individuals in the marginalized sectors who experience the economic outcomes at a personal level in their ability or inability to access the basic health resources of life.

The culture-centered approach creates discursive openings for listening to these voices and their very real stories of oppression and poverty. The opening story of Sumirah presented in this chapter provides a human element to the case of a plummeting Indonesian economy. As Gershman and Irwin (2000) put it in their piece, these stories "remind us that the manipulation of money, even in its 'hottest' and most disembodied forms, has consequences for real human bodies: for the health and indeed the very survival of vulnerable individuals, families, and communities . . . for the poor, the stakes in the economic casino are infinitely higher. Financial and political fortunes can be, and routinely are, won back again after an initial defeat. The life of a child is a different sort of gambling chip. Once lost, it is gone forever" (pp. 41–2).

It is through the interpellation of narratives that the culture-centered approach draws our attention to the local contexts within which the effects of structure are played out. It is in the realm of day-to-day lives of community members that problems of inequity and inaccess are faced. The structural deprivation of communities in the global economic realm becomes meaningful in these stories, which capture the experiences of members of marginalized communities.

The introduction of the voice of the subaltern participant in the discursive space elucidates the interaction between structure and agency. It demonstrates the active engagement in meaning-making in marginalized contexts. Not only does the life experience of the narrator draw our attention to the inequity of the structural distribution of resources under projects of globalization and development, but it also demonstrates the active participation of subaltern communities in making sense of the inequities that are central to their lived experience, and in resisting the dominant discursive constructions of development. This resistance to the dominant discursive framings of the neoliberal project is further articulated in the following example provided in Farmer and Bertrand's article:

> I don't know what is meant by "structural adjustment," but it sounds to me like even less for poor people. How could we possibly live on less? If privatization goes forward, they might as well just dig a big pit and shove us all into it. (peasant farmer from Kay, June 1996, quoted in Farmer and Bertrand 2000: 81).

The narrative presented here attests to agency in the interpretation of the structural impediments in subaltern contexts. Through this narrative we come to understand the context within which health is constituted in poverty-stricken contexts. It draws our attention to the agency of the participant in engaging with the structure and drawing interpretations about the implications of structural adjustments. The notion that privatization would further marginalize the poor directly contradicts the neoliberal discourse, which suggests that further growth at a national level would lead to improvement in the conditions of the poor. In doing so, the voice of the subaltern participant suggests an alternative understanding of a neoliberal policy that has been traditionally framed in terms of its universal good for underdeveloped or developing economies. It is through this rearticulation of dominant framings of key structural issues that resistance is enacted at a global level.

Global Resistance and Activism

Where capital operates globally to create markets and to sustain them, resistance to the capitalization and commoditization of health is also being articulated in the global realm. Increasingly, writers and activists are addressing the issue of globalization, particularly in the realm of fore-grounding the interests of the pharmaceutical industry and the ways in which such interests have created unhealthy conditions within the global economy. Resistance is embodied in the very act of documenting the unhealthy nature of global policies and the ways in which such policies create and sustain conditions of poverty and inequality.

The articulation of criticism to the global policies and to its hypocrisies offers resistance to the humanitarian rhetoric within which global poli-cies have been placed. That the policies serve the interests of the global capital, further contributing to the lack of access among the underserved segments of the population, is a critical piece of information, which holds the capacity to transform global politics. Furthermore, the critical explo-ration of the hypocrisies of the global policies provides an entry point for alternative discourses. This is in itself a form of resistance, as it creates vistas for alternative policies and alternative frameworks for exploring issues of global health. For instance, the documentation concerning the link between global agricultural policies and health outcomes provides new openings for action. Increasingly, the public discursive space has opened up to the possibilities of social change through the voicing of the fundamental problems of the neoliberal model. Authors such as Paul Farmer and Arundhati Roy continue to draw public attention to the global injustices that are played out by the neoliberal ideology.

Furthermore, resistance has been offered globally through the mobi-lization of activist publics on a global scale. The growth in the uses of the Internet among activist publics has opened up new possibilities of com-municating with audiences worldwide. The Internet has created a discur-sive space for activist groups to communicate with each other and to mobilize themselves globally. The platform has opened up avenues for organizing that can connect publics across geographically dispersed loca-tions; it has also opened up opportunities for voicing critical stances about key policy issues without needing to depend upon the traditional gatekeepers in the mass media. This can be seen in the collective uses of the medium to mobilize against the meetings of the World Trade Organization (WTO). In this instance, the Internet created a space for communication among various activist groups, a communicative plat-form for mobilizing group action against powerful policy-makers, and then for organizing on cyberspace to enact resistance in the geographical space.

The Internet has also created new opportunities for connecting the local and the global. Forms of resistance at local levels are communicated today to global publics; thus publics are mobilized globally on the basis of local examples of empowered action. One such instance of local action that has created a global impact is the Narmada Bachao Andolan (NBA – also known as "Save the River Narmada" project). In order to protest against the building of dams that would displace thousands of indigenous families living on the banks of the river Narmada, the movement started through the participation of local men and women in the threatened communities (Dutta and Pal, in press). Community members used a variety of communicative strategies in order to oppose the building of the dam, including letter-writing campaigns, *gheraoing* (surrounding) the precincts of local administrative centers, street protests, hunger strikes, meeting with politicians at the national level, organizing nationwide rallies and so on. Furthermore, through the use of the Internet, the movement was connected with global publics interested in resisting the building of large dams that threaten the health of the displaced communities.

Currently, using the ability of the Internet to mobilize multiple stakeholder groups beyond geographical boundaries, the movement has created participatory opportunities for global publics. Such opportunities include: signing a petition to the prime minister of India; participating in hunger strikes individually or in dispersed global communities; globally dispersed candlelight vigils and rallies organized around certain time zones on certain days. Through its building of global resistance centered on a local issue, the NBA demonstrates the ways in which activism in a globalized context connects the global and the local. Practices of resistance now include a variety of new media platforms along with the traditional modes of resistance. Future scholarship in health communication ought to examine the avenues through which social change might be communicated on a global scale. Also, health communication activism is a topic of inquiry that has barely been interrogated in the realm of global politics.

Discussion point 10.4

- What are the possibilities of engaging in healthcare activism in the context of globalization?
- How would you go about developing a culture-centered approach to activism in your work as a health communication scholar?

Conclusion

Chapter 7 discussed the postcolonial logic of health communication, documenting how the dominant health communication discourse continues to create an "other" who exists outside the realm of normalcy and serves as the site of enactment of the colonial agenda of transnational hegemony. This chapter delved further into the discussion of colonization in the realm of the global processes of the twenty-first century. Whereas some of the threads of colonization continue to dominate the globalization discourse, our examination of globalization here further documents the ways in which power is fragmented, multifaceted, and fluid as it is played out in the realm of international networks that might be physically or virtually connected. The commoditization of healthcare in the global marketplace ensures that health is traded and exchanged as a commodity on the basis of market principles; this exchange takes place in a global realm on the basis of demand for the commodity and the capacity of the involved actors to pay for the commodity. One of the critical tasks ahead of health communicators is the examination of the role of communication, as it is deployed in supporting and sustaining unhealthy global policies that breed inequity. Of particular importance is the task of interrogating the ways in which discourse is mobilized globally to support the neoliberal project. As suggested by Zoller (2005, 2006), one of the critical tasks awaiting health communication scholars is the articulation of communication strategies that draw public attention to global policies and locate health within the realm of the structural roles played by these global policies.

11 Culture as Praxis

Chapter objectives

In this chapter, we will:

- understand the practical implications of the culture-centered approach
- connect culture-centered theory with research methodology and practical applications
- understand evaluative criteria for examining the culture-centered approach
- suggest directions for engaging health communication praxis

So far in the book we have discussed the culture-centered approach and the ways in which it brings forth its commitment to voice and agency in the study of health communication. In these chapters, we have explored the ways in which the culture-centered approach offers us theoretical and methodological insights into the study of culture in healthcare settings, drawing these insights from the interactions between structure, culture, and agency. We have learned that health is constituted in local contexts and health meanings are articulated through the voices of cultural members; that health is embedded within the structural constraints that shape it; and that centralizing the agency of cultural members offers an entry point for re-theorizing health communication. We have also learned that the primary commitment of the culture-centered approach is to create a dialogical space for the co-construction of problems on the basis of the engagement of the community in problem definition, articulation of solutions, and mobilization to implement the co-constructed solution. How, then, does the culture-centered approach suggest entry points for praxis?

This final chapter will summarize the basic principles of the culture-centered approach and connect the study of culture in health communication to the development and reconfiguration of praxis in health communication. More specifically, we will discuss how health communication applications that engage in the culture-centered approach might look, and we will provide suggestions for the development of culture-centered applications in health communication. Ultimately, the goal of this chapter is to suggest applications for health communication practitioners who work with diverse cultures in proposing, implementing, and evaluating health solutions.

A heuristic response that is typically provoked by the culture-centered approach concerns the practical value of such an approach. What are the contributions of the culture-centered approach to the practice of health communication? What are the ways in which health communication theorists, researchers, and practitioners might go about applying the culture-centered approach in their works? This concluding chapter underscores the pragmatic value of the culture-centered approach; provides guidelines regarding the possible conceptualizations, implementations, and evaluations of the culture-centered approach in health communication efforts; and suggests directions for engaging the culture-centered approach in the scholarship and practice of health communications.

To begin with, the chapter will elucidate the practice of the culture-centered approach through a case study of the SHIP. Building on this case study, it will then summarize the key arguments put forth in the book and suggest ways of linking them to applications in health communication applications. The chapter will conclude by suggesting applications that embody the culture-centered approach to the study of health communication.

Culture-Centered Praxis: The Case of SHIP

Throughout the chapter, the case of the Sonagachi HIV/AIDS Intervention Program (SHIP) will be used as a case study for elucidating the practical value of the culture-centered approach (Jana et al. 2004). Since its launch in 1992, the SHIP has successfully been able to increase the rate of condom usage among sex workers in Sonagachi, changing the percentage usage of condoms among commercial sex workers (CSWs) from 3 percent in 1992 to 90 percent in 1999. Located in the eastern part of India, in the city of Kolkata, Sonagachi is Kolkata's largest red-light area. Along with other sex worker sites in India, it has been the testing ground for several HIV/AIDS campaigns driven by the dominant framework. In their early years, most of these HIV/AIDS campaigns were formulated as top-down health promotion efforts and they promoted a condom use-based model for HIV/AIDS prevention, on the basis of the notion that providing information to CSWs would bring about change in their knowledge, attitudes, and behaviors. The basic assumption guiding these campaigns is that spreading awareness about the high risk of being infected with HIV/AIDS, the life-threatening dangers associated with such an infection, and how using condoms can help prevent such infections will lead to condom-use compliance among CSWs (Chattopadhyay and McKaig 2004; Jana et al. 2004). That this approach has not traditionally worked is evident in the UNAIDS (2002) and NACO (2003) figures, which indicate that, despite condom promotion efforts, HIV sero-prevalence rates among CSWs has been on the rise – rates of 50 percent to 90 percent have been reported in cities like Mumbai, Delhi, and Chennai. In contrast, the success at Sonagachi in bringing down the rate of HIV infection among sex workers has been attributed to the SHIP, which applies a culture-centered approach that builds on the networks of solidarity among CSWs.

According to the campaign planners of SHIP (Jana et al. 2004), the underlying principle was the belief that CSWs ought to take the leading role in a campaign that seeks to improve their health. It acknowledged the ability of the sex workers to resist and act within the constraints of their marginalized spaces, and to shape the course of action of the health promotion effort. Aligned with the goals of the culture-centered approach, steps were also taken to ensure that the structural factors surrounding HIV/AIDS were addressed, so that there was adequate access to condoms, STD (sexually transmitted disease) treatment, HIV testing, information on the diseases, and financial opportunities for the CSWs not to be constrained by their economic situation to engage in unsafe practices. As the campaign progressed, the participation of the CSWs on the programming committee led to the emergence of economic programs as a vital component of the campaign. Earlier, when sex workers were in need of money, banks or wealthy individuals would typically charge the CSWs 50 percent interest, fostering circumstances where the CSWs would be constrained to forego condom use in an attempt to earn a living. To combat this situation, a cooperative loan service (Usha) was established for sex workers. The cooperative bank granted small loans at 15 percent interest with feasible payment arrangements. It provided the CSWs with a security they could call their own and trust, which meant that they could resist clients who insisted on not using condoms. The SHIP also organized the CSWs into a quasi-trade union. The Durbar Mahila Samnwaya Committee (DMSC) was born in 1995 to help the sex workers exercise collective power and articulate their demands (Newman 2003). The case of the SHIP elucidates that a campaign that began as an attempt to address HIV/AIDS in a CSW community emerged as a community-based collective effort at addressing the structural features surrounding the lives of the CSWs.

The SHIP demonstrates how the agency of cultural participants may be actively mobilized in culture-centered health communication efforts (Dutta-Bergman 2004a; Dutta and Basu 2007). The SHIP passes the core criteria of the culture-centered approach because (a) it involves the local community in the identification of a health problem and in the development of relevant health solutions to address the problem through active participation; (b) it locates the health communication effort in the local context, articulated through the voices of community members participating in the project; and (c) it addresses the structures surrounding the health problem through the mobilization of community members. The CSWs actively participated in defining the key problems facing the community, and then formed a community organization that would respond to the community needs. In this process, an HIV/AIDS prevention campaign emerged that was responsive to the basic problems within the community and to the needs felt by community members; the problem and the emergent solution were contextually defined and structurally situated.

Not only has the SHIP campaign generated greater adoption rates of condoms, but it has also created a safe space for negotiating the structural forces around sex workers. The sex workers in Sonagachi today are able to mobilize resources in order to prevent and collectively resist the pressure put by clients on the sex workers to have sex without condoms. Furthermore, through the creation of a sex workers' cooperative, the Durbar Mahila Swamanaya Committee (DMSC), the sex workers are able to resist the structural pressures put on them by the police, politicians, and local goons. Therefore, in essence, the SHIP documents the intersections of structure, culture, and politics in the realm of health communication, as outlined by the culture-centered approach (Dutta-Bergman 2005a, 2005b). It demonstrates the ways in which change in a health-related behavior (the use of condoms in the realm of sex work) is embedded within the structural context and is enacted through the active participation of local community members. The participation of sex workers in the campaign and their engagement in securing change within the social system were critical to the improvement of health within the community. Health here was located within the structure, and it was by mobilizing themselves to create a cooperative that the sex workers were able to create an alternative structure which would be more accessible for securing better health within the community. Drawing upon the example of SHIP and other similar campaigns that have responded to the voices of cultural members, this chapter outlines the ways in which the culture-centered approach might be directed toward social change in the realm of health communication.

Culture as a Concept: From Theory to Research to Praxis

As presented in the introductory section of this book, culture is conceptualized in various ways in existing health communication theories and applications. These different approaches to culture can be primarily conceptualized within the realms of the cultural sensitivity approach and of the culture-centered approach. As we have observed earlier in this chapter, whereas the cultural sensitivity approach seeks to create health communication solutions that are sensitive to the characteristics of the culture and are tailored to these characteristics, the culture-centered approach highlights the notion of identifying problems and accompanying solutions from within the culture, through the active participation of cultural members in the project. Whereas one approach responds to the cultural characteristics to create communication that is conducive to the elements of the culture, the other approach foregrounds the agency of cultural participants in defining problems and solutions that are meaningful to them.

Both of these approaches offer unique entry points for the development of health communication solutions, and both offer ways of engaging with cultural participants in order to suggest solutions that are meaningful to them. As outlined in the introduction, one of the primary objectives of the book was to present the culture-centered approach as a strategy for

Box 11.1   The story of Doug

Doug works on projects funded by the United States Agency for International Development (USAID) and is posted as the HIV/AIDS program coordinator for the South African sector of Family Communications International. He recently came across the literature on the culture-centered approach to health communication and became very interested in this concept. However, after having read about the approach, Doug had a sense of paralysis. He didn't really quite know how to proceed with his work, as he came to see that anything he did ultimately served the status quo and the powerful actors in the global healthcare system.

What recommendations would you have for Doug in the realm of engaging in health communication work for FCI (Family Communications International)? Would it be possible for Doug to use the culture-centered approach in his work on HIV/AIDS? If so, how? How would you recommend he go about utilizing the culture-centered approach in his work?

engaging in theory-building, research, and practice of health communication. In the next few sections, we will identify specific elements of theory, research, and practice involved in conducting culture-centered health communication scholarship.

Culture in theory

Theoretically, the culture-centered approach conceptualizes culture in terms of the contextually situated life experiences of its members. In this sense, culture is dynamic and is enacted in the daily lives of its members, shifting with the contexts within which it is formed. The values, beliefs, and practices that constitute the culture become meaningful when articulated in the context within which they are realized. In other words, culture is represented in the everyday practices of its members. For instance, the value of individualism in US culture becomes meaningful when presented in the context of the health communication choices of privacy and disclosure in the physician–patient setting. The expectations of privacy articulated by the patient become meaningful when articulated in the realm of the local contexts surrounding these expectations. Communication here is the shared exchange of messages among cultural members; it is within the mutually meaningful cultural space that contextually rich choices are made among physicians, patients, and their families, and the space is meaningful when juxtaposed in the backdrop of the cultural expectations. Similarly, in the example of the CSWs presented earlier in this chapter, the use of condoms is negotiated within the contexts of economic needs and client pressures; the use of condoms becomes meaningful when articulated through the voices of cultural members that bring forth this contextually embedded nature of their day-to-day practices.

It is also important to highlight that cultural meanings become possible within the elements of structure in the social system where meanings are continuously created and recreated. In the situation of disclosure discussed earlier, the communication between the physician, patient, and his/her family is rendered meaningful when looked at in the light of the values of the actors, the setting within which the decision is made, and the structural choices within which the involved actors make the choices. For instance, the issue of patient privacy takes on new meaning when examined within the structural context of mobile clinics looking after underserved populations. Similarly, the meaning of eating fruits and vegetables is structurally situated when considered in the context of marginalized populations, who have too limited financial resources to afford fruits and vegetables. In the case of the CSWs in the SHIP, the negotiation of condom use is located within the broader structures constituting sex work; the ability of the CSWs to negotiate condom use is constrained by their structural dependence on their clients to earn a living. It is worth noting that much of the emphasis of the culture-centered approach has traditionally been directed toward marginalized contexts because of the interest of this framework in understanding conditions at the margins that are marked by limited access to basic infrastructural resources. Furthermore, with its emphasis on listening to subaltern voices that have typically been placed outside the realm of the discursive space, the culture-centered approach becomes theoretically interesting when considered in the context of marginalized experiences, left out of mainstream discourse. The presence of the subaltern voices in the discursive space creates openings for structure-based changes.

As theorized in chapters 1 and 2, structure exists in a dialectical relationship with agency. Agency refers to the capacity of individuals to participate in a relationship with the structure and to work with structural constraints in order to secure resources and ensure health for the individual, his or her family, and the community. Agency is presented in the health choices made by individuals as they respond to the very structures that constrain them. Within settings of resource inaccess, community members discuss ways of challenging the structures that constrain their lives, with the goal of obtaining better resources. In addition, they discuss participating in actions that respond to the constraints imposed by the structure on a daily basis. Once again, in the SHIP example discussed earlier in this chapter, agency is enacted in the organizing efforts of the CSWs to put together a trade union (the DMSC) that would provide protection and bargaining power for its members, and to create a cooperative loan service for the CSWs such that they could now negotiate safer sex practices with clients from a sense of financial security.

In the culture-centered framework, agency becomes meaningful and gains mobilizing capacity in the realm of culture. Culture connects individual action to collective communication about social change by providing the context within which meanings are exchanged, constructed, and reconstructed. It is through these co-constructed meanings that cultural members act toward securing resources. Agency played out at the level of community is typically rendered meaningful through the participation of community members in communication of shared values, beliefs, and practices. Take for instance the agency of the Sonagachi Sex Workers Movement in response to the constraining structure that imposed barriers on the use of condoms. Within such a context, agency was enacted through the participation of sex workers in developing community norms regarding client practices and in enforcing these norms within the community. The development of such norms was a cultural process, as cultural symbols and practices were negotiated by the participants, and new meanings were created around sex work, attaching it to the values of health and well-being.

Discussion point 11.1

- What are the key elements of culture-centered theorizing?
- What is the value of culture-centered theory to the ways in which we practice health communication today?
- How would you apply the culture-centered theory in your own work?

Culture in research

In applying the culture-centered approach to the research they engage in, scholars foreground the voices of cultural members in articulating community-specific problems and solutions and in developing theoretical understandings that look beyond the constructions of the dominant paradigm. Essential to the development of a culture-centered research strategy are the commitment to the voices of cultural members and the emphasis on dialogue as a way of articulating alternative understandings of phenomena situated outside the realm of the dominant paradigm. It is through the voices of subaltern groups that the culture-centered approach creates new theoretical opportunities; it simultaneously foregrounds the value-laden nature of the universalistic theories of health constituted under the dominant paradigm. Because the culture-centered approach is in essence set in opposition to the dominant paradigm, culture-centered research methodology looks for the possibilities for articulating these alternatives that have traditionally been silenced. For instance, what are the alternatives to the biomedical model in the ways in which health is constructed and applied? What are the ways in which health meanings can be understood beyond the modernist framework?

Dialogue provides the entry point to the presence of subaltern voices in the discursive space, voices that have typically been absent from the discussions of policy and its manner of implementation; it also offers the entry point for articulating understandings of health that have typically been silenced by the dominant paradigm. Given the relevance of these voices of subaltern groups, typically absent from the dominant health communication platforms, the emphasis of the dialogue is on constructing health meanings seen as relevant and critical by local community members. For instance, the SHIP campaign demonstrates the relevance of understanding the meanings of condom use as voiced by the CSWs; these meanings are embedded in the local context, constituted within the structure, and directed toward alternative sets of solutions, such as formation of cooperatives and sex worker unions, as opposed to the individual-behavior efforts evident in the dominant paradigm of health campaigns; the former promote awareness-based efforts targeted toward CSW communities.

Given its focus on opening up spaces for alternative epistemologies, the culture-centered research method is both deconstructive and constitutive. As a deconstructive exercise, the approach focuses on examining that which is absent from the discursive space; the emphasis here is on writing the narratives of culture from below. In other words, the focus is on the erasures and the silences, on exploring the gaps and fissures in the dominant paradigms of health, and on bringing about change through the examination of these absences in the dominant discursive space. The constitutive element of the culture-centered approach involves reflexive engagement with local communities in order to create spaces for dialogue. The researcher is an active participant who co-constructs narratives together with cultural members, and the discursive space is built upon the sharing of stories between the researcher and the cultural participants. These stories offer the bases for building alternative narratives of health to those that have hitherto been told.

Method as deconstruction. In the deconstructive element of the culture-centered approach, therefore, the researcher begins by starting to question the basic assumptions that are inherent in his or her position of expertise; "knowledge" becomes the very object of interrogation. Culture-centered scholars ask questions such as: Who creates knowledge? For what purposes? What are the assumptions that go into the creation of knowledge? What are the values embedded in the assumptions of knowledge made by the dominant paradigm? What remains silent and untold in the articulations of knowledge? How does power play out in the constructions of knowledge?

As health communication students and scholars, we are trained into certain sets of assumptions that we typically take for granted and consider as universally applicable. The deconstructive exercise draws attention to these assumptions and seeks to examine them for their erasures. For instance, Dutta-Bergman's critical interrogation of health communication campaigns (2006) demonstrates that these campaigns are built upon the Eurocentric logic of individualism, based on the assumption that the individual is the unit of decision-making in health situations, and is not reflective of cultural contexts where health decisions are negotiated in relational and familial contexts and the family plays a critical role in deciding about treatment options. The emphasis on targeting the individual as a point of behavior change reflects the individualistic ideology at its core. Bringing forth this individualistic value driving theories of health campaigns ruptures the logic of universal rationality that underlies the formulation of theoretical frameworks in health communication.

Similarly, in the context of the SHIP, the deconstruction of the dominant paradigm of health campaigns demonstrates their central emphasis on individual knowledge and behavior in the realm of safe sex, and the simultaneous absence of discussions about the structural constraints within which safe sex is negotiated. Therefore the deconstructive component of the culture-centered methodology focuses on looking for erasures by bringing forth the dominant assumptions under investigation. Through this deconstructive exercise, it brings to attention the moments of epistemic violence, where the ways of knowing of subaltern groups are undermined as primitive and the dominant knowledge frameworks are imposed upon subaltern communities. It is important to note that essential to the dominance of the Eurocentric frameworks of knowledge is the articulation of the primitiveness of the subaltern sectors. That the subaltern "needs" interventions from the dominant actors is crucial to maintaining the control of the dominant actors. As demonstrated by postcolonial scholars, the dominant hegemony is deeply intertwined with the economic interests of these powerful actors and helps sustain new forms of colonialism (also referred to as neocolonialism). The national elite is complicit in creating and sustaining positions of marginality, as they too benefit economically and are able to continue to exert their control on the subaltern sectors. In the sphere of health campaigns, for instance, the ability to demonstrate the ignorance of the subaltern sectors is critical to the articulation of a "need" and to the procurement of funding. In other words, the political economy of health campaigns is fundamentally built upon the constructions of the subaltern as primitive and in need of interventions. The culture-centered method looks for the ways in which power plays out in the enunciative value of certain knowledge positions, on the basis of questions such as: Who is included in the processes of knowledge production and who is excluded from these processes? It also looks for the underlying ideologies driving health campaigns, with particular emphasis on the political and economic interests that are tied to them.

As articulated earlier, the logic of the rational scientific discourse that dominates much of the health communication scholarship is based on the universal appeal of science and of the tools of modernity. For instance, when faced with the question of whether to immunize a child or not, the rational scientific discourse supplies a ready-made and obvious answer, and it is on the basis of this answer that health communicators continue to develop interventions on immunization. What gets left out of the discursive space matters such as the contested nature of immunizations, their efficacy, their unintended side effects, and the like. Similarly, a chronic disease such as cancer is constructed in the realm of the modern medical technologies that can fight it, simultaneously backgrounding alternative constructions that explore spiritually and culturally situated meanings of cancer.

In summary, the blind emphasis on the rational scientific discourse in health communication limits possibilities for articulating other meanings of health, and hence other possibilities for conceptualizing disease and illness. The culture-centered approach calls into question the viability of the dominant paradigm and interrogates its limits in understanding human health, disease, and illness. A culture-centered research method, therefore, begins by being continuously reflexive about the viability of health problems and solutions as conceptualized within the dominant paradigm. It interrogates the underlying ideologies connected with the very conceptualization of problems, and the configurations of solutions proposed by health communicators. In this realm, what is needed, then, is a detailed interrogation of the basic applicability of the health solutions which are typically proposed for underserved communities. The proposed solution itself needs to be questioned, and in doing this, the researcher needs to bring under scrutiny his or her own biases and the assumptions that drive the type of work that he or she does, and the types of solutions that he or she is funded to investigate and disseminate. In essence, the very position of expertise becomes a point of interrogation in the deconstructive phase of culture-centered research because it brings under scrutiny the role of the researcher as a producer of knowledge, thus contesting the sacredness of that knowledge.

It is also critical for the researcher at this point to question his or her privilege and the ways in which such privilege is maintained by working on specific health communication solutions deployed in underserved communities. To the extent that I receive funding from a federal agency to carry on a campaign in an underserved community (say, for instance, on a 'Five-A-Day' campaign promoting the consumption of five or more servings of fruits and/or vegetables in a rural African American community), the basic logic about the nature of the problem in the community serves as the economic rationale for the campaign work that I would engage in. In other words, the political economy of the research enterprise is built on certain fundamental assumptions that are typically erased from the discursive space when considering issues such as effectiveness of health interventions. Therefore, the culture-centered approach suggests greater need for research that examines the fundamental necessity of the health solutions that are promoted within communities.

Research method as co-construction.   Culture-centered research, however, does not end with deconstruction, as it becomes deeply aware of the absences in the dominant epistemic spaces through the deconstructive exercise. Deconstruction offers an opening for engaging with the possibilities for articulating the voices of subaltern participants through dialogue. The culture-centered approach examines the intersection between structure, agency, and culture, and therefore needs to respond to the shifting nature of the context within which such interactions are situated through the presence of subaltern voices that bring forth these interactions. The intersection between culture and agency is articulated in dialogue with cultural members. These dialogues open up spaces for co-constructing knowledge in ways that not only challenge the epistemic assumptions of the dominant paradigm, but also open up new opportunities for conceptualizing health and for constituting health communication practice. Practical applications are co-constructed through this dialogue with cultural members. What, then, are the key elements for approaching dialogue in culture-centered method? The culture-centered research method (a) examines the power structures inherent in the dialogical process; (b) develops communicative openings (listening, participating, encouraging) based on the awareness of power; (c) builds a network of solidarity with cultural members, with a deep sense of commitment to the communicative openings; and (d) participates in the co-construction of narratives with these cultural members.

The dialogue suggested by the co-constructive approach is built upon an awareness of the power structures within which it is situated. The co-constructive exercise articulated in the culture-centered method begins with a profound awareness of the power structures that constrain the opportunities for dialogue rather than being oblivious to these power structures.

Central to the co-constructive approach is the reflection that engaging in the very practice of research creates conditions of marginality; voices are silenced as particular sets of narratives get narrated and re-narrated by culture-centered researchers in mainstream academic journals, where knowledge is played out and contested. Being a culture-centered researcher embodies the realization that there is really no way out of this predicament; that the very privilege embodied in the position of the researcher is a marker of the marginalizing practices of the dominant paradigm. For instance, the very publishing of Dutta-Bergman's (2004a) work on Santali theories of health in a major communication journal, *Communication Theory*, is an act of marginalization that "others," "dichotomizes," and "fixes." Being reflexive means continuously engaging with this reality of the work that we do as culture-centered researchers. A culture-centered researcher can't write off her/his privilege by going through a standard set of rituals, but rather must be deeply aware of the ways in which his/her practices continue to embody the privilege, and create discursive closures just as it creates openings. The very practice of researching and reporting our work creates positions of subalternity, as they mark out the subaltern and fix him/her within the discursive space.

Discussion point 11.2

- What are the connections between culture-centered theory and culture-centered research method?
- What are the similarities and differences between the cultural deconstruction and cultural co-construction methods? How would you use these methods in your own work?
- Is it possible truly to engage in a culture-centered method that gives voice to marginalized communities? Why? Why not?

Culture in practice

In conceptualizing culture as a concept that informs practice, the culture-centered approach begins by highlighting the relevance of developing communication processes that open up the discursive space to the participation of those voices which have not been present in the traditional discursive spaces of health applications (Dutta-Bergman 2004a; 2004b). Communication here is envisioned not simply in the realm of messages, but as a process that brings forth dialogical spaces where multiple voices can be heard. Therefore a key practical contribution of the culture-centered approach is the development of processes for articulating the voices of cultural members. Also relevant is the application of the culture-centered approach as an evaluative framework for health communication applications, serving as an indicator of the extent to which the health communication program is constitutive of the voices of the cultural members. The steps of the process-based framework offer criteria for examining whether a health communication effort is culture-centered or not. This evaluative framework may be applied to health campaigns, physician–patient interactions, healthcare organizations, and so on.

Culture-centered process.   The example of the SHIP elucidates the workings of the culture-centered approach and outlines steps for putting it into practice. The culture-centered approach creates a discursive space for engaging with cultural members. In order to do so, (a) it identifies structural inequities in communication platforms in which cultural members may articulate their voices; (b) it creates opportunities for making accessible those communication tools that are essential for community members to articulate their voices; and (c) it creates a facilitating environment for the use of communicative tools by community members. The approach to dialogue here is intertwined with analyses of structural inequities that foster or prevent the possibilities of dialogue, and it addresses these structural inequities through the creation of community-specific communication spaces that are embedded within the local context. A plethora of communication strategies and tools may be fostered in marginalized communities in order to create openings for subaltern voices in the discursive space. It is crucial that these communicative platforms for community dialogues be situated within the local contexts of communities.

   In the example of SHIP, the health promotion effort initially went about creating community meetings involving CSWs, so that they had opportunities to articulate their needs and concerns. In this context, the community meetings served as mobilizing platforms that brought the CSWs together under the broader agenda of improving their health and well-being; these meetings served as initial spaces for getting organized into a community. Furthermore, CSWs were involved in the campaign early on and were given leadership roles in spearheading the campaign. In doing so, efforts were put into place for making sure that the CSWs had access to the communication resources they needed in order to lead the campaign; the community was equipped with communicative tools (such as workshops on folk performances, street theaters, and the like) which were critical to the articulation of the voices of the CSWs.

These communication resources developed in the community were instrumental in mobilizing the CSW community; this was evident in the formation of the DMSC, which became a key element in the ability of the CSWs to negotiate their health choices. The initial investment into the communication platforms became a conduit for fostering and sustaining additional communicative exchanges. For instance, the investment in formal community-wide meetings triggered greater communication through informal networks and word-of-mouth communication; this resulted in more sustained efforts of organizing, evident in the formation of the DMSC. Furthermore, structural resources were presented in the communities in order to provide the CSWs with opportunities for enacting the changes they deemed relevant to the program. An example of such structural resources is the cooperative loan program, which supported the ability of the sex workers to negotiate their choices.

Yet another example of the culture-centered approach is the photo-voice project, which draws upon the life experiences of local community members to impact broader policy. Photo-voice is a participatory action research method that involves placing cameras in the hands of community members, so that they may visually represent and communicate their lived experiences to internal and external stakeholders. With its emphasis on providing venues for voices that are typically silenced in the mainstream discourse, the photo-voice method enables participants to share their emotions, feelings, and insights about issues that are important to them through photographs. In doing so, the method (a) records the key issues faced by the community and community strengths as constructed by community members, (b) promotes critical dialogue and builds new knowledge through the discussion of the photographs, and (c) influences positive social change by reaching policy-makers and decision-makers through public fora and showings of the photographs. The photo-voice method was originally applied by Caroline Wang and her colleagues in China's Yunnan province, to create a platform for rural women who had minimal access to the policy-makers who made decisions that affected their lives (Wang and Burris 1994). Through the showings of the photographs and through their interpretations by the women in public fora, a discursive space was created for social change, through the enactment of women's agency. The women were able to share their stories and identify the issues that were most important to them, and hence to have control over "the ways in which their perspectives and life situations were depicted, discussed and communicated to others" (Lopez et al. 2005: 327). The photographs, coupled with the critical discussions they generated, led to structural changes in the communities, for instance the construction of day-care facilities and water tanks in villages, and the establishment of educational scholarships for rural girls (Wang and Burris 1994).

Similar applications of the photo-voice method have involved residents of homeless shelters in Ann Arbor, Michigan, who countered stereotypes and stigmas about homeless people by documenting their everyday life, work and health conditions through photographs (Wang, Cash and Powers 2000), and Latino adolescents in North Carolina who examined their lives in the context of immigration. The Inspirational Images Project engaged African American breast cancer survivors in rural eastern North Carolina, to create a discursive space for identifying the needs of the women and for developing an action plan for addressing these needs on the basis of a public showing of the photographs and of a public forum that brought the women and policy-makers together (Lopez et al. 2005).

The photo-voice method meets the three criteria of the culture-centered approach: (a) it engages culture through the articulation of the local contexts within which the lived experiences of the cultural members are enacted; (b) it addresses structural issues through the emphasis on policy and decision-making processes that influence the health of the local communities; (c) it creates a space for the enactment of agency by shifting the discursive control over the narratives, representations, identification of issues and respective solutions in the hands of local community members; and (d) it resists the dominant structures through the voices of community members. Ultimately, through the application of photo-voice, the health needs and corresponding solutions are developed from within the community, through dialogue with policy-makers and other decision-makers, rather than emerging from outside the realm of the community. The photo-voice method resists the dominant discourses of health interventions by displacing the expert voices of health communicators with the voices of cultural members, represented through the photographs and their interpretations by community members. As in the case of the SHIP, the community is invested with communicative resources (the actual tools as well as the skills) in order to foster a space for articulating community needs in mainstream discourse and for creating an opening for the addressing of community-specific problems. Also, the child reporters of the Koraput project in India harness the participatory capacity of local communities by creating and sustaining community potential in the form of media reports of local issues written by child reporters; these reports are made available to the media, policy-makers, development workers, and bureaucrats. In addition to creating and implementing processes for the articulation of community voices, the culture-centered approach suggests evaluative criteria for health communication programs.

Culture-centered evaluative criteria.   The application of such evaluations is driven by the conceptualization of communication as a process that creates openings for voices. The primary question driving such evaluation is: to what extent does the communicative space create openings for those voices that have traditionally been silenced by mainstream health communication projects?

For instance, in the realm of health communication campaigns, Dutta and Basnyat (in press) have applied the culture-centered approach to examine the participatory claims of the Radio Communication Project (RCP) in Nepal. In this project, the researchers demonstrated that, although the RCP claimed to be participatory, it really did not provide a discursive space for the voices of the cultural participants. Instead, it used participatory tools such as community meetings and folk performances to diffuse the health problem and corresponding solutions, which were decided by the campaign planners and funding agencies before engaging in dialogue with the community.

Furthermore, an analysis of the RCP discourse demonstrated that the campaign materials embodied a colonial lens imbued with the top-down ideology of the campaign, which was based on the dichotomy of tradition and modernity. Whereas the subaltern spaces in Nepal were portrayed as traditional and undeveloped, the solutions proposed by the campaign planners (mainly population control) were portrayed as developed and modern. Applying the culture-centered approach to this case allowed the researchers to evaluate the intervention with respect to the question of voices of subaltern participants in the discourse, and the analysis demonstrated that, in spite of its claims of participation, the discursive space of the RCP did not really provide opportunities for listening to subaltern voices.

The forms of evaluation applied to the RCP might also be extended to healthcare interactions such as physician–patient relationships and healthcare organizations. In the area of physician–patient relationships, specific interactions might be evaluated with respect to their culture-centeredness. A culture-centered interaction would move toward a dialogical space that would allow for the raising of issues and concerns by both parties and would open up the discourse to the free flow of communication. For instance, when the interactions described in Fadiman's book *The Spirit Catches you and you Fall* are evaluated from a culture-centered perspective, what is revealed is that the communication between the physician and patient was deeply steeped in the logical scientific discourse of the physician and did not really create any openings for articulating the voices of the patient's family.

The absence of a legitimate discursive opening for the patient's family in this case might also be extended to the organizational structure, raising questions such as: To what extent do hospitals, as modern organizations, provide discursive openings for the voices of patients? What are the processes through which such discursive openings are closed? The application of the culture-centered approach in evaluating healthcare organizations might focus on questions of organizational structure and organizational communication process which provide possibilities for listening to other voices or which limit such possibilities. For instance, the ways in which hospital rooms are structurally constituted, or the organization of examination rooms, might suggest that the creation of such spaces follows individualistic values that emphasize privacy, simultaneously limiting the discursive space for other cultures, where family ties play a critical role, particularly in the context of healthcare and medical interactions.

In addition to serving as an evaluative tool, the culture-centered approach provides a conceptual basis for developing health communication solutions that are responsive to the voices of communities. In developing a process-based application for culture-centered solutions, the primary objective of the culture-centered approach is connected with the question of the voices of community members: To what extent are community members articulating the problems and participating in developing the solutions that they consider to be relevant for them? Note that the question of participation of community members here is not simply a token that can be measured in terms of the number of community members present at discussions focused on problem identification and solution development.

Therefore culture-centered applications begin by working on communication processes that open up spaces for listening to voices of cultural members. The emphasis here is on assessing and creating communication infrastructures that are responsive to the voices of community members and are legitimately concerned with the critical issues in the communities, as these are constructed by the members. The initial phases of the application therefore focus on assessing community communication infrastructures in terms of the communication avenues available to community members for communicating with a variety of outside stakeholders, particularly those stakeholder groups actively involved in making and in implementing policy decisions. With an emphasis on listening, the subsequent steps of the health communication application are focused on creating avenues that would present opportunities for listening to the subaltern voices.

Culture-centered applications focus on building listening skills within the communities of researchers and practitioners who, traditionally, have been trained to offer health communication solutions for marginalized communities on the basis of the expertise and knowledge they have. Questioning this very basic expertise of supplying knowledge, the culture-centered approach calls for a very different type of expertise: the ability to build meaningful relationships with subaltern communities on the basis of listening to their members. This procedure suggests a critical change in how health communication solutions are proposed and executed: the focus shifts, from teaching necessary skills to target communities, to building necessary skills such as listening and participating in dialogue within expert groups. This also shifts the emphasis of health communication scholarship, from simply focusing on developing messages for effective dissemination, to examining ways of developing effective listening skills within research communities. Therefore the culture-centered approach would initially focus on teaching skills such as listening, dialogue, and relationship-building to the health communication practitioners. Ultimately, at this stage of application development, the focus would be on preparing the community of researchers and practitioners to engage in culture-centered practices.

Once the community has been engaged in dialogical platforms and spaces which offer opportunities for the exchange of communication between the researcher and community members, the next step is to engage policy-makers in the health issues that have been articulated by the community. At this stage, the culture-centered approach emphasizes the development of community mobilizing strategies that would allow opportunities for the community to come together and question the taken-for-granted assumptions of health communication policies that continue to ignore the basic issues of structural inequities and inaccess. In terms of constructing research agendas around praxis, the emphasis here is on developing appropriate strategies and tools for communicating with policy-makers, which would bring about opportunities for structural change.

Culture in Social Change

As documented in chapter 9, culture provides a lens for resisting dominant structures, and yet it is also itself contested through communicative practices within the culture – practices which challenge the status quo privileged by the culture. In this section I will outline specific strategies for engaging culture in addressing issues of structural change. The ultimate goal here is to address those unhealthy structures which create the conditions at the margins.

Influencing individual-level praxis

Individual-level praxis refers to the solutions that are developed by way of addressing individual values, attitudes, and behaviors in health communication contexts. In the dominant paradigm of health communication scholarship, applications have typically focused on extracting certain aspects of the culture at the individual level that are typically categorized as beliefs of the target audience, which is to serve as a receiver of the campaign messages. In such instances, cultural beliefs are operationalized as negative traits, to be overcome by campaigns targeting these traits. For instance, campaigns targeting the Latino population have often discussed the external locus of control in the population and therefore have sought to build an internal locus of control through campaign messages. In other instances, campaigns have been designed and developed with the sense of being culturally sensitive, that is, of responding to the salient characteristics of the culture. In these situations, the goal of the campaign designers is to develop messages that are responsive to the characteristics of the culture targeted by the message.

The individual-level praxis of the culture-centered approach, however, differs substantively from the dominant approach of identifying cultural beliefs and attempting to modify them through strategic campaign messages. It is also different from the emphasis on cultural sensitivity, which seeks to develop culturally meaningful persuasive messages that would correspond to the characteristics of the culture. The culture-centered approach focuses on creating discursive spaces for listening to the voices of individual cultural members. The emphasis is on developing partnerships with individual members that open up avenues for social change. The personal experiences of individual members provide an epistemological basis for articulating health problems and corresponding solutions responsive to these problems.

Therefore the application of the culture-centered approach in health communication projects suggests a fundamental shift in how the individual is conceptualized, both as a research participant and as a target member of health interventions. The focus is on developing avenues and skills for listening in the community of researchers and practitioners, so that the stories of health may be articulated. It is through these narratives that health communication becomes a site for cultural practice. Cultural members articulate contextually relevant health solutions, and these solutions need to be supported through praxis. Appropriate and adequate resources need to be identified that would facilitate the development of culturally meaningful solutions to health problems.

At the individual level, the culture-centered approach legitimizes the experiences of the individual as points of application for health communication. These narratives of individual identity, relationships, and daily experiences in the realm of healthcare point out the ways in which individual actors make sense of their day-to-day lives in accessing and securing healthcare. It is only through these stories that health communicators can come to understand the ways in which health is constituted and communicated, thus being able to understand the questions and issues of marginalization in underserved communities.

Influencing organizational praxis

At the level of the organization, the culture-centered approach suggests that healthcare organizations need to be fundamentally influenced in the way they understand culture and conceptualize it in the delivery of healthcare. Culture is not simply a set of categorical variables that might be included in training programs to make providers more culturally competent. Culture is manifested in the context and becomes meaningful in the realm of the lives of its members. Yet most health organizations responding to the need to be culturally adaptive have sought to extract categorical variables that might be used in developing training programs. In such programs, the notion of culture is restrictive and static, and does not really create openings for the local voices.

Although cultural sensitivity programs might focus on teaching the providers the relevant characteristics of certain cultures that constitute the target audience, being culture-centered means more than having organizational training in a core set of cultural characteristics, because training in these characteristics still does not ensure that the culture finds legitimacy as a co-participant in the discursive space. For instance, a training program that suggests the development of a certain set of communication skills directed toward collectivistic cultures misses out on the many nuances of the interactions between individualist and collectivist tendencies in varying contexts. In order to create spaces for cultural legitimacy, health communicators ought to develop a fundamental orientation toward respecting multiple contexts and the meanings embodied in these contexts. This sort of commitment is process-based and is not directly tied to a set of categorical outcomes, derived from a set of categorical variables. Rather, it is a shift in paradigmatic orientation within the medical community, one that calls for a questioning of the very arrogant stance of "expert," which comes with the profession, and for a willingness to take a dialogical stance.

Culture is dynamic and enacted in the local context; hence it cannot really be translated into a list of variables that might then be used to train healthcare providers. Instead, to be culture-centered, the organization needs to be fundamentally oriented toward listening to the voices of patients, and legitimately to open up communicative spaces for these voices. Culture-centered health communication begins with a commitment to solidarity with cultural members, and this solidarity is built upon an emphasis on mutual respect. Therefore health organizations ought to invest in health communication approaches that focus on building respect, in the community of providers, toward alternative worldviews and in ways of experiencing the world that might not always coincide with the biomedical model. Being respectful of these alternatives is not a matter of tolerating them, but a matter of learning to acknowledge them as legitimate ways of knowing, which provide meaningful access points for interpreting disease and illness.

Influencing social praxis

The culture-centered approach explores the intersection of structure, agency, and culture. The engagement with structure is intended to bring about social adjustments that would allow opportunities for engaging with questions of inaccess faced by marginalized communities. In other words, one of the goals of the culture-centered approach is to engage with the structures that impede access to healthcare in marginalized communities. How can communication be mobilized toward changing the structures that create inequitable healthcare and sustain pockets of healthcare inaccess? What role can communicators play in the realm of altering unhealthy social structures that impede access to the basic capabilities of healthcare? Here the culture-centered approach explores the role of communication in bringing about structural change and in opening up avenues for fundamentally altering an unhealthy healthcare system.

Instead of being directed at modifying individual behaviors that embody a preventive approach, the goal is to communicate in culturally meaningful ways, so as to alter those structures that impeded basic access to healthcare systems. Within this framework, it is once again critical that the structural points of change emerge from within the community, through its members and through their participation in the processes of change. Structural adjustments become meaningful only when articulated in the day-to-day context of the community and of its needs. For instance, structurally situated programs that seek to build basic food capabilities in underserved communities need to attend to the cultural constructions of food and to what is considered healthy food within the community.

It is through the participatory engagement of community members that appropriate points of structural change can be identified and structurally meaningful changes can be carried on within the social system. Furthermore, the channels and modalities of social change become meaningful when articulated within the social context of the culture. The emphasis on engaging with the structure suggests the relevance of developing programs of communicative activism that offer avenues for changing unhealthy structures. Also worth exploring are the ways in which communicators might participate in media agenda-setting functions. What are the communicative strategies that would draw media attention to key health issues faced by the community? What communicative processes might be put into place to create discursive openings within civil society platforms that have been traditionally neglectful of subaltern voices and instead served hegemonic configurations? How could communicators create open spaces for listening to subaltern voices? These are key questions facing health communication researchers and practitioners working with the culture-centered approach to health communication.

Influencing global praxis

Structural systems that impeded access to basic healthcare are connected with national level politics, which is furthermore embedded within the realm of global politics. The local is played out in the context of the global, and this local–global connection is critical for health communicators. The health effects and inaccess experienced at the local level is played out in the domain of global politics. Unhealthy global policies create conditions of inaccess and further support these unhealthy conditions. Therefore a vital goal of culture-centered health communication is to address the global policies that sustain the unhealthy conditions in underserved communities and create conditions of inaccess.

In the realm of global politics, health communicators ought to highlight the ways in which global policies create conditions of inaccess and poor health. The growing research on the healthcare disparities brought about by global policies needs to be placed on the media agendas and articulated within the public discursive space. Furthermore, the articulation of such policies in the public discursive space ought to provide openings for exploring the ways in which healthcare activism serves as a communicative avenue for social change. How could communicators use meaningful health communication strategies to shift unhealthy structures globally? How could policy-makers and global publics be targeted with communication that seeks to alter policies? This calls for an emphasis, within the discipline of health communication, on scholarship that examines strategies for impacting policy-making processes at local, national, and global levels.

- How would you go about implementing the culture-centered approach in your own health communication work?
- How would you go about developing applications using the culture-centered approach?
- In what respects would these applications be similar to, or different from, other applications?

Conclusion

In conclusion, this chapter brings us back to the conceptualization that culture is complex and intertwined with structure and agency. The interactions between structure and agency are embodied in the norms, beliefs, and shared practices of the culture. Culture supplies the meanings, communicative symbols, and communicative spaces that are mobilized in the daily practices of individuals, as they interact with the structures within which they live their lives. The lived experiences of the individual provide the lens through which agency is enacted in cultural communities and the structures of inaccess are resisted by community members.

Ultimately, the chapter suggests that the notion of culture as dynamic and constituted through the participation of its members is central to the culture-centered approach. In its commitment to research and practice, the culture-centered approach highlights the relevance of listening to the voices of cultural members. Ultimately, it claims that health communication is more responsive to the needs of community members at local levels when it privileges the voices of cultural participants and seeks to listen to them. Future research building on the culture-centered approach ought to explore the ways in which the voices of cultural members are silenced, and the communicative processes through which spaces might be created for listening to the voices of community members.

Points for reflection

- What are the possibilities for engaging in culture-centered research?
- Compare culture-centered research with other forms of health communication research which involve the concept of culture. What are the similarities and differences between these different approaches?
- How would you go about connecting culture-centered research to the development of culture-centered applications in the field?
- What are the ethical dilemmas faced by culture-centered researchers? How would you recommend that a health communication scholar navigate these dilemmas?

References

Abraham, L. (1993). *Mama Might Be Better Off Dead: The Failure of Healthcare in Urban America.* Chicago: The University of Chicago Press.

Agency for Healthcare Research and Quality (2004). *National Healthcare Disparities Report, 2004.* AHRQ, Rockville, MD. http://www.ahrq.gov/qual/nhdr04/nhdr04.htm>.

Airhihenbuwa, C. (1994). "Health promotion and the discourse on culture: Implications for empowerment." *Health Education and Behavior,* 21, 345–53.

Airhihenbuwa, C. (1995). *Health and Culture: Beyond the Western Paradigm.* Thousand Oaks, CA: Sage.

Airhihenbuwa, C. and Obregon, R. (2000). "A critical assessment of theories/models used in health communication for AIDS." *Journal of Health Communication,* 5 (Suppl.), 5–15.

Airhihenbuwa, C., Makinwa, B. and Obregon, R. (2000). "Toward a new communication framework for HIV/AIDS." *Journal of Health Communication,* 5 (Suppl.), 101–11.

Ajzen, I. and Fishbein, M. (1974). "Factors influencing intentions and the intention–behavior relation." *Human Relations,* 27, 1–15.

Ajzen, I. and Fishbein, M. (1980). *Understanding Attitudes and Predicting Social Behavior.* Englewood Cliffs, NJ: Prentice Hall.

Albrecht, T. L. and Goldsmith, D. (2003). "Social support, social networks, and health." In T. L. Thompson, A. M. Dorsey, K. I. Miller, and R. Parrott (eds), *Handbook of Health Communication* (pp. 263–84). Mahwah, NJ: Lawrence Erlbaum.

Alford, L. and Van Pelt, E. (2000). *The Scalpel and the Silver Bear.* New York: Bantam Books.

Amin, S. (1989). *Eurocentrism,* tr. R. Moore. New York: Monthly Review Press.

Anderson, L. A. and Sharpe, P. A. (1991). "Improving patient and provider communication: A synthesis and review of communication interventions." *Patient Education and Counseling,* 17, 99–134.

Arcury, T. A., Austin, C. K., Quandt, S. A. and Saavedra, R. (1999). "Enhancing community participation in intervention research: Farmworkers and agricultural chemicals in North Carolina." *Health Education and Behavior,* 26, 563–78.

Atkinson, A. and Micklewright, J. (1992). *Economic Transformation in Eastern Europe and the Distribution of Income.* Cambridge: Cambridge University Press.

Babrow, A., Kline, K. and Rawlins, W. (2005). "Narrating problems and problematizing narratives: Linking problematic integration and narrative theory in telling stories about health." In L. Harter, P. Japp, and C. Beck (eds), *Narratives, Health and Healing: Communication Theory, Research, and Practice* (pp. 31–60). Mahwah, NJ: Lawrence Erlbaum.

Baer, H. (1986). "The replication of the medical division of labor in medical anthropology: Implications for the field." *Medical Anthropology Quarterly,* 17, 63–5.

Baer, H., Singer, M., and Susser, I. (2003). *Medical Anthropology and the World System.* Westport, CT: Praeger.

Bain, D. J. (1979). "The content of physician/patient communication in family practice." *Journal of Family Practice,* 8, 745–53.

Baker, E. and Motton, F. (2005). "Creating understanding and action through group dialogue." In B. Israel, E. Eng, A. Schulz and E. Parker (eds), *Methods in Community-Based Participatory Research for Health* (pp. 307–25). San Francisco, CA: Jossey-Bass.

Bakhtin, M. (1981). *The Dialogic Imagination. Four Essays by M. M. Bakhtin*, ed. M. Holquist, trs Caryl Emerson and Michael Holquist. Austin: University of Texas Press.

Bandura, A. (1977). "Self-efficacy: Toward a unifying theory of behavioral change." *Psychological Review*, 84, 191–215.

Bandura, A. (1986). *Social Foundations of Thought and Action: A Social Cognitive Theory*. London: Prentice-Hall.

Baquet, C. (2002). "What is 'health disparity?'" *Public Health Report*, 17, 426–9.

Baum, F. (1999). "The role of social capital in health promotion: Australian perspectives." *Health Promotion Journal of Australia*, 9, 171–8.

Bauman, Z. (2000). *Culture as Praxis*. Thousand Oaks, CA: Sage.

Bearinger, L. H. and Blum, R. W. (1997). "The utility of locus of control for predicting adolescent substance use." *Research in Nursing and Health*, 20, 229–45.

Beck, C. (2005). "Becoming the story: Narratives as collaborative, social enactments of individual, relational and public identities." In L. Harter, P. Japp, and C. Beck (eds), *Narratives, Health and Healing: Communication Theory, Research, and Practice* (pp. 61–81). Mahwah, NJ: Lawrence Erlbaum.

Becker, E. (1975). *Escape From Evil*. New York: Collier Macmillan.

Beisecker, A. E. and Beisecker, T. D. (1990). "Patient in information-seeking behaviors when communicating with doctors." *Medical Care*, 28, 19–28.

Bellah, R. N., Madsen, R., Sullivan, W. M., Swidler, A. and Tipton, S. M. (1985). *Habits of the Heart*. Berkeley, CA: University of California Press.

Berger, G. (2002). "Theorizing the media-democracy relationship in Southern Africa. *Gazette: The International Journal for Communication Studies*, 64(1), 21–45.

Beverley, J. (1999). *Subalternity and Representation: Arguments in Critical Theory*. Durham, NC: Duke University Press.

Beverley, J. (2004). *Testimonio: On the Politics of Truth*. Minneapolis: University of Minnesota Press.

Bird, C. (1979). *What Women Want*. New York: Simon and Schuster.

Bond, G. G., Aiken, L. S. and Somerville, S. C. (1992). "The health belief model and adolescents with insulin dependent diabetes mellitus." *Health Psychology*, 11, 190–8.

Bordo, S. (1987). *The Fight to Objectivity: Essays on Cartesianism and Culture*. Buffalo, NY: SUNY.

Bosticco, C. and Thompson, T. L. (2005). "The role of narratives in coping during the grieving process." In L. Harter, P. Japp, and C. Beck (eds) *Narratives in Health and Illness*. Mahwah, NJ: Erlbaum.

Boston Women's Health Book Collective. (1973). *Our Bodies, Ourselves*. Boston, MA: Boston Women's Health Book Collective.

Bourdieu, P. (1993). *La Misère du monde*. Pana: Éditions du Seuil.

Brashers, D. E. (2001). "Communication and uncertainty management." *Journal of Communication*, 51, 477–97.

Brislin, R. (1993). *Understanding Culture's Influence on Behavior*. Orlando, FL: Harcourt Brace.

Brislin, R. and Yoshida, T. (eds) (1994). *Improving Intercultural Interactions: Modules for Cross-Cultural Training Programs*. Thousand Oaks, CA: Sage.

Brodie, M., Flournoy, R. E., Altman, D. E., Blendon, R. J., Benson, J. M. and Rosenbaum, M. D. (2000). "Health information, the Internet, and the digital divide." *Health Affairs*, 19, 255–65.

Brody, H. (1987). *Stories of Sickness*. New Haven: Yale University Press.

Bronner, Y. (1994). "Cultural sensitivity and nutrition counseling." *Topics in Clinical Nutrition*, 9, 13–19.

Brown, R. (1979). *Rockefeller Medicine Men: Medicine and Capitalism in America*. Berkeley, CA: University of California Press.

Burgess, D. J., Fu, S. S., and van Ryn, M. (2004). "Why do providers contribute to disparities and what can be done about it?" *Journal of General Internal Medicine*, 19, 1154–9.

Burke, A. W. (1976). "Attempted suicides among Asian immigrants in Birmingham." *The British Journal of Psychiatry*, 128, 528–33.

Butler, J. (1990). *Gender Trouble: Feminism and the Subversion of Identity*. New York: Routledge.

Campbell, C. and Gillies, P. (2001). "Conceptualizing 'social capital' for health promotion in small local communities: A micro-qualitative study." *Journal of Community and Applied Social Psychology*, 11, 329–46.

Campbell, C. and Jovchelovitch, S. (2000). "Health, community, and development: Towards a social psychology of participation." *Journal of Community and Applied Social Psychology*, 10, 255–70.

Campinha-Bacote, J. (1994). "Cultural competence in psychiatric mental health nursing: A conceptual model." *Nursing Clinics of North America*, 29, 1–8.

Carr, D. (1986). *Time, Narrative and History*. Bloomington: Indiana University Press.

Carrasquillo, O., Himmelstein, D., Woolhandler, S. and Bor, D. (1999). "Trends in health insurance coverage, 1989–1997." *International Journal of Health Services*, 29, 467–83.

Casey, D. (1994): "Depression in the elderly." *South Medical Journal*, 87 (5), 559–63.

Castro, F. G., Cota, M. K. and Vega, S. (1999). "Health promotion in Latino populations: Program planning, development, and evaluation." In R. M. Hough and M. V. Kline (eds), *Promoting Health in Multicultural Populations: A Handbook for Practitioners* (pp. 137–68). Thousand Oaks, CA: Sage.

Cegala, D. (1997). "A study of doctors' and patients' patterns of information exchange and relational communication during a primary care consultation: Implications for communication skills training." *Journal of Health Communication*, 2, 169–94.

Cegala, D. and Broz, S. (2003). "Provider and patient communication skills training." In T. L. Thompson, A. M. Dorsey, K. I. Miller, and R. Parrott (eds), *Handbook of Health Communication* (pp. 95–120). Mahwah, NJ: Lawrence Erlbaum.

Cegala, D., Coleman, M., and Warisse, J. (1998). "The development and partial test of the Medical Communication Competence Scale (MCCS)." *Journal of Health Communication*, 10, 261–88.

Cegala, D., Marinelli, T., and Post, D. (2000). "The effect of patient communication skills training on treatment compliance in primary care." *Archives of Family Medicine*, 9, 57–64.

Cegala, D. J., Post, D. M., and McClure, L. (2001). "The effects of patient communication skills training on the discourse of elderly patients during a primary care interview." *Journal of the American Geriatrics Society*, 49, 1505–11.

Cegala, D., McClure, L., Marinelli, T., and Post, D. (2000). "The effects of communication skills training on patients' participation during medical interviews." *Patient Education and Counseling*, 41, 209–22.

Cegala, D., McNeilis, K., Socha McGee, D., and Jonas, A. (1995). "A study of doctors' and patients' perceptions of information processing and communication competence during the medical interview." *Health Communication*, 7, 179–203.

Centers for Disease Control and Prevention. (2001). *Protecting the Nation's Health in an Era of Globalization: CDC's Global Infectious Disease Strategy*. Atlanta, GA: US Department of Health and Human Services, Public Health Service, CDC.

Chamberlain, T. and Hall, C. (2001). *Realized Religion*. West Conshohocken, PA: Templeton Foundation Press.

Charmaz, K. (1991). *Good Days, Bad Days: The Self in Chronic Illness and Time*. Berkeley, CA: University of California Press.

Chattopadhyay, A. and McKaig, R. G. (2004). "Social development of commercial sex workers in India: An essential step in HIV/AIDS prevention." *AIDS Patient Care Studies*, 18, 159–68.

Cheney, G. (2000). "Interpreting interpretive research: Toward perspectivism without relativism." In S. R. Corman and M. S. Poole (eds), *Perspectives on Organizational Communication: Finding Common Ground* (pp. 17–45). New York: Guilford.

Chenoweth, D. (1994). "Positioning health to make an economic impact." In J. P. Opatz (ed.), *Economic Impact of Worksite Health Promotion* (pp. 33–49). Champaign, IL: Human Kinetics.

Chuengsatiansup, K. (2001). "Civil society and health: Broadening the alliance for Health Development." Paper prepared for the Ministry of Public Health, Thailand.

Clarkson, S. (1999). "The global–continental–national dynamic: Some hypotheses on comparative continentalism." In S. Nagel (ed.), *Global Public Policy: Among and Within Nations*. New York: St. Martin's.

Coleman, J. S. (1988). "Social capital in the creation of human capital." *American Journal of Sociology*, 94 (Suppl.), 95–120.

Coleman, J. S. (1990). *Foundations of Social Theory*. Cambridge, MA: Harvard University Press.

Comaroff, J. (1982). "Medicine: Symbol and ideology." In P. Wright and A. Treacher (eds), *The Problem of Medical Knowledge* (pp. 49–68). Edinburgh: Edinburgh University Press.

Comaroff, J. (1985). *Body of Power, Spirit of Resistance: The Culture and History of a South African People*. Chicago: University of Chicago Press.

Comaroff, J. and Comaroff, J. (1991). *Of Revelation and Revolution*. Vol. 1: *Christianity, Colonialism, and Consciousness in South Africa*. Chicago: University of Chicago Press.

Comaroff, J. and Comaroff, J. (1992). *Ethnography and the Historical Imagination*. Boulder, CO: Westview Press.

Conquergood, D. (1982a). "Communication as performance: dramaturgical dimensions of everyday life." In J. I. Sisco (ed.), *The Jensin Lectures: Contemporary Communication Studies* (pp. 24–43). Tampa: University of South Florida Press.

Conquergood, D. (1982b). "Performing as a moral act: Ethical dimensions of the ethnography of performance." *Literature in Performance*, 5, 1–13.

Conquergood, D. (1988). "Health theater in a Hmong refugee camp." *The Drama Review*, 32, 174–208.

Conquergood, D. (1989). "Poetics, play, process, and power: The performative turn in anthropology." *Text and Performance Quarterly*, 9, 82–8.

Conquergood, D. (1991a). "Rethinking ethnography: Towards a critical cultural politics." *Communication Monographs*, 58, 179–94.

Constantelos, D. (1991b). "The interface of medicine and religion." In J. T. Chirban (ed.), *Health and Faith: Medical, Psychological and Religious Dimensions* (pp. 13–24). New York: University Press of America.

Das, V. (1989). "Subaltern as perspective." In R. Guha (ed.), *Subaltern Studies VI* (pp. 310–24). Delhi: Oxford University Press.

Das, V. (1993). "Moral orientations to suffering: Legitimation, power, and healing." In L. C. Chen, A. Kleinman and N. C. Ware (eds), *Health and Social Change in International Perspective*. Oxford: Oxford University Press.

Das, V. (1995). *Critical Events: An Anthropological Perspective on Contemporary India*. Delhi: Oxford University Press.

Das, V. (1997). "Language and body: Transactions in the construction of pain." In A. Kleinman, V. Das and M. Lock (eds), *Social Suffering* (pp. 67–91). Berkeley, CA: University of California Press.

Das, V. and Kleinman, A. (2000). "Introduction." In V. Das, A. Kleinman, M. Ramphele, and P. Reynolds (eds), *Violence and Subjectivity* (pp. 1–18). Berkeley, CA: University of California Press.

Das, V., Kleinman, A., Ramphele, M., and Reynolds, P. (2000). *Violence and Subjectivity*. Berkeley, CA: University of California Press.

Davenport Sypher, B., McKinley, M., Ventsam, S., and Valdeavellano, E. (2002). "Fostering reproductive health through entertainment–education in the Peruvian Amazon: The social construction of Bienvenida Salud!" *Communication Theory*, 12, 192–205.

Delia, J. 1987. "Commmunication research: A history". In: C. R. Berger and S. H. Chaffee, eds, *Handbook of Communication Science* (20–98). Beverly Hill, CA: Sage Publications.

Dennis, R. E. and Giangreco, M. F. (1996). "Creating conversation: Reflections of cultural sensitivity in family interviewing." *Exceptional Children*, 63, 103–16.

Dervin, B. (2005). "Libraries reaching out with health information to vulnerable populations: Guidance from research on information seeking and use." *Journal of Medical Library Association*, 93(S1), S64–S80.

DeSouza, R., Basu, A., Kim, I. Basnyat, I., and Dutta, M. (in press). "Who agreed to the neoliberal trade agreements? A discussion of the impact of 'fair trade' on the health of marginalized communities." In H. Zoller and M. Dutta (eds), *Emerging Perspectives in Health Communication: Interpretive, Critical, and Cultural Approaches*.

Dirlik, A. (1994). "The postcolonial aura: Third World criticism in the age of global capitalism." *Critical Inquiry*, 20, 328–56.

Dow, M., Verdi, M. and Sacco, W. (1991). "Training psychiatric patients to discuss medication issues: Effects on patient communication and knowledge of medications." *Behavior Modification*, 15, 3–21.

Dube, N. and Wilson, D. (1996). "Peer education programmes among HIV-vulnerable communities in southern Africa." In B.Williams and C. Campbell (eds), *HIV/AIDS in the South African Mining Industry*. Johannesburg, South Africa: ERU.

Dugdale, D. C., Epstein, R. and Pantilat, S. Z. (1999). "Time and the physician–patient relationship." *Journal of General Internal Medicine*, 14, 34–40.

Dutta, M. J. (2006). "Theoretical approaches to entertainment education campaigns: A subaltern critique." *Health Communication*, 20(3), 221–31.

Dutta, M. J. (2007). "Communicating about culture and health: Theorizing culture-centered and cultural sensitivity approaches." *Communication Theory*, 17, 304–28.

Dutta, M. J. and Basnyat, I. (in press). "The Radio Communication Project in Nepal: A critical analysis." *Health Education and Behavior*.

Dutta, M. J. and Basu, A. (2007). "Health among men in rural Bengal: Exploring meanings through a culture-centered approach." *Qualitative Health Research*, 17(1), 38–48.

Dutta, M. J. and Pal, M. (in press). "The Internet as a site of resistance: the case of the Narmada Bachao Andolan." In S. Duhe (ed.), *New Media and Public Relations*. New York: Peter Lang.

Dutta, M., Bodie, G. and Basu, A. (in press). "Health disparity and the racial divide among the nation's youth: Internet as a site for change." In A. Everett (ed.), *The MacArthur Series on Digital Media and Learning: Race and Ethnicity*. Boston, MA: MIT.

Dutta-Bergman, M. J. (2004a). "The unheard voices of Santalis: Communicating about health from the margins of India." *Communication Theory*, 14, 237–63.

Dutta-Bergman, M. J. (2004b). "Poverty, structural barriers and health: A Santali narrative of health communication." *Qualitative Health Research*, 14, 1–16.

Dutta-Bergman, M. J. (2004c). "Primary sources of health information: Comparison in the domain of health attitudes, health cognitions, and health behaviors." *Health Communication*, 16, 273–88.

Dutta-Bergman, M. (2004d). "Demographic and psychographic antecedents of community participation: Applying a social marketing model." *Social Marketing Quarterly*, 9, 17–31.

Dutta-Bergman, M. J. (2004e). "The impact of completeness and Web use motivation on the credibility of e-Health information." *Journal of Communication*, 54, 253–69.

Dutta-Bergman, M. J. (2004f). "Health attitudes, health cognitions and health behaviors among Internet health information seekers: Population-based survey." *Journal of Medical Internet Research*, 6, e15. Retrieved June 2, 2004, from http://www.jmir.org/2004/2/e15/index.htm.

Dutta-Bergman, M. J. (2004g). "A descriptive narrative of healthy eating: A social marketing approach using psychographics." *Health Marketing Quarterly*, 20, 81–101.

Dutta-Bergman, M. J. (2005a). "Theory and practice in health communication campaigns: A critical interrogation." *Health Communication*, 18(2), 103–22.

Dutta-Bergman, M. J. (2005b). "Access to the internet in the context of community participation and community satisfaction." *New Media and Society*, 17, 89–109.

Dutta-Bergman, M. J. (2006). "Media use theory and Internet use for health care." In M. Murero and R. E. Rice (eds), *The Internet and Health Care: Theory, Research, and Practice* (pp. 83–103). Mahwah, NJ: Lawrence Erlbaum.

Dutta-Bergman, M. J. and Doyle, K. (2001). "Money and meaning in India and Great Britain." *American Behavioral Scientist*, 45, 205–22.

Erwin, D. (1987). "The military medicalization of cancer treatment." In H. Baer (ed.), *Encounters with Biomedicine: Case Studies in Medical Anthropology* (pp. 201–227). New York, NY: Gordon and Breach.

Escobar, A. (1995). *Encountering Development: The Making and Unmaking of the Third World.* Princeton, NJ: Princeton University Press.

Estes, C. L. (1999). "Critical gerontology and the new political economy of aging." In M. Minkler and C. L. Estes (eds), *Critical Gerontology: Perspectives from Political and Moral Economy.* Amityville, NY: Baywood, pp. 17–35

Estes, C. L. and Binney, E. A. (1997). "The restructuring of home care." In Daniel M. Fox and Carol Raphael (eds), *Home Based Care For A New Century* (pp. 5–21). New York: Co-published Milbank Memorial Fund and Blackwell.

Fadiman, A. (1998). *The Spirit Catches You and You Fall Down.* New York: Farrar, Straus and Giroux.

Fair, J. E. (1989). "29 years of theory and research on media and development: The dominant paradigm impact." *Gazette*, 44, 129–50.

Fair, J. E. and Shah, H. (1997). "Continuities and discontinuities in communication and development research since 1958." *Journal of International Communication*, 4(2), 3–22.

Farmer, P. (1988a). "Bad blood, spoiled milk: Bodily fluids as moral barometers in rural Haiti." *American Ethnologist*, 15, 131–51.

Farmer, P. (1988b). "Blood, sweat, and baseballs: Haiti in the West Atlantic system." *Dialectical Anthropology*, 13, 83–99.

Farmer, P. (1992). *AIDS and Accusation: Haiti and the Geography of Blame.* Berkeley, CA: University of California Press.

Farmer, P. (1994). *The Uses of Haiti.* Monroe, Maine: Common Courage Press.

Farmer, P. (1996). "On suffering and structural violence: A view from below." *Daedalus*, 125, 261–83.

Farmer, P. (1999). *Infections and Inequalities: The Modern Plagues.* Berkeley, CA: University of California Press.

Farmer, P. (2003). *Pathologies of Power: Health, Human Rights, and the New War on the Poor.* Berkeley, CA: University of California Press.

Farmer, P. and Bertrand, D. (2000). "Hypocrisies of development and the health of the Haitian poor." In J. Kim, J. Millen, A. Irwin and J. Gershman (eds), *Dying for Growth: Global Inequality and the Health of the Poor* (pp. 65–89). Monroe, Maine: Common Courage Press.

Fawcett, S. B., Paine, A. L., Francisco, V. T., and Vliet, M. (1993). "Promoting health through community development." In D. Glenwick and L. A. Jason (eds), *Promoting Health and Mental Health in Children, Youth, and Families.* New York: Springer Publishing.

Fawcett, S. B., Paine, A. L., Francisco, V. T., Richter, K. P., Lewis, R. K., Williams, E. L., Harris, K. J., and Winter-Green, K. (1992). *Preventing Adolescent Substance Abuse: An Action Planning Guide for Community-Based Initiatives.* Lawrence, KS: Work Group on Health Promotion and Community Development, University of Kansas.

Feather, N. T. (1967). "Valence of outcome and expectation of success in relation to task difficulty and perceived locus of control." *Journal of Personality and Social Psychology*, 7, 372–86.

Ferguson, B. (1991). "Concepts, models and theories for immigrant health care." In B. Ferguson and E. Browne (eds), *Health Care and Immigrants: A Guide to the Helping Professions.* Sydney, Australia: MacLennan and Petty.

Ferrence, R. (2001). "Diffusion theory and drug use: Environmental factors." *Addiction*, 96, 165–73.

Finnegan, J., Bracht, N., and Viswanath, K. (1989). "Community power and leadership analysis in lifestyle campaigns." In C. Salmon (ed.), *Information Campaigns: Balancing Social Values and Social Change* (pp. 54–83). Newbury Park, CA: Sage.

Fishbein, M. and Ajzen, I. (1975). *Belief, Attitude, Intention, and Behavior: An Introduction to Theory and Research*. Reading, MA: Addison-Wesley.

Flowers, P., Duncan, B., and Frankis, J. (2000). "Community, responsibility and culpability: HIV-risk management among Scottish gay men." *Journal of Community and Applied Social Psychology*, 10, 285–300.

Food First (2005). "Democratizing market." Retrieved April 12, 2006, from http://www. foodfirst.org/programs.

Food Research Action Center (2005). "Health consequences of hunger." Retrieved April 12, 2006, from http://www.frac.org/html/hunger_in_the_us/health.html.

Ford, L. A. and Yep, G. A. (2003). "Working along the margins: Developing community-based strategies for communicating about health with marginalized groups." In T. Thompson, A. Dorsey, K. Miller, and R. Parrot (eds), *Handbook of Health Communication* (pp. 241–61). Hillsdale, NJ: Lawrence Erlbaum.

Foss, S. K. and Griffin, C. L. (1995). "Beyond persuasion: A proposal for an invitational rhetoric." *Communication Monographs*, 62, 2–18.

Foucault, M. (1972). *The Archaeology of Knowledge and the Discourse on Language*. New York: Pantheon.

Foucault, M. (1988). *The History of Sexuality, III: The Care of the Self*, tr. R. Hurley. New York: Vintage Books.

Foucault, M. (1995). *Discipline and Punish: The Birth of the Prison*. New York: Vintage Books.

Frank, A. (1991). *At the Will of the Body: Reflections on Illness*. Boston: Houghton Mifflin.

Frank, A. (1995). *The Wounded Storyteller: Body, Illness, and Ethics*. Chicago: University of Chicago.

Freidson, E. (1961). *Patients' Views of Medical Practice*. New York: Russell Sage Foundation.

Freidson, E. (1970). *Profession of Medicine: A Study of the Sociology of Applied Knowledge*. New York: Dodd, Mead, and Co.

Freire, P. (1970). *Pedagogy of the Oppressed*. New York: Seabury.

Freire, P. (1973). *Education for Critical Consciousness*. New York: Continuum.

French, B. N., Kurczynski, T. W., Weaver, M. T., and Pituch, M. J. (1992). "Evaluation of the health belief model and decision making regarding amniocentesis in women of advanced maternal age." *Health Education and Behavior*, 19, 177–86.

Freudenberg, N., Rogers, M., Ritas, C., and Nerney, M. (2005). "Policy analysis and advocacy: An approach to community-based participatory research." In B. Israel, E. Eng, A. Schulz, and E. Parker (eds), *Methods in Community-Based Participatory Research for Health* (pp. 349–370). San Francisco, CA: Jossey-Bass.

Garro, L. (1992). "Chronic illness and the construction of illness." In M. J. Good, P. Brodwin, B. Good, and A. Kleinman (eds), *Pain as Human Experience* (pp. 100–37). Berkeley, CA: University of California Press.

Garro, L. C. (2000). "Cultural knowledge as resource in illness narratives: Remembering through accounts of illness." In C. Mattimgly and L. C. Garro (eds), *Narrative and the Cultural Construction of Illness and Healing* (pp. 70–87). Berkeley, CA: University of California Press.

Garro, L. C. and Mattingly, C. (2000). "Narrative as construct and construction." In C. Mattingly and L. C. Garro (eds), *Narrative and the Cultural Construction of Illness and Healing* (pp. 1–49). Berkeley, CA: University of California Press.

Geertz, C. (1973). "Thick description: Toward an interpretive theory of culture." In C. Geertz (ed.), *The Interpretation of Cultures*. London: Hutchinson.

Geist-Martin, P., Horsley, K., and Farrell, A. (2003). "Working well: Communicating individual and collective wellness initiatives." In T. Thompson, A. Dorsey, K. Miller, and R. Parrot (eds), *Handbook of Health Communication* (pp. 423–43). Hillsdale, NJ: Lawrence Erlbaum.

Geist-Martin, P., Ray, E. B., and Sharf, B. F. (2003). *Communicating Health: Personal, Social and Political Complexities*. Wadsworth Publishing Co: Belmont, CA.

Gershman, J. and Irwin, A. (2000). "Getting a grip on the global economy." In J. Kim, J. Millen, A. Irwin, and J. Gershman (eds), *Dying for Growth: Global Inequality and the Health of the Poor* (pp. 11–43). Monroe, Maine: Common Courage Press.

Giddens, A. (1984). *The Constitution of Society*. Berkeley, CA: University of California Press.

Giddens, A. (1986). *The Constitution of Society: Outline of the Theory of Structuration*. Berkeley, CA: University of California Press.

Giddens, A. (1989). "A reply to my critics". In D. Held and J. B. Thompson (eds), *Social Theory of Modern Societies: Anthony Giddens and His Critics*. Cambridge: Cambridge University Press.

Giddens, A. (1990). "Structuration theory and sociological analysis." In J. Clark, C. Modgil, and S. Modgil (eds), *Anthony Giddens: Consensus and Controversy* (pp. 297–315). London, UK: The Falmer Press.

Giddens, A. (1991). *Modernity and Self-Identity: Self and society in the late modern age*. Cambridge: Polity.

Giddens, A. (2004). *The Progressive Manifesto: New Ideas for the Centre-Left*. Cambridge: Polity.

Gillam, S. J. (1991). "Understanding the uptake of cervical cancer screening: The contribution of the health belief model". *British Journal of General Practice*, 41, 510–3.

Gonsalez, C. (2002). "Institutionalizing inequality: The WTO agreement on agriculture, food security, and developing countries." *Columbia Journal of Environmental Law*, 27(433).

Good, B. (1994). *Medicine, Rationality, and Experience: An Anthropological Perspective*. Cambridge: Cambridge University Press.

Goold, S. D. and Lipkin, M. (1999). "The doctor–patient relationship: Challenges, opportunities, and strategies." *Journal of General Internal Medicine*, 14, S26–33.

Gordon, R. (1988). "Tenacious assumptions in Western medicine." In M. Lock and D. Gordon (eds), *Biomedicine Examined* (pp. 11–56). Dordrecht and Boston: Kluwer Academic Publishers.

Gramsci, A. (2003). *The Antonio Gramsci Reader: Selected Writings, 1916–1935*. New York: The New York University Press.

Gronemeyer, M. (1993). "Helping." In Wolfgang Sachs (ed.), *The Development Dictionary: A Guide to Knowledge as Power*. London: Zed Books, pp. 51–69.

Gropper, R. C. (1996). *Culture and the Clinical Encounter: An Intercultural Sensitizer for the Health Professions*. Yarmouth, ME: Intercultural Press.

Guha, R. (ed.) (1982). *Subaltern Studies I*. Delhi: Oxford University Press.

Guha, R. (1988). "The prose of counter-insurgency." In R. Guha and G. Spivak (eds), *Subaltern Studies* (pp. 37–44). Delhi, India: Oxford University Press.

Guha, R. and Spivak, G. (eds). (1988). *Selected Subaltern Studies*. New Delhi, India: Oxford University Press.

Haffner, S. M., Hazuda, H. P., Mitchell, B. D., Patterson, J. K., and Stern, M. P. (1991). "Increased incidence of type II diabetes mellitus in Mexican Americans." *Diabetes Care*, 14, 102–8.

Hahn, R. (1983). "Biomedical practice and anthropological theory: Frameworks and directions." *Annual Review of Anthropology*, 12, 305–33.

Hahn, R. A. (1995). *Sickness and Healing: An Anthropological Perspective*. New Haven: Yale University Press.

Hahn, R. (1999). *Anthropology in Public Health: Bridging Differences in Culture and Society*. Oxford: Oxford University Press.

Hahn, B. and Flood, A. B. (1995). No insurance, public insurance, and private insurance – do these options contribute to differences in general health? *Journal of Health Care for the Poor and Underserved*, 69(1), 41–59.

Hamelink, C. J. (1994). *The Politics of World Communication*. Thousand Oaks, CA: Sage Publications.

Hammerschlag, C. (1988). *The Dancing Healers: A Doctor's Journey of Healing with Native Americans*. San Francisco: Harper.

Harris, J. S. (1994). "The health benefits of health promotion." In M. P. O'Donnell and J. S. Harris (eds), *Health Promotion in the Workplace*, 2nd edn, (pp. 3–40). Albany, NY: Delmar.

Harris, R. and Seid, M. (2004). *Globalization and Health in the New Millennium*. Boston, MA: Brill.

Harris, K. J., Ahluwalia, J. S., Okuyemi, K. S., Turner, J. R., Woods, M. N., Backinger, C. L., and Resnicow, K. (2001). "Addressing cultural sensitivity in a smoking cessation intervention: Development of the Kick It at Swope project." *Journal of Community Psychology*, 29, 447–58.

Harter, L., Kirby, E., Edwards, A., and McClanahan, A. (2005). "Time, technology and meritocracy: The disciplining of women's bodies in narrative constructions of age-related infertility." In L. Harter, P. Japp, and C. Beck (eds), *Narratives, Health and Healing: Communication Theory, Research, and Practice* (pp. 83–106). Mahwah, NJ: Lawrence Erlbaum.

Hawe, P. and Shiell, A. (2000). "Social capital and health promotion: A review." *Social Science and Medicine*, 51, 871–85.

Hayden, S. (1997). "Re-claiming bodies of knowledge: An exploration of the relationship between feminist theorizing and feminine style in the rhetoric of the Boston Women's Health Book Collective." *Western Journal of Communication*, 61, 127–163.

Haynes, D. E. and Prakash, G. (1992). *Contesting Power: Resistance and Everyday Social Relations in South Asia*. Berkeley, CA: University of California Press.

Hegel, G. W. F. (1991). *Elements of the Philosophy of Right*. Cambridge: Cambridge University Press.

Hellander, I., Moloo, J., Himmelstein, D. U., Woolhandler, S., and Wolfe, S. (1995). "The growing epidemic of uninsurance: new data on the health insurance coverage of Americans." *International Journal of Health Services*, 25(3), 377–92.

Helman, C. (1986). *Culture, Health and Illness*. Bristol: Wright.

Helman, C. (2001). *Culture, Health and Illness*. London: Arnold.

Hornik, R. and McAnany, E. (2001). "Theories and evidence: Mass media effects and fertility change." *Communication Theory*, 11(4), 454–71.

Huff, R. and Kline, M. (1999a). "Health promotion in the context of culture." In R. Huff and M. Kline (eds), *Promoting Health in Multicultural Populations: A Handbook for Practitioners* (pp. 3–22). Thousand Oaks, CA: Sage.

Huff, R. and Kline, M. (eds) (1999b). *Promoting Health in Multicultural Populations: A Handbook for Practitioners*. Thousand Oaks, CA: Sage.

Institute of Medicine (1997). *America's Vital Interest in Global Health: Protecting our People, Enhancing our Economy, and Advancing our International Interests*. Washington, DC: National Academy Press.

Institute of Medicine. (2002). *Unequal Treatment: Confronting Racial and Ethnic Disparities in Healthcare*. Washington, DC: National Academy Press.

Israel, B., Eng, E., Schulz, A., and Parker, E. (2005). *Methods in Community-Based Participatory Research for Health*. San Francisco, CA: Jossey-Bass.

Iyengar, B. K. S. (1996). *Light on the Yoga Sutras of Patanjali*. London: Thorsons.

Iyengar, B. K. S. (2005). *Light on Life*. London: Rodale.

Jackson, C. and Haynes, T. (1992). *Cultural Sensitivity: A Working Model*. Atlanta, GA: Southern Council for Collegiate Education in Nursing.

Jacobson, T. L. (2003). "Participatory communication for social change: The relevance of the theory of communicative action." In P. Kalbfleisch (ed.), *Communication Yearbook 27* (pp. 87–124). Mahwah, NJ: Erlbaum.

Jacobson, T. L. and Storey, J. D. (2004). "Development communication and participation: Applying Habermas to a case study of population programs in Nepal." *Communication Theory*, 14, 99–121.

Jana, S., Basu, I., Rotheram-Borus, M. J., and Newman, P. A. (2004) "The Sonagachi project: A sustainable community intervention program." *AIDS Education and Prevention*, 16(5), 405–14.

Jana, S., Bandyopadhyay, N., Mukherjee, S., Dutta, N., Basu, I., and Saha, A. (1998). "STD/HIV intervention with sex workers in West Bengal, India." *AIDS*, 12(Suppl. B), 101–8.

Janz, N. and Becker, M. (1984). "The health belief model: A decade later." *Health Education Quarterly*, 11, 1–47.

Jewson, N. (1976). "The disappearance of the sick man from medical cosmology, 1770–1870." *Medical Sociology*, 10, 225–44.

Johns Hopkins University/ Center for Communication Programs (JHU/CCP) (1998). *Design Document: Cut Your Coat According to Your Cloth*. Radio Drama Serial Phase III for the General Audience. NHEIC, NHTC, DHS/MH, JHU/CCP and USAID.

Kagawa-Singer, M. (2001). "From genes to social science: Impact of the simplistic interpretation of race, ethnicity, and culture on cancer outcome." *Cancer*, 91(S1), 226–32.

Kamins, M., Marks, L. J., and Skinner, D. (1991). "Television commercial evaluation in the context of mood: Congruency versus consistency effects." *Journal of Advertising*, 20(2), 1–14.

Kaplan, G. (1996). "People and places: Contrasting perspectives on the association between social class and health." *International Journal of Health Services*, 26, 507–19.

Kaplan, S. H., Greenfield, S., and Ware, J. E., Jr. (1989). "Assessing the effects of physician–patient interactions on the outcomes of chronic disease." *Medical Care*, 27(Suppl.), S110–S127.

Kawachi, I. and Kennedy, B. (1999). "Income inequality and health: Pathways and mechanisms." *Health Services Research*, 34, 215–27.

Kawachi, I., Kennedy, B., and Wilkinson, R. (1999). *The Society and Population Health Reader: Income Inequality and Health*. New York: The New Press.

Kawachi, I., Kennedy, B., Gupta, V., and Prothrow-Stith, D. (1999). "Women's status and the health of women and men: A view from the States." *Social Science and Medicine*, 48(1), 21–32.

Kawachi, I., Levine, S., Miller, S., Lasch, K., and Amick, B. (1994). *Income Inequality and Life Expectancy: Theory, Research, and Policy*. Boston: Health Institute, New England Medical Center.

Kennedy, B. (2001). "Community involvement at what cost? – Local appraisal of a pan-European nutrition promotion programme in low income neighborhoods." *Health Promotion International*, 16(1), 35–45.

Kennedy, B., Kawachi, I., and Prothrow-Stith, D. (1996). "Income distribution and mortality: Cross-sectional ecological study of the Robin Hood Index in the United States." *British Medical Journal*, 312, 1004–7.

Kim, J., Millen, J., Irwin, A., and Gershman, J. (2000). *Dying for Growth: Global Inequality and the Health of the Poor*. Monroe, Maine: Common Courage Press.

King, N. B. (2002). "Security, disease, commerce: Ideologies of postcolonial global health." *Social Studies of Science*, 32, 763–89.

Kleinman, A. (1973). "Medicine's symbolic reality." *Inquiry*, 16, 206–13.

Kleinman, A. (1974). "Cognitive structures of traditional medical systems." *Ethnomedicine*, 3, 27–49.

Kleinman, A. (1980). *Patients and Healers in the Context of Culture: An Exploration of the Borderland Anthropology, Medicine, and Psychiatry*. Berkeley, CA: University of California Press.

Kleinman, A. (1995). *Writing at the Margin*. Berkeley, CA: University of California Press.

Kleinman, A. (1997). *Writing at the Margin: Discourse between Anthropology and Medicine*. Berkeley, CA: University of California Press.

Kleinman, A. (2000). "The violence of everyday life: The multiple forms and dynamics of social violence." In V. Das, A. Kleinman, M. Ramphele, and P. Reynolds (eds), *Violence and Subjectivity* (pp. 26–241). Berkeley, CA: University of California Press.

Kleinman, A. and Kleinman, J. (1991). "Suffering and its professional transformation: Toward an ethnography of interpersonal experience." *Culture, Medicine, and Psychiatry*, 15, 275–301.

Kleinman, A. and Kleinman, J. (1994). "Cultural revolution. How bodies remember: Social memory and bodily experience of criticism, resistance, and delegitimation following China's cultural revolution." *New Literary History*, 25, 707–23.

Kleinman, A., Das, V. and Lock, M. (eds). (1997). *Social Suffering*. Berkeley, CA: University of California Press.

Klessig, J. (1992). "The effect of values and culture on life-support decisions." *Journal of Western Medicine*, 157, 316–22.

Kline, K. (2003). "Popular media and health: Images, effects, and institutions." In T. Thompson, A. Dorsey, K. Miller, and R. Parrot (eds), *Handbook of Health Communication* (pp. 557–82). Hillsdale, NJ: Lawrence Erlbaum.

Koller, J. M. and Koller, P. J. (1991). *A Sourcebook in Asian Philosophy*. Englewood Cliffs, NJ: Prentice Hall.

Korten, D. (1995). *When Corporations Ruled the World*. London: Earthscan.

Korten, D. (1999). *The Post-Corporate World*. San Francisco, CA: Kumarian.

Kotler, P., Roberto, N., and Lee, N. (2002). *Social Marketing: Improving the Quality of Life*. Thousand Oaks, CA: Sage.

Kreps, G. (2002). "Enhancing access to relevant health information." In R. Carveth, S. Klichmer, and D. Schuler (eds), *Shaping the Network Society: Patterns for Participation, Action and Change* (pp. 149–152). Palo Alto, CA: Computer Professional for Social Responsibility.

Kreps, G. (2003). "The impact of communication on cancer risk, incidence, morbidity, mortality, and quality of life." *Health Communication*, 15, 163–71.

Kreps, G. (2005a). "Disseminating relevant information to underserved audiences: Implications from the Digital Divide Projects." *Journal of the Medical Library Association*, 93, S68–S73.

Kreps, G. (2005b). "Narrowing the digital divide to overcome disparities in care." In E. B. Ray (ed.), *Health Communication in Practice: A Case Study Approach* (pp. 357–64). Mahwah, NJ: Lawrence Erlbaum.

Kreps, G. (2006). "Communication and racial inequalities in health care." *American Behavioral Scientist*, 49, 760–74.

Kumar, K. (1993). "Civil society: An inquiry into the usefulness of a historical term." *The British Journal of Sociology*, 44(3), 375–95.

Labonte, R. (2001). "Globalization and reform of the World Trade Organization." *Canadian Journal of Public Health*, 92(4), 248–9.

Labonte, R. and Torgerson, R. (2002). *Frameworks for Analyzing the Links between Globalization and Health*. Saskatoon: University of Saskatchewan.

Lammers, J. C., Barbour, J. B., and Duggan, A. P. (2003). "Organizational forms and the provision of healthcare." In T. Thompson, A. Dorsey, K. Miller and R. Parrot (eds), *Handbook of Health Communication* (pp. 319–45). Hillsdale, NJ: Lawrence Erlbaum.

Lefcourt, H. M. and Wine, J. (1969). "Internal versus external control of reinforcement and the deployment of attention in experimental situations." *Canadian Journal of Behavioral Science*, 1, 167–81.

Lefebvre, R. C. and Flora, J. A. (1988). "Social marketing and public health intervention." *Health Education Quarterly*, 15, 299–315.

Lerner, D. (1968). *The Passing of Traditional Society*. Glencoe, IL: Free Press.

Leslie, C. (1976). *Asian Medical Systems: A Comparative Study*. Berkeley, CA: University of California Press.

Leslie, C. and Young, A. (1992). *Paths to Asian Medical Knowledge*. Berkeley, CA: University of California Press.

Lochner, K. (1999). *State Income Inequality and Individual Mortality Risk: A Prospective Multilevel Study*. Harvard University: PhD Dissertation.

Locke, D. (1992). *Increasing Multicultural Understanding: A Comprehensive Model*. Newbury Park, CA: Sage.

Lopez, E., Eng, E., Robinson, N., and Wang, C. (2005). "Photovoice as a community-based participatory research method: A case study with African American breast cancer survivors in rural Eastern North Carolina." In B. Israel, E. Eng, A. Schulz, and E. Parker, *Methods in Community-Based Participatory Research for Health* (pp. 326–48). San Francisco, CA: Jossey-Bass.

Lorde, A. (1980). *The Cancer Journals*. Argyle, NY: Spinsters Ink.

Lupton, D. (1994). "Toward the development of a critical health communication praxis." *Health Communication*, 6(1), 55–67.

Lupton, D. (1995a). *Medicine as Culture*. Thousand Oaks, CA: Sage.

Lupton, D. (1995b). *The Imperative of Health: Public Health and the Regulated Body*. London: Sage.

Lupton, D. (2003). *Medicine as Culture*, 1st edn. Thousand Oaks, CA: Sage.

Lupton, D. (2006). *Medicine as Culture: Illness, Disease, and the Body in Western Science*, 2nd edn. Thousand Oaks, CA: Sage.

McMichael, A. J. and Beaglehole, R. (2000). "The changing global context of public health." *Lancet*, 356, 495–9.

McMichael, C. and Manderson, L. (2004). "Somali women and well-being: Social networks and social capital among immigrant women in Australia." *Human Organization*, 63, 88–99.

MacStravic, S. (2000). "Missing links in Social Marketing." *Journal of Health Communication*, 5, 255–63.

Mainous, A. G., III, Hueston, W. J., Love, M. M., and Griffith, C. H., III (1999). "Access to care for the uninsured: Is access to a physician enough?" *American Journal of Public Health*, 89, 910–12.

Mairs, N. (1993). *Ordinary Times: Cycles in Marriage, Faith, and Renewal*. Boston: Beacon Press.

Marcovich, A. (1988). "French colonial medicine and colonial rule: Algeria and Indochina." In R. Macleod and M. Lewis (eds), *Disease, Medicine, and Empire: Perspectives on Western Medicine and the Experience of European Expansion*. London and New York: Routledge, pp. 100–19.

Marcovich, M. and Manderson, L. (2002). "Crossing national boundaries: Social identity formation among recent immigrant women in Australia from former Yugoslavia. *Identity: An International Journal of Theory and Research*, 2(4): 303–16.

Markos, P. A. Allen, D. N. (2001). "A model of primary healthcare service delivery for individuals who are homeless." *Guidance and Counselling*, 16, 127–31.

Marmot, M. (2004) *Status Syndrome: How Your Social Standing Directly Affects Your Health and Life Expectancy*. London: Bloomsbury.

Marshall, A. A. and McKeon, J. K. (1996). "Reaching the 'unreachables': Educating and motivating women living in poverty." In E. B. Ray (ed.), *Communication and Disenfranchisement: Social Health Issues and Implications* (pp. 137–55). Mahwah, NJ: Lawrence Erlbaum Associates.

Martin, E. (1987). *The Woman in the Body: A Cultural Analysis of Reproduction*. Boston: Beacon Press.

Marx, K. (1975). *Early Writings*. London: Penguin Books.

Mattingly, C. and Garro, L. (eds) (2000). *Narrative and the Cultural Construction of Illness and Healing*. Berkeley, CA: University of California Press.

Mattson, M. (1999). "Toward a reconceptualization of cues to action in the Health Belief Model: HIV test counseling." *Communication Monographs*, 66, 240–65.

Mehmet, O. (1995). *Westernizing the Third World: The Eurocentricity of Economic Development Theories*. London: Routledge.

Melkote, S., Muppidi, S., and Goswami, D. (1995). "Social and economic factors in an integrated behavioral and societal approach to communications in HIV/AIDS." *Journal of Health Communication*, 5, 17–27.

Merzel, C. and D'Afflitti, J. (2003). "Reconsidering community-based health promotion: Promise, performance, and potential." *American Journal of Public Health*, 93(4), 557–74.

Millen, J. and Holtz, T. (2000). "Dying for growth, Part I: Transnational corporations and the health of the poor." In J. Kim, J. Millen, A. Irwin, and J. Gershman (eds), *Dying for Growth: Global Inequality and the Health of the Poor* (pp. 177–223). Monroe, Maine: Common Courage Press.

Millen, J., Irwin, A., and Kim, J. (2000). "Introduction: What is growing? Who is dying?" In J. Kim, J. Millen, A. Irwin, and J. Gershman (eds), *Dying for Growth: Global Inequality and the Health of the Poor* (pp. 3–10). Monroe, Maine: Common Courage Press.

Millen, J., Lyon, E., and Irwin, A. (2000). "Dying for growth, Part II: The political influence of national and transnational corporations. In J. Kim, J. Millen, A. Irwin, and J. Gershman (eds), *Dying for Growth: Global Inequality and the Health of the Poor* (pp. 225–44). Monroe, Maine: Common Courage Press.

Miller, E. and Kehler, R. (1996). "Mischievous myths about money in politics." *Dollars and Sense*, July/August, 22–7.

Minkler, M. and Wallerstein, N. (eds) (2003). *Community-Based Participatory Research for Health*. San Francisco, CA: Josey-Bass.

Mitchell, M. (2001). "Risk, threat, and information seeking about genital herpes: The effects of mood and message framing." *Communication Studies*, 52, 141–52.

Mittelmark, M. B. (2001). "Promoting social responsibility for health: Health impact assessment and healthy public policy at the community level." *Health Promotion International*, 16, 269–74.

Mokros, H. B. and Deetz, S. (1996). "What counts as real? A constitutive view of communication and the disenfranchised in the context of health." In E. B. Ray (ed.), *Communication and Disenfranchisement: Social Issues and Implications* (pp. 29–44). Mahwah, NJ: Lawrence Erlbaum.

Mony, T., Salan, E., Youthy, E., Piseth, E. S., and Brown, E. (1999). *Crossing Borders, Crossing Realities: The Vulnerability of Vietnamese Sexworkers in Cambodia*. Kuala Lumpur, Malaysia: CARAM Cambodia.

Morgan, John D. 2002. "Dying and grieving are journeys of the spirit." In R. B. Gilbert (ed.), *Health Care and Spirituality: Listening, Assessing, and Caring*. Amityville, NY: Baywood.

Mudimbe, V. Y. (1988). *The Invention of Africa: Gnosis, Philosophy, and the Order of Knowledge*. Bloomington, IN: Indiana University Press.

Muhiuddin, H. and Kreps, G. (2004). "Forty years of diffusion of innovations: Utility and value in public health." *Journal of Health Communication*, 9, 3–11.

Murray-Johnson, L. and Witte, K. (2003). "Looking toward the future: Health message design strategies." In T. L. Thompson, A. M. Dorsey, K. I. Miller, and R. Parrott (eds), *Handbook of Health Communication* (pp. 473–96). Mahwah, NJ: Lawrence Erlbaum Associates.

Musick, K. (1997). "The politics of implants for breast cancer survivors: Feminist issues for counsel and action." *Women and Therapy*, 20, 39–50.

"Naco: Facts and figures" (2003). National AIDS Control Organization. Retrieved March 8, 2005, from http://www.nacoonline.org/facts_hivestimates.htm.

Naditch, M. P., Gargan, M. A., Michael, L. B. (1975). "Denial, anxiety, locus of control, and the discrepancy between aspirations and achievements as components of depression." *Journal of Abnormal Psychology*, 84, 1–9.

Nandy, A. (ed.) (1996). *Science, Hegemony, and Violence*. New Delhi, India: Oxford University Press.

Narayan, D. and Petesch, P. (2002). *Voices of the Poor: From Many Lands*. Washington, DC: The World Bank.

Narayan, D., Patel, R., Schafft, K., Rademacher, A., and Koch-Schulte, S. (2000). *Voices of the Poor: Can Anyone Hear Us?* Washington, DC: The World Bank.

Nelson, G. (1982). "Social class and public policy for the elderly." *Social Science Review*, 56, 85–107.

Newman, P. A. (2003). "Reflections on Sonagachi: An empowerment-based HIV-preventive intervention for female sex workers in West Bengal, India." *Women's Studies Quarterly*, 31(1/2), 1–2.

Nichter, M. and Nichter, M. (1996). *Anthropology and International Health: Asian Case Studies*. New York: Gordon and Breach Publishers.

Nir, Z. and Neumann, L. (1991). "Self-esteem and internal locus of control, and their relationship to weight reduction." *Journal of Clinical Perspectives*, 47, 568–75.

Noah, D. and Fidas, G. (2000, January). *The Global Infectious Disease Threat and its Implications for the United States*. Washington, DC: US Department of State and National Security Council, National Intelligence Council.

O'Hanlon, R. (2000). "Recovering the subject: Subaltern studies and histories of resistance in colonial South Asia." In V. Chaturvedi (ed.), *Mapping Subaltern Studies and the Postcolonial* (pp. 72–115). London: Verso.

Oldenburg, B. F., Hardcastle, D., and Kok, G. (1997). "Diffusion of health education and health promotion innovations." In K. Glanz, B. F. Lewis, and B. Rimer (eds), *Health Behaviour and Health Education: Theory, Research and Practice* (2nd edn, pp. 270–86), Jossey-Bass, San Francisco, CA: Jossey-Bass.

Pandey, G. (1991). "In defense of the fragment: Writing about Hindu–Muslim riots in India today." *Economic and Political Weekly*, 26, 559–72.

Pandey, G. (2000). "Voices from the edge: The struggle to write subaltern histories." In V. Chaturvedi (ed.), *Mapping Subaltern Studies and the Postcolonial* (pp. 281–99). London: Verso.

Papa, M. J., Singhal, A., and Papa, W. H. (2006). *Organizing for Social Change*. New Delhi: Sage Publications.

Papa, M., Singhal, A., Law, S., Pant, S., Sood, S., Rogers, E., and Shefner-Rogers, C. (2000). "Entertainment–education and social change: An analysis of parasocial interaction, social learning, collective efficacy, and paradoxical communication." *Journal of Communication*, 50, 31–55.

Parker, R. and Kreps, G. L. (2005). "Library outreach: Overcoming health literacy challenges." *Journal of the Medical Library Association*, 93(S1), S81–S85.

Paul, J. (1978). "Medicine and imperialism." In J. Ehrenreich (ed.), *The Cultural Crisis of Modern Medicine* (pp. 271–86). Madison, NJ: Fairleigh Dickinson University Press.

Pavalko, R. M. (1988). *Sociology of Occupations and Professions*. Itasca, IL: F. E. Peacock Publishers.

Payer, L. (1988). *Medicine and Culture: Varieties of Treatment in the United States, England, West Germany and France*. New York: H. Holt.

Pérez-Stable, E. J., Sabogal, F., Otero-Sabogal, R., Hiatt, R. A., and McPhee, S. J. (1992, Dec. 9). "Misconceptions about cancer among Latinos and Anglos." *JAMA*, 268(22), 3219–23.

Perloff, R. (2006). "Introduction: Communication and health care disparities." *American Behavioral Scientist*, 49, 755–9.

Person, B. and Cotton, D. (1996). "A model for community mobilization for the prevention of HIV in women and infants." *Public Health Reports*, 3(1), 89–98.

Petersen, A. and Lupton, D. (1996). *The New Public Health*. New Delhi, India: Sage Publications.

Pilkington, P. (2002). "Social capital and health: Measuring and understanding social capital at a local level could help to tackle health inequalities more effectively." *Journal of Public Health Medicine*, 24, 156–9.

Piotrow, P., Kincaid, D., Rimon, J. and Rinehart, W. (1997). *Health Communication Lessons from Family Planning and Reproductive Health*. Westport, CT: Praeger.

Porkert, M. (1976). "The intellectual and social impulses behind the evolution of traditional Chinese medicine." In C. Leslie (ed.), *Asian Medical Systems: A Comparative Study* (pp. 63–81). Berkeley, CA: University of California Press.

Prakash, G. (1992). "Postcolonial criticism and Indian historiography." *Social Text*, 31, 8–19.

Prakash, G. (2000). "Can the subaltern ride? A reply to O'Hanlon and Washbrook." In V. Chaturvedi (ed.), *Mapping Subaltern Studies and the Postcolonial* (pp. 220–38). London: Verso.

Putnam, R. (1993). *Making Democracy Work*. Princeton, NJ: Princeton University Press.

Putnam, R. (1995). "Bowling alone: America's declining social capital." *Journal of Democracy*, 6, 65–78.

The Quran (1880). Translated by E. H. Palmer, Oxford: The Clarendon Press.

Ramirez, A., Villarreal, R., and Chalela, P. (1999). "Community-level diabetes control in a Texas barrio: A case study." In R. M. Huff and M. V. Kline (eds), *Promoting Health in Multicultural Populations: A Handbook for Practitioners* (p. 554). Thousand Oaks, CA: Sage Publication.

Ramirez, A., Villarreal, R., Suarez, L., and Flores, E.T. (1995). "The emerging Hispanic population: A foundation for cancer prevention and control." *Journal of National Cancer Institute Monographs*, 18, 1–9.

Rappaport, J. (1987). "Terms of empowerment/exemplars of prevention: Toward a theory of community psychology." *American Journal of Community Psychology*, 15, 121–48.

Rawlins, W. K. (2005). "Our Family's Physician." In Lynn Harter, Phyllis Japp, and Christina Beck (eds), *Narratives, Health, and Healing: Communication Theory, Research, and Practice*. Mahwah, NJ: Lawrence Erlbaum Associates, pp. 197–216.

Reese, William. L. 1980. *Dictionary of Philosophy and Religion: Eastern and Western Thought*. Atlantic Highlands, NJ: Humanities Press.

Regush, N. (1992). "Toxic breasts." *Mother Jones*, Jan/Feb, 26–31.

Repucci, N. D., Woolard, J. L., and Fried, C. S. (1999). "Social, community, and preventive interventions." *Annual Review of Psychology*, 50, 387–418.

Resnicow, K., Braithwaite, R. L., Dilorio, C., and Glanz, K. (2002). "Applying theory to culturally diverse and unique populations." In K. Glanz, B. K. Rimer, and F. M. Lewis (eds), *Health Behavior and Health Education: Theory, Research, and Practice* (3rd edn, pp. 485–509). San Francisco, CA: Jossey-Bass.

Rimal, R., Lapinski, M., Cook, R., and Real, K. (2005). "Toward a theory of normative influences: How perceived benefits and similarity moderate the impact of descriptive norms on behaviors." *Journal of Health Communication*, 10, 433–50.

Robinson, E. J. and Whitfield, M. J. (1985). "Improving the efficiency of patients' comprehension monitoring: A way of increasing patients' participation in general practice consultations." *Social Science and Medicine*, 21, 915–19.

Robinson, K. L. and Elliott, S. J. (1999). "Community development approaches to heart health promotion: A geographical perspective." *Professional Geographer*, 51, 283–95.

Rogers, E. M. (1995). *Diffusion of Innovations*. New York: Free Press.

Rogers, E. M. (2000). "Introduction." *Journal of Health Communication*, 5(1), 1–3.

Rogers, E. M. and Kincaid, D. L. (1981). *Communication Networks: Toward a New Paradigm for Research*. New York: Free Press.

Rogers, E. M. and Storey, D. (1987). "Communication campaigns." In C. Berger and S. Chaffee (eds), *Handbook of Communication Science*, pp. 817–46. Newbury Park, CA: Sage.

Rosenberg, C. (1962). *The Cholera Years*. Chicago: University of Chicago Press.

Rosenberg, C. (1988). "Disease and social order in America: Perceptions and expectations." In E. Fee and D. Fox (eds), *AIDS: The Burdens of History* (pp. 12–32). Berkeley, CA: University of California Press.

Rosenstock, I. M. (1966). "Why people use health services." *Milbank Memorial Fund Quarterly*, 44, 94–124.

Rosenstock, I. M. (1974). "Historical origins of the health belief model." *Health Education Monographs*, 2, 328–35.

Rost, K. M., Flavin, K. S., Cole, K., and McGill, J. B. (1991). "Change in metabolic control and functional status after hospitalization: Impact of patient activation intervention in diabetic patients." *Diabetes Care*, 14, 881–9.

Roter, D. L. (1977). "Patient question-asking in physician patient interaction." *Health Psychology*, 3, 395–409.

Rotter, J. (1966). "Generalized expectancies for internal versus external control of reinforcement." *Psychological Monographs*, 80, 1–28.

Rotter, J. (1975). "Some problems and misconceptions related to the construct of internal versus external control of reinforcement." *Journal of Consulting and Clinical Psychology*, 43, 56–67.

Rudy, K. (1997). "Ethics, reproduction, utopia: Gender and childbearing in women on the edge of time and the left hand of darkness." *NSWA Journal*, 9, 22–39.

Said, E. (1978). *Orientalism*. New York: Vintage Books.

Salmon, C. T. and Atkin, C. (2003). "Using media campaigns for health promotion." In T. L. Thompson, A. M. Dorsey, K. I. Miller, and R. Parrott (eds), *Handbook of Health Communication* (pp. 449–72). Mahwah, NJ: Lawrence Erlbaum Associates.

Sandler, I. and Lakey, B. (1982). "Locus of control as a stress moderator: The role of control perceptions and social support." *American Journal of Community Psychology*, 10, 65–80.

Sarkar, S., Durnadin, F., Jana, S., Hassan, R., Hoque, E., Quddus, M. A. (1997). "A community-based survey of commercial sex workers in a brothel of Bangladesh on knowledge, intent, trial, and practice for use of condoms." Paper presented at the Sixth Annual Scientific Conference, Dhaka, Bangladesh.

Schaef, A. (1981). *Women's Reality*. Minneapolis, MN: Winston Press.

Schafer, R. (1981). "Narration in the psychoanalytic dialogue." In W. Mitchell (ed.), *On Narrative*. Chicago: University of Chicago Press.

Schafer, R. (1992). *Retelling a Life: Narration and Dialogue in Psychoanalysis*. New York: Basic Books.

Schank, R. C. (1990). *Tell Me a Story: A New Look at Real and Artificial Memory*. New York: Scribner.

Scheper-Hughes, N. (1992). *Death without Weeping: The Violence of Everyday Life in Brazil*. Berkeley, CA: University of California Press.

Scheufele, D. A. and Shah, D. V. (2000). "Personality strength and social capital: The role of dispositional and informational variables in the production of civic participation." *Communication Research*, 27, 107–31.

Seaman, G. (1992). "Winds, waters, seeds, and souls: Folk concepts of physiology and etiology in Chinese geomancy." In C. Leslie and A. Young (eds), *Paths to Asian Medical Knowledge* (pp. 74–97). Berkeley, CA: University of California Press.

Sen, A. (1999). *Development as Freedom*. New York: Anchor Books.

Shain, M. and Groenveld, J. (1980). *Employee-Assistance Programs: Philosophy, Theory, and Practice*. Lexington, MA: Lexington Books.

Shakow, A. and Irwin, A. (2000). "Terms reconsidered: Decoding development discourse." In J. Kim, J. Millen, A. Irwin, and J. Gershman (2000), *Dying for Growth: Global Inequality and the Health of the Poor* (pp. 44–61). Monroe, Maine: Common Courage Press.

Shapiro, M. (1988). *The Politics of Representation: Writing Practices in Biography, Photography, and Policy Analysis*. Madison, WI: University of Wisconsin Press.

Shapiro, S., MacInnis, D. and Park, C. W. (2002). "Understanding program-induced mood effects: Decoupling arousal from valence." *Journal of Advertising*, 31(4), 15–26.

Sharf, B. (2005). "How I fired my surgeon and embraced an alternate narrative." In L. Harter, P. Japp and C. Beck (eds), *Narratives, Health and Healing: Communication Theory, Research, and Practice* (pp. 325–42). Mahwah, NJ: Lawrence Erlbaum.

Sharf, B. and Kahler, J. (1996). "Victims of the franchise: A culturally-sensitive model of teaching patient–doctor communication in the inner city." In E. B. Ray (ed.), *Communication and Disenfranchisement: Social Health Issues and Implications* (pp. 95–115). Mahwah, NJ: Lawrence Erlbaum.

Sharf, B., Geist-Martin, P. and Ray, E. B. (2003). *Communicating Health: Personal, Cultural, and Political Complexities*. Belmont, CA: Wadsworth.

Shavers, V. L. and Brown, M. L. (2002). "Racial and ethnic disparities in the receipt of cancer treatment." *Journal of the National Cancer Institute*, 94, 334–57.

Shilling, C. (1993). *The Body and Social Theory*. London: Sage.

Shiva, V. (1988). "Reductionist science as epistemic violence." In A. Nandy (ed.), *Science, Hegemony, and Violence*. New Delhi, India: Oxford University Press.

Short, P. F. and Lair, T. J. (1994). Health insurance and health status: Implications for financing health care reform." *Inquiry*, 31, 425–37.

Silberman, I. (2005). "Religion as a meaning system: Implications for the new millennium." *Journal of Social Issues*, 61, 641–63.

Silverman, J. (1967). "Shamanism and acute schizophrenia." *American Anthropologist*, 69, 21–31.

Singer, M. (1989). "The coming of age of critical medical anthropology." *Social Science and Medicine*, 30, 179–87.

Singer, M. and Baer, H. (1995). *Critical Medical Anthropology*. Amityville, NY: Baywood Press.

Singhal, A. and Brown, W. J. (1996). "The entertainment–education communication strategy: Past struggles, present status, future agenda." *Jurnal Komunikasi*, 12, 19–36.

Singhal, A. and Rogers, E. (1999). *Entertainment–Education: A Communication Strategy for Social Change*. Mahwah, NJ: Lawrence Erlbaum Associates.

Singhal, A. and Rogers, E. (2002). "A theoretical agenda for entertainment–education." *Communication Theory*, 12, 117–35.

Singhal, A., Rogers, E. and Brown, W. (1993). "Harnessing the potential of entertainment–education telenovelas." *Gazette*, 51, 1–18.

Slater, M. (1996). "Theory and method in health audience segmentation." *Journal of Health Communication*, 1, 267–83.

Slater, M. (1999). "Integrating application of media effects, persuasion, and behavior change theories to communication campaigns: A stages-of-change framework." *Health Communication*, 11, 335–54.

Socha McGee, D. and Cegala, D. J. (1998). "Patient communication skills training for improved communication competence in the primary care medical consultation." *Journal of Applied Communication Research*, 26, 412–30.

Soffa, V. (1994). *The Journey Beyond Breast Cancer, from the Personal to the Political*. Rochester, VT: Healing Arts Press.

Sonnenstuhl, W. J. and Trice, H. M. (1986). *Strategies for Employee Assistance Programs: The Crucial Balance*. Ithaca, NY: ILR Press.

Sontag, S. (1977). *Illness as Metaphor*. New York: Vintage.

Sontag, S. (1988). *AIDS and its Metaphors*. New York: Farrar Straus Giroux.

Spence, D. (1982). *Narrative Truth and Historical Truth: Meaning and Interpretation in Psychoanalysis*. New York: Norton.

Spivak, G. (1988). "Can the subaltern speak?" In G. Nelson and L. Grossberg (eds), *Marxism and the Interpretation of Culture* (pp. 271–313). Urbana: University of Illinois Press.

Spivak, G. (1990). *The Post-Colonial Critic: Interviews, Strategies and Dialogues*. New York: Routledge.

Spivak, G. (2000). "The new subaltern: A silent interview." In V. Chaturvedi (ed.), *Mapping Subaltern Studies and the Postcolonial* (pp. 324–340). London: Verso.

Stark, R. (1971). "Psychopathology and religious commitment." *Review of Religious Research*, 12: 165–76

Starr, P. (1982). *The Social Transformation of American Medicine*. New York, NY: Basic Books.

Stein, H. (1990). *American Medicine as Culture*. Boulder, CO: Westview Press.

Stephens, K., Rimal, R., and Flora, J. (2004). "Expanding the reach of health campaigns: community organizations as eta-channels for the dissemination of health information." *Journal of Health Communication*, 9, 97–111.

Stewart, M. (1984). "What is a successful doctor–patient interview? A study of interactions and outcomes." *Social Science and Medicine*, 19, 167–75.

Stewart, D. E. and Streiner, D. L. (1995). "Cigarette smoking during pregnancy." *Canadian Journal of Psychiatry*, 40, 603–7.

Storey, D. and Jacobson, T. (2004). "Entertainment–education and participation: Applying Habermas to a population program in Nepal." In A. Singhal, M. Cody, E. Rogers, and M. Sabido, *Entertainment Education and Social Change* (pp. 377–97). Mahwah, NJ: Lawrence Erlbaum.

Storey, D., Boulay, M., Karki, Y., Heckert, K., and Karmacharya, D. (1999). "Impact of the intergrated Radio Communication Project in Nepal, 1994–1997." *Journal of Health Communication*, 4, 271–94.

Street, R. L. (1991). "Information-giving in medical consultations: The influence of patients' communicative styles and personal characteristics." *Social Science and Medicine*, 32, 541–8.

Street, R. L. (2003). "Communication in medical encounters: An ecological perspective." In T. L. Thompson, A. M. Dorsey, K. I. Miller, and R. Parrott (eds), *Handbook of Health Communication* (pp. 63–89). Mahwah, NJ: Lawrence Erlbaum Associates.

Street, R. L., Voigt, B., Geyer, C., Manning, T., and Swanson, G. (1995). "Increasing patient involvement in choosing treatment for early breast cancer." *Cancer*, 76, 2275–85.

Sunwolf, Frey, L., and Keranen, L. (2005). "Rx story-prescription: The healing effects of storytelling and storylistening in the practice of medicine." In L. Harter, P. Japp, and C. Beck (eds), *Narratives, Health and Healing: Communication Theory, Research, and Practice* (pp. 237–57). Mahwah, NJ: Lawrence Erlbaum.

The Synergy Project (2002). *Room for Change: Preventing HIV Transmission in Brothels.* University of Washington, Center for Health Education and Research.

Thompson, T. L. (2003). "Introduction". In T. L. Thompson, A. M. Dorsey, K. I. Miller, and R. Parrott (eds), *Handbook of Health Communication* (pp. 1–5). Mahwah, NJ: Lawrence Erlbaum Associates.

Tocqueville, A. D. (1999). *Democracy in America.* New York: Westvaco.

Tomlinson, J. (1991). *Cultural Imperialism.* Baltimore: Johns Hopkins University Press.

Tong, R. (2002). "Love's labor in the health care system: Working toward gender equity." *Hypatia*, 17, 200–13.

Trawick, M. (1992). "Death and nurturance in Indian systems of healing." In C. Leslie and A. Young (eds), *Paths to Asian Medical Knowledge* (pp. 129–59). Berkeley, CA: University of California Press.

Triandis, Harry C. (1995). *Individualism and Collectivism.* Boulder, CO: Westview.

Ulrey, K. L. and Amason, P. (2001). "Intercultural communication between patients and health care providers: An exploration of intercultural communication effectiveness, cultural sensitivity, stress, and anxiety." *Health Communication*, 13, 449–63.

UNAIDS (2000). *Female Sex Worker HIV Prevention Projects: Lessons Learnt from Papua New Guinea, India, and Bangladesh.* Geneva: Author.

UNAIDS (2002, June). "Technical Update. Sex work and HIV/AIDS."

Underwood, S. M. (2003). "Reducing the burden of cancer borne by African Americans: If not now, when?" *Cancer Epidemiology Biomarkers and Prevention*, 12, 270S–6S.

Unschuld, P. (1992). "Epistemological issues and changing legitimation: Traditional Chinese medicine in the twentieth century." In C. Leslie and A. Young (eds), *Paths to Asian Medical Knowledge* (pp. 44–61). Berkeley, CA: University of California Press.

USAID (1999). *US Overseas Loans and Grants.* Washington, DC: USAID.

USAID (2002). *Foreign Aid in the National Interest.* Washington, DC: Author.

USAID (2004). *US Foreign Aid: Meeting the Challenges of the Twenty-First Century.* Washington, DC.

Vaughan, P., Regis, A., and St. Catherine, E. (2000). "Effects of an entertainment–education radio soap opera on family planning and HIV prevention in St. Lucia." *International Family Planning Perspectives*, 26, 148–57.

Vaughan, P., Rogers, E., Singhal, A. and Swahele, R. (2000). "Entertainment–education and HIV/AIDS prevention: A field experiment in Tanzania." *Journal of Health Communication*, 5, 81–100.

Veenstra, G. (2000). "Social capital, SES and health: An individual-level analysis." *Social Science and Medicine*, 50, 619–29.

Viswanath, K. and Finnegan, J. R. (1996). "The knowledge gap hypothesis: Twenty-five years later." In B. Burleson (ed.), *Communication Yearbook*, 19 (pp. 187–227). Thousand Oaks, CA: Sage.

Viswanath, K. and Finnegan, J. R. (2002). "Community health campaigns and secular trends: Insights from the Minnesota Heart Health Program and community trials in heart disease prevention." In R. Hornik (ed.), *Public Health Communication: Evidence for Behavior Change* (pp. 289–312). New York: Lawrence Erlbaum.

Voelker, R. (1995). "Speaking the languages of medicine and culture." *Journal of the American Medical Association*, 273, 1639–41.

Waitzkin, H. (1981). "The social origins of illness: A neglected history." *International Journal of Health Services*, 11, 77–103.

Waitzkin, H. (1983). *The Second Sickness: Contradictions of Capitalist Health Care*. New York: Free Press.

Waitzkin, H. (1984). "The micropolitics of medicine: A contextual analysis." *International Journal of Health Services*, 14, 339–78.

Waitzkin, H. (1991). *The Politics of Medical Encounters: How Patients and Doctors Deal with Social Problems*. New Haven, CT: Yale University Press.

Wallack, L. (1989). "Mass communication and health promotion: A critical perspective." In R. Rice and C. Atkin (eds), *Public Communication Campaigns*, 2nd edn (pp. 353–68). Newbury Park, CA: Sage.

Wallack, L. (1990). "Mass media and health promotion: Promise, problem, and challenge." In C. K. Atkin and L. Wallack (eds), *Mass Communication and Public Health: Complexities and Conflicts* (pp. 147–63). Newbury Park, CA: Sage.

Wallack, L. and Dorfman, L. (2001). "Putting policy into health communication: The role of media advocacy." In R. Rice and C. Atkin (eds), *Public Communication Campaigns*, 3rd edn (pp. 389–401). Thousand Oaks, CA: Sage.

Wallack, L., Dorfman, L., Jernigan, D., and Themba, M. (1993). *Media Advocacy and Public Health: Power for Prevention*. Newbury Park, CA: Sage.

Wallerstein, N., Duran, B., Minkler, M., and Foley, K. (2005). "Developing and maintaining partnerships with communities." In B. Israel, E. Eng, A. Schulz, and E. Parker (eds), *Methods in Community-Based Participatory Research for Health* (pp. 31–51). San Francisco, CA: Jossey-Bass.

Wang, C. (1999). "Photovoice: A participatory action research strategy applied to women's health." *Journal of Women's Health*, 8, 185–92.

Wang, C. and Burris, M. (1994). "Empowerment through photo novella: Portraits of participation." *Health Education Quarterly*, 21, 171–86.

Wang, C., Cash, J., and Powers, L. (2000). "Who knows the streets as well as the homeless? Promoting personal and community action through photovoice." *Health Promotion Practice*, 1, 81–9.

Weitzman, E. and Kawachi, I. (2000). "Giving means receiving: The protective effect of social capital on binge drinking on college campuses." *American Journal of Public Health*, 90, 1936–9.

West, C. (1984). *Routine Complications: Troubles with Talk between Doctors and Patients*. Bloomington: Indiana University Press.

Wilkinson, R. G. (1994). *Unhealthy Societies: The Afflictions of Inequality*. London: Routledge.

Wilkinson, R. G. (1996). *Unhealthy Societies. The Afflictions of Inequality* (2nd edn). London: Routledge.

Willis, E. (1989). *Medical Dominance: The Division of Labor in Australian Health Care*. Sydney: Allen and Unwin.

Wilson, B. (ed.) (1971). *Rationality*. New York: Harper and Row.

Witte, K. (1992). "Putting the fear back into fear appeals: The extended parallel process model." *Communication Monographs*, 59, 329–49.

Witte, K. (1995). "Fishing for success: Using the persuasive health message framework to generate effective campaign messages." In E. Maibach and R. Parrott (eds), Designing Health Messages: Approaches from Communication Theory and Public Health Practice (pp. 145–66). Thousand Oaks, CA: Sage.

Witte, K. (1998a). "How to motivate protective action." *Health Risk Communicator*, 2(1), 1–2.

Witte, K. (1998b). "A theoretically based evaluation of HIV/AIDS prevention campaigns along the Trans-Africa Highway in Kenya." *Journal of Health Communication*, 3(4), 345–63.

Witte, K. and Morrison, K. (1995). "Intercultural and cross-cultural health communication: Understanding people and motivating healthy behaviors." *International and Intercultural Communication Annual*, 19, 216–46.

Witte, K., Stokols, D., Ituarte, P., and Schneider, M. (1993). "A test of the perceived threat and cues to action constructs in the health belief model: A field study to promote bicycle safety helmets." *Communication Research*, 20, 564–86.

Woolf, S. H., Johnson, R. E., Fryer, G. E., Rust, G. and Satcher, D. (2004). "The health impact of resolving racial disparities: An analysis of US mortality data." *American Journal of Public Health*, 94, 2078–81.

Wrightson, K. and Wardle, J. (1997). "Cultural variation in health locus of control." *Ethnicity and Health*, 2, 13–20.

Wu, L., Kouzis, A., and Leaf, P. (2003). "Influence of comorbid alcohol and psychiatric disorders on utilization of mental health services in the National Comorbidity Survey." *American Journal of Psychiatry*, 156, 1230–6.

Yoder, P. S., Hornik, R. and Chirwa, B. C. (1996). "Evaluating the program effects of a radio drama about AIDS in Zambia." *Studies in Family Planning*, 27, 188–204.

Zoller, H. M. (2003). "Health on the line: Identity and disciplinary control in employee occupational health and safety discourse." *Journal of Applied Communication Research*, 31(2), 118–39.

Zoller, H. M. (2004). "Dialogue as global issue management: Legitimizing corporate influence in the Transatlantic Business Dialogue." *Management Communication Quarterly*, 18(2), 204–40.

Zoller, H. M. (2005). Health activism: Communication theory and action for social change. *Communication Theory*, 15, 341–64.

Zoller, H. M. (2006). "Suitcases and swimsuits: On the future of organizational communication." *Management Communication Quarterly*, 19, 661–6.

Zones, J. S. (1992). "The political and social context of silicone breast implant use in the United States." *Journal of Long-Term Effects of Medical Implants*, 1(3), 225–41.

Index

CPSIA information can be obtained at www.ICGtesting.com
Printed in the USA
LVOW02*0558040614

388478LV00006B/44/P

9 780745 634913